ORTHOPAEDIC
BIOMATERIALS
IN **RESEARCH**
AND **PRACTICE**

SECOND EDITION

Kevin L. Ong
Scott Lovald
Jonathan Black

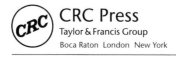

CRC Press
Taylor & Francis Group
Boca Raton London New York

CRC Press is an imprint of the
Taylor & Francis Group, an **informa** business

CRC Press
Taylor & Francis Group
6000 Broken Sound Parkway NW, Suite 300
Boca Raton, FL 33487-2742

First issued in paperback 2017

© 2014 by Taylor & Francis Group, LLC
CRC Press is an imprint of Taylor & Francis Group, an Informa business

No claim to original U.S. Government works

ISBN-13: 978-1-4665-0350-2 (hbk)
ISBN-13: 978-1-138-07486-6 (pbk)

Library of Congress Cataloging-in-Publication Data

Black, Jonathan, 1939- author.
  Orthopaedic biomaterials in research and practice / Kevin L. Ong, Jonathan Black, Scott Lovald. -- Second edition.
    p. ; cm.
  Jonathan Black's name appears first in the previous edition.
  Includes bibliographical references and index.
  ISBN 978-1-4665-0350-2 (hardcover : alk. paper)
  I. Ong, Kevin L., author. II. Lovald, Scott (Scott T.), author. III. Title.
  [DNLM: 1. Biocompatible Materials--therapeutic use--Examination Questions. 2. Orthopedic Procedures--methods--Examination Questions. 3. Prostheses and Implants--Examination Questions. WE 18.2]

RD755
617.9--dc23   2013045981

Visit the Taylor & Francis Web site at
http://www.taylorandfrancis.com

and the CRC Press Web site at
http://www.crcpress.com

ORTHOPAEDIC
BIOMATERIALS
IN RESEARCH
AND PRACTICE

SECOND EDITION

Kevin Ong:

To my loving family (Shawna, Tyler, and Natalie) for supporting me in my endeavors and pursuit of knowledge; my parents (George and Irene) for teaching me about drive and persistence; and my mentors for educating and training me.

Scott Lovald:

To my parents, John and Roberta, for their wonderful example.

Contents

3 Mechanical properties   53

4 Viscoelasticity   77

13 Fixation   **317**

14 Host response   **339**

16 Materials retrieval and analysis   395

17 Self-test   415

Preface—1st edition

Orthopaedics, the treatment of disorders of the musculoskeletal system, represents a peculiar union of the physical and biological sciences. The body is alive, formed of metabolically active cells and their elaborate products, the tissues and organs. Nevertheless, the function of the resulting structures depends strongly on mechanical and materials properties.

Recognition of the role of physical properties in body functions led to early and fruitful collaboration between orthopaedists and engineers. Much of this collaboration has focused on mechanical aspects and falls into the field of *biomechanics*. However, all mechanical structures derive their extrinsic physical properties from intrinsic or materials properties. Much of the work in biomechanics takes these intrinsic materials properties as given, resting on the achievements of materials science. However, the materials aspects of tissues and the materials used to support or replace damaged tissues—collectively called *biomaterials*—should be as important to the orthopaedist as biomechanics.

Fifteen years ago, in *An Introduction to Orthopaedic Materials* (Charles C Thomas, Springfield, Illinois, 1975), John H. Dumbleton and I laid out the principles of biomaterials relevant to orthopaedic practice and described the then current understanding of clinical phenomena related to intrinsic properties of natural and fabricated biomaterials. While the principles have remained the same since that book was published, there has been explosive growth in research and clinical applications of orthopaedic biomaterials—hence, the need for this new book.

Orthopaedic Biomaterials in Research and Practice is designed to serve three primary functions. First, it can be used as a textbook for a course of lectures for orthopaedic residents. Each chapter, with additional reading, can be the basis for a 45- to 60-minute discussion. Second, this book can be used as a self-paced review for the Orthopaedists In-Training Examination (OITE), the Orthopaedic Self-Assessment Examination, or the Orthopaedic Board Examination. To this end, the book includes both worked problems in the text and a complete self-evaluation test with annotated answers. Third, this book can be used as a self-contained survey of biomaterials aspects of orthopaedics. The first 10 chapters, which introduce principles of materials science, will open the field to the medical student or practitioner who lacks primary engineering training. A selective annotated bibliography is provided, which, with the text, provides a contemporary overview of orthopaedic biomaterials for researchers in other fields.

This book deals with three central aspects of biomaterials, viewed relative to the problems and requirements of orthopaedics: the properties of tissues, the properties of fabricated materials, and the interaction between natural and fabricated materials. The last topic is commonly called "biocompatibility," but in this work, it is referred to as *biologic performance of materials*, thus covering both host response (biological response) and material or implant response (material degradation). In addition, the two final chapters deal with design and introduction of new materials and with analysis of device failure.

To make this book more useful as a study aid, a glossary of engineering terms is included.

It is hoped that *Orthopaedic Biomaterials in Research and Practice* will serve as a useful daily tool in increasing the knowledge of materials science as it bears on orthopaedic research, education, and practice. The author welcomes comments and criticism, and looks forward with hope to future editions incorporating them.

Jonathan Black

Preface—2nd edition

In the more than 25 years since the first edition of this work appeared, there have been many changes in biomaterials science and engineering and in the application of its principles and conclusions to orthopaedic research and clinical practice. Much to my surprise, the original work has proven durable, remaining on bookshelves over many desks, being utilized in teaching situations, and, amazingly, maintaining value in the secondary book market. Thus, it seemed timely and proper that when the subject came up, agreement should be made with Taylor & Francis for a second, revised edition.

This work is made possible by the collaboration and leadership of two co-authors, Kevin Ong and Scott Lovald. I owe a great debt to them for agreeing to the project and for retaining both the aims and the essential plan of the original work. The three central aspects of the field of orthopaedic materials—the properties of tissues, the properties of fabricated materials, and the interaction between natural and fabricated materials—continue to be present, with extensive revision and modernization, reflecting the progress by engineers, biologists, researchers, and clinicians in understanding and treating musculoskeletal disorders. New chapters deal with the emerging topics of hybrid, combination, and replant materials as well as the emerging field of tissue engineering. Worked problems, an annotated bibliography, and a self-test have been revised and renewed. Errors and omissions have also been addressed.

Much has been achieved but much remains to be learned and applied in the clinic and the operating room. Joint replacement is now properly recognized as one of the great medical achievements of the 20th century, with both individual patients and significant case series well into their third decades of clinical experience. However, we seem to be approaching a period of uncertainty. With the changing patient demographics, recent clinical experiences of some patients with surface replacement, metal-on-metal articulation, and increased component modularity suggest just how hard further progress in improving outcomes will be.

I suggest that it is only with a firm grounding in the basic and applied sciences underlying clinical practice will this and the next generations of orthopaedists be able to provide optimal and effective care to patients. It is my intention that, as the baton is passed to my able co-authors, *Orthopaedic Biomaterials in Research and Practice* will continue as an accessible tool in gaining such understanding.

Jonathan Black

Acknowledgments

We would like to acknowledge Greta Hambke and Eric Wysocki for contributing toward the new figures in this edition.

Authors

Kevin L. Ong, PhD, PE, is a senior managing engineer in E^{x}ponent® Engineering and Scientific Consulting's Biomedical Engineering Practice. He holds degrees in mechanical engineering (BS and PhD, Cornell University). Prior to joining E^{x}ponent, Dr. Ong was a research assistant in the Department of Mechanical and Aerospace Engineering at Cornell University in the Cornell University Hospital for Special Surgery Program in Biomedical Mechanics.

With over 15 years of research in biomechanics, his area of interest is in product design evaluation and failure analysis of medical devices, with a focus on evaluating how patient, surgical, and design factors influence performance. He also has background in nonlinear finite element analysis, solid mechanics, and orthopaedic biomechanics. Dr. Ong has directed preclinical and postmarket mechanical testing experiments of bone and soft tissue to evaluate and characterize biomaterials and medical devices, including wear testing and retrieval (explant) analysis. He has designed experiments for standard tests (e.g., ASTM, ISO), as well as developed nonstandard or novel testing protocols.

Dr. Ong has melded his product development interests with health care services research, specifically using administrative claims data and hospital records to examine utilization, outcomes, economic burden, comparative effectiveness, and health care technology assessment. He has received awards from the American Association of Hip and Knee Surgeons for his research in clinical outcomes and from the British Orthopaedic Research Society and the British Orthopaedic Trainees Association for his research in hip resurfacing. Dr. Ong also currently holds a visiting research professor appointment at the Drexel University School of Biomedical Engineering, Science and Health Systems, Philadelphia, Pennsylvania.

Scott Lovald, PhD, MBA, holds degrees in mechanical engineering (BS and PhD, University of New Mexico), manufacturing engineering

(ME, University of New Mexico), and business (MBA, University of New Mexico). He is currently a senior associate in E^{x}ponent's Biomedical Engineering Practice. His past experience has included various positions focused on medical implant design and research.

Immediately prior to working at E^{x}ponent, Dr. Lovald initiated and directed the research, seed funding, design, manufacturing, FDA 510(k) clearance, and postmarket study Institutional Review Board approval of a novel trauma system that has been the subject of numerous peer-reviewed journal publications and subsequently introduced into a Level I trauma center.

He has also previously worked in the area of clinical research by designing and managing postmarket studies that investigated the clinical outcomes of total knee arthroplasty, total hip arthroplasty, atrial fibrillation, knee resurfacing, and degenerative disc disease patients.

Dr. Lovald specializes in outcomes, performance optimization, and failure analysis of orthopaedic, trauma, and cardiovascular devices. With 10 years of biomechanics and biomaterials experience, he has published work on the design and optimization of bone fracture internal fixation devices, blood flow through the atherosclerotic carotid artery, wall shear on abdominal aortic aneurysms, airflow through a resected nasal cavity, bioabsorbable polymer fixation devices, design and optimization of local skin flap designs for reconstructive surgery, and a number of clinical outcomes studies from both disease-specific and general (Medicare, Nationwide Inpatient Sample) medical databases.

Jonathan Black, PhD, FBSE, is Hunter Professor Emeritus of Bioengineering, Clemson University, Clemson, South Carolina. He holds degrees in physics (BS, Cornell University), engineering science (ME, Pennsylvania State University), and metallurgy (biomaterials) (PhD, University of Pennsylvania). Before his appointment as the first occupant of the Hunter Chair of Bioengineering at Clemson in 1988, for 17 years he was a member of the Department of Orthopaedic Surgery at the University of Pennsylvania with a secondary appointment in the Department of Bioengineering. During 1992–1995, he was a senior visiting fellow in the IRC for Biomaterials at Queen Mary and Westfield College (London, UK), with support from a SERC Fellowship. In 2011, he was appointed adjunct professor of biomedical engineering at Cornell University, Ithaca, New York.

Professor Black has long been active in research and teaching in several areas of biomaterials science and engineering, with special reference to the biological performance of metallic implants and to the needs of orthopaedic clinical practice. He is the author of many articles and several textbooks, including *Biological Performance of Materials* (1981, 1992, 1999, 2006), *Orthopaedic Biomaterials in Research and Practice* (1988), *Handbook of Biomaterial Properties* (with G. Hastings) (1998), and *Orthopaedic Research: Why? What? How?* (2009, 2011). He has a long-term interest in implant registries and implant retrieval and analysis and is the author of a major 1992–1993 study of the field commissioned by the US Food and Drug Administration.

He has been involved in professional activities in biomaterials for more than 40 years and is a Charter Fellow of Biomaterials Science and Engineering (FBSE). He is a charter member and past president of the Society for Biomaterials (US), was a frequent presenter and session chair at the Gordon Research Conferences on Biomaterials (US), and was an organizer of the triennial Biointeractions conference series in the UK. He has served on a number of advisory and editorial boards and was an assistant editor of the *Journal of Biomedical Materials Research* from 1978 to 1995. He is an associate member of the American Academy of Orthopaedic Surgeons and recipient of the Presidential Gold Medal from the British Orthopaedic Association.

In 1992, Prof. Black established IMN Biomaterials, a professional consultancy in biomaterials and orthopaedic engineering, in which he serves as principal. He was chair of the Scientific Advisory Board for Stryker Orthopaedics (SO) (previously Osteonics then Howmedica Osteonics), 1990–2007, and continues to serve as a member of this and other SO advisory boards.

Forces and equilibrium

The orthopaedic surgeon uses materials to multiple and various ends in treating disabilities of the musculoskeletal system. There are many requirements that these materials must meet if they are to form either a temporary or a lasting union with the part of the body being treated, and the recipe for each material is often unique and tailored to the particular application. Considerations for the ideal material for orthopaedic applications include its material strength and stiffness, biologic response, toxicity, and conductivity, just to name a few. All of these factors derive from the structure and composition of materials, and their study constitutes the materials science called *biomaterials*.

Frequently, the first questions asked about a material are in relation to its strength. Mechanical behavior holds a position of primacy among these factors: the materials being used must have sufficient integrity to sustain the forces placed upon them. Before it can be discussed whether a material is strong enough, it is important to know exactly for what it needs to be strong enough. In other words, what is the mechanical environment to which the material will be subjected? Discussion of mechanical behavior requires a language suitable first for dealing with the position and motion of objects acted on by external forces and then for examining the internal effects of these forces.

The external description of the position and motion of objects has been a traditional problem for philosophers, physicists, and engineers. In the modern era, we speak of the field of *statics* as dealing with the relationships between objects that are in *equilibrium*—that is, objects that are seen to be either at rest or moving with a constant velocity—whereas the field of *dynamics* deals with objects undergoing a change in velocity, called *acceleration*.

Units

Both fields, which are analytic and quantitative, require the use of units of measurement to permit exact comparison of physical quantities. We can describe the weight of a patient by deciding which unit of weight

Table 1.1 Systems of basic units

Units	British (or English)		CGS (centimeter–gram–second)		SI[a] (International System)
Length	foot (ft)		centimeter (cm)		meter (m)
	1	=	30.48	=	0.3048
	0.03281	=	1	=	0.01
	3.281	=	100	=	1
Mass	pound (lb)		gram (g)		kilogram (kg)
	1	=	453.6	=	0.4536
	0.002205	=	1	=	0.001
	2.205	=	1000	=	1
Time	second (s)		second (s)		second (s)
Temperature	degree Fahrenheit (°F)		degree Centigrade (°C)		degree Celsius (°C)
	1	=	0.5556[b]	=	0.5556[b]
	1.8	=	1	=	1

[a] All examples and problems in this book will use SI metric units since this is the *Journal of Bone and Joint Surgery* editorial standard.

[b] 5/9 exact fraction.

Table 1.2 Prefixes for metric units

Prefix	Abbreviation	Multiply unit by
giga-	G-	10^9
mega-	M-	10^6
kilo-	k-	10^3
deca-	da-	10
deci-	d-	10^{-1}
centi-	c-	10^{-2}
milli-	m-	10^{-3}
micro-	μ-	10^{-6}
nano-	n-	10^{-9}
pico-	p-	10^{-12}

measurement to use and then by specifying the number of units required to equal the patient's weight. In common terms, the "standard" patient weighs 70 kg or 154 lb or even 11 stone.* The units and the quantity of each required are different, but each combination gives us a quantitative description of the patient's weight. To permit calculations to be done, these units must be used together in compatible groups that will yield correct results. The common systems in use and the basic units (and

---

* However, with the obesity epidemic in the United States and also in other countries, what is considered a "standard" patient has changed.

their abbreviations) from which all others can be derived are shown in Table 1.1.

The British or English system is still in common use, whereas the metric system (based on the meter or fraction of a meter) (CGS and SI) units are coming into wider use, especially in Europe and in journals with international circulations. However, as each physical measurement is discussed, the units and equivalents in all three systems will be provided.

It is useful at this time to review the common modifying prefixes that are used with metric terms; these are given in Table 1.2.

Force

We can know about forces only by observing the motion of objects. When an object is at rest or moving with a constant velocity, it is said to be in equilibrium, which is a shorthand way of saying that the sum of forces or the *net force* on that object is zero. This is the substance of Newton's first principle or law, sometimes called the law of inertia. The relationship between force and change in velocity (acceleration) is called Newton's second law and will be discussed later in this chapter. For the time being, we shall simply accept that such a relationship exists.

The units of force magnitude are the pound (British), the dyne (CGS), and the newton (SI) (Table 1.3). Since the pound is defined as the force exerted on a mass of one pound in the Earth's gravitational field, it is also convenient to define a companion but unofficial unit, the kilogram-force (kgf), as the gravitational force on a mass of one kilogram.

In addition to the magnitude of a force, the direction must be specified. This arises since velocity has both magnitude (speed) and direction and forces can act to change both aspects. Any quantity that has both magnitude and direction is called a *vector* quantity and is represented by an arrow, whose length is proportional to the magnitude of the quantity, pointing in the direction of action. The direction of a force is called its *line of action*.

In Figure 1.1, we see a cube of material resting on a smooth surface and acted on by a horizontally directed force $\bar{A}$ (a bar over a letter,

Table 1.3 Units of force

Units	System		
	British	CGS	SI
Force[a]	pound (lb)	dyne (dyne)	Newton (N)
	1	$= 4.448 \times 10^5$	$= 4.448$
	2.248×10^{-5}	$= 1$	$= 10^{-5}$
	2.248	$= 10^5$	$= 1$

[a] 1 kgf = 0.4536 lb = 9.807×10^5 dynes = 9.807 N.

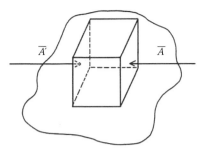

FIGURE 1.1   Applied force and reaction force.

as $\bar{A}$, denotes a vector quantity). We see that in this case, the force is not large enough to make the cube move; thus, the cube is said to be in equilibrium, and there must be an equal force opposing $\bar{A}$. That is, there must be a force $\bar{A}' = (-\bar{A})$ that has the same magnitude as $\bar{A}$ ($|\bar{A}|$ or A indicates the magnitude of $\bar{A}$) and the opposite direction, so that the sum of the forces (the net force) is zero. In this case, the opposing force is a *reaction* force, which is produced by friction between the cube and the surface on which it rests (see Chapter 11 for a discussion of frictional forces). There are limits to the frictional reaction force; if $|\bar{A}|$ is increased until it is greater than $|\bar{A}'|$ (without changing the direction of either force), the cube will no longer be in static equilibrium and will begin to move.

Working with vectors

Although vectors have both magnitude and direction, it is possible to add and subtract them in much the same way as simple numbers. There are two principal techniques for this: *direct* and *after resolution*.

In Figure 1.2, we see that vectors are added directly by placing the tail of the second vector to the head of the first vector and so on and then connecting the free head and tail with a new vector. Thus, $\bar{C} = \bar{A} + \bar{B}$, $\bar{D} = \bar{A} + \bar{B} + \bar{C}$. Subtraction is performed by reversing the direction of the second vector, so that $\bar{E} = \bar{A} - \bar{B}$ or $\bar{E} = \bar{A} + (-\bar{B})$. When multiple vectors are present, the order of addition and subtraction has no effect on the result, as is the case for regular numbers. ("Regular" numbers possess only magnitude and are called *scalars*.)

PROBLEM 1.1

In Figure 1.2, if $|\bar{A}| = 15$ N, what is $|\bar{C}|$? Assume 1 cm = 5N.

ANSWER:

A scale rule shows that $\bar{A}$ is 3 cm long; thus, 1 cm = 5 N.* Since $\bar{D}$ is 5 cm long, $|\bar{D}| = 5 \times 5 = 25$ N.

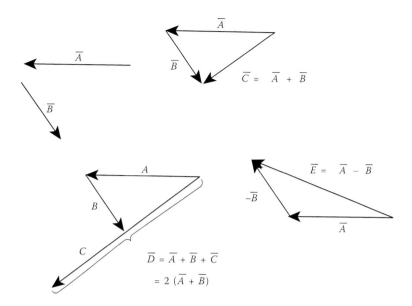

FIGURE 1.2 Addition and subtraction of vectors.*†

Resolution of vectors

Since vectors may be added together to make new vectors, it is reasonable to suppose that any vector may be broken down or *resolved* into a set of smaller vectors. Resolution of vectors is a very useful technique for answering problems in statics and dynamics.

Although any set of vectors may be added together to form a new vector, such as $\bar{A}$, $\bar{B}$, and $\bar{C}$ adding to form $\bar{D}$, in Figure 1.2, they are said to be *components* of the new vector; components are particularly useful when they are defined as *orthogonal* components.

Any two vectors that add to form a third *and* have a right angle between them are said to be (in two dimensions) *orthogonal* components of the new vector. Thus, in Figure 1.3, $\bar{G}$ and $\bar{H}$ are orthogonal components of $\bar{J}$. The direction and magnitude of any vector in two dimensions can alternatively be described using the resolved components in a conveniently defined orthogonal coordinate system. The traditional x–y coordinate system is the most famous example of an orthogonal system. There are an infinite number of such pairs of orthogonal components for any vector. For example, an x–y system can be rotated by any angle in its plane to form a new orthogonal system.

---

* For ease of graphic analysis, all figures are drawn to scale. For force, four scales are used, depending on the size of the problem: 1 cm = 5 N, 1 cm = 10 N, 1 cm = 500 N, or 1 cm = 500 N. The force scale as well as other scale information is noted in a box in the lower right corner of each succeeding figure.

† Reference is made here and elsewhere to two dimensions (or directions). Certainly, we live in a three-dimensional world, but for simplicity, all of the problems and examples in this book are presented and solved in two dimensions. However, all of the principles discussed may be generalized to three dimensions. It is also possible, in most cases, to solve three-dimensional problems as a sequence of two-dimensional ones. Such solutions are left to the reader; they are not necessary to a satisfactory understanding of orthopaedic biomaterials.

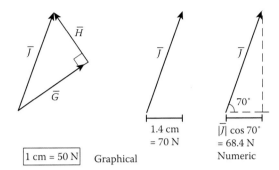

FIGURE 1.3   Resolution of vectors.

PROBLEM 1.2

In Figure 1.3, what is the magnitude of the component of $\bar{J}$ in the horizontal direction?

ANSWER:

Graphic. Place an object with a square edge, such as an envelope, over $\bar{J}$ so that the bottom edge is horizontal and just touches the tail of $\bar{J}$, while the right edge just touches the point of $\bar{J}$. Mark the location of the corner of the envelope and measure the distance from the tail of $\bar{J}$ to this point. This is 1.4 cm; since the scale is 1 cm = 50 N, the answer is 1.4 × 50 = 70 N.

Numeric. Measure the angle between $\bar{J}$ and the horizontal (= 70°). Measure $|\bar{J}|$; this is equal to 4 cm or 200 N. The desired result is: $|\bar{J}| \times \cos 70° = 200 \times 0.342 = 68.4$ N.

The two results are somewhat different; however, the graphic one is accurate enough for most purposes. All of the problems in this book are designed to be solved graphically; a simple plastic scale/protractor, such as given away by device salesmen, is all that is required to do the graphic solutions. For those who wish to solve them numerically, Table 1.4 gives values of the trigonometric functions most commonly used. A simple pocket calculator will provide values for angles not given. Graphic and numeric solutions will be provided to all problems.

Table 1.4   Useful values of trigonometric functions

Angle θ (°)	Sin θ	Cos θ
0	0	1
15	0.259	0.966
30	0.5	0.867
45	0.707	0.707
60	0.867	0.5
75	0.966	0.259
90	1	0

Trigonometric relationships

To solve Problem 1.2 and later ones, it is useful to remember some simple trigonometry. The principal functions for a triangle with a right angle are shown in Figure 1.4.

A useful mnemonic device for understanding trigonometric functions is the short phrase "soh-cah-toa." Referring to the definitions given in Figure 1.4, expanding this phrase reveals the following:

sin = **o**pposite side length/**h**ypotenuse

cos = **a**djacent side length/**h**ypotenuse

tangent = **o**pposite side length/**a**djacent side length

A more formal expansion reveals the following trigonometric identities:

$$\sin \alpha = \frac{o}{h}$$

$$\cos \alpha = \frac{a}{h}$$

$$\tan \alpha = \frac{o}{a}$$

$$(\sin \times \sin) + (\cos \times \cos) = \sin^2 + \cos^2 = 1$$

The values of these trigonometric functions for frequently occurring angles are given in Table 1.4.

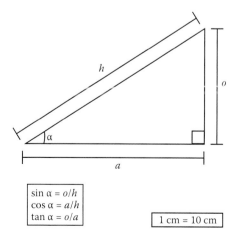

$$\sin \alpha = o/h$$
$$\cos \alpha = a/h$$
$$\tan \alpha = o/a$$

1 cm = 10 cm

FIGURE 1.4 Trigonometric relationships in a right-angle triangle.

Resultant force

When a number of forces act on an object, the effect is the same as the action of a single force called the *resultant*. The resultant force is equal to the sum of the forces, acting at a point where they intersect. Any multiple of non-parallel forces may have a single and unique point of intersection.

Since the effect of the forces may be replaced by the effect of the resultant, a first condition for equilibrium is described with the following rule:

> Translational equilibrium exists if the resultant of forces on an object is equal to zero.

Equilibrium may be investigated in two ways. The first is through inspection of the direct forces without decomposition into their component forces. When this is not possible because of non-orthogonal forces, it is often convenient to resolve the forces into orthogonal components before determining their sum in any direction.

PROBLEM 1.3

If a limb is placed in split Russell's traction (Figure 1.5), what are the magnitude and direction of the force on the distal femur?

A. 8 kgf horizontally to the left

B. 45 N horizontally to the left

C. 45 N inclined 35° from the horizontal, proximal to distal

D. 29.4 N vertically up

E. None of the above

Is the limb in Figure 1.5 in equilibrium? It does not appear to be by this calculation, since the resultant force is not equal to zero. More careful consideration leading to a complete solution must include the

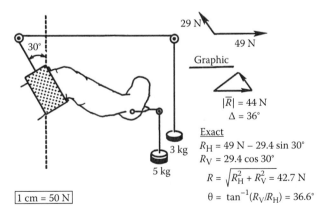

FIGURE 1.5   Split Russell's traction (Problem 1.3).

gravitational forces exerted on the mass of the limb segments and the
frictional resistance of the patient's trunk on the bed.

ANSWER:

The best answer is *C*, since the graphic solution is 44 N at an angle of
36°, proximal to distal. Note that cables, such as traction lines or tendons, exert their force in the direction that they leave the initial point of
attachment.

Moments

It is possible for the resultant of a group of forces acting on an object to
be zero and yet for equilibrium not to be present. This occurs when the
directions of action of all of the forces do not pass through a single point.
The result is the presence of a *net moment*.

Forces cause *translational* movement, whereas moments cause *rotational* movement. Another way of stating this is to say that the moment
of a force about a point is the tendency of the force to cause rotation
about that point.

Moments have the dimension of force times distance (Table 1.5).
They are obtained by multiplying the magnitude of the force by the
length of the perpendicular from the force's line of action to the point in
question. This *perpendicular* distance is often called the *moment arm*.
The direction of the force is retained in the sign of the moment: forces
that tend to cause counterclockwise motion are positive, whereas those
that cause clockwise motion are negative, as shown in Figure 1.6. This
is commonly known as the right-hand rule. After aligning the fingers of
your right hand with the position vector, rotate your palm so that your
fingers curl toward the force vector. If your thumb is pointing out of the
plane of the page, then it is a positive moment. If it is pointing into the
plane of the page, then it is a negative moment.

The moment of $\bar{L}$ at P is much smaller than that of $\bar{K}$ at P, even
though L is larger than K, since the moment is the product of the magnitude of the force and the moment arm. The results shown in Figure 1.6

Table 1.5 Units of moment

Units	System		
	British	CGS	SI
Moment	foot-pound (ft·lb)[a]	cm-dyne (cm·dyne)	newton-meter (N·m)
	1	$= 1.356 \times 10^7$	$= 1.356$
	1.376×10^{-8}	$= 1$	$= 10^{-7}$
	0.7376	$= 10^7$	$= 1$

[a] It is conventional practice to separate unit abbreviations with a "·" as in N·m, signify-
ing multiplication.

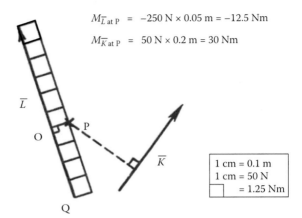

$M_{\bar{L} \text{ at P}} = -250 \text{ N} \times 0.05 \text{ m} = -12.5 \text{ Nm}$

$M_{\bar{K} \text{ at P}} = 50 \text{ N} \times 0.2 \text{ m} = 30 \text{ Nm}$

1 cm = 0.1 m	
1 cm = 50 N	
□ = 1.25 Nm	

FIGURE 1.6 Moments.

may be obtained graphically by constructing a rectangle with the length equal to the length of each force vector and the width equal to the length of the moment arm and then by dividing the area up into squares of known moment. Thus, the rectangle constructed on $\bar{L}$ contains 10 squares, each with an area of 0.25 cm², representing a moment of 1.25 N·m, for a total moment of 12.5 N·m. It is noted from the example that the moment arm is always drawn perpendicular in a line normal to the force vector to the point on which the moment is being taken around. For example, the moment arm of force L around P is drawn from point O to P, as opposed to point Q to P, or any other point. The force vector can be graphically translated in a direction parallel to its vector direction without changing the problem. In more complicated problems, it may be convenient to utilize the trigonometric relationships described above to construct a set of equations that will allow solving for the unknown reactions in a structure at equilibrium. Finally, it is obvious that a force that passes through a point may exert no moment at that point.

The existence of moments imposes a second condition for equilibrium:

Rotational equilibrium exists if the sum of moments about any point on an object is equal to zero.

Moment calculations may be greatly simplified since it can be shown that if the sum of the moments is equal to zero at *any point* on an object, it is equal to zero at *all points* on the object. When an object is in rotational equilibrium, a point may be selected that eliminates the moment of one force (i.e., is on the line of action of that force), which may reduce the number of equation unknowns for which to solve.

If the conditions for both translational and rotational equilibrium are met, then Newton's first law is satisfied and the object is either at rest or moving with a constant velocity.

PROBLEM 1.4

Is the boomerang in Figure 1.7 in equilibrium?

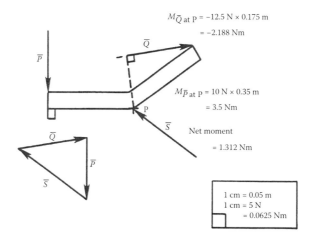

FIGURE 1.7   Boomerang (Problem 1.4).

ANSWER:

The boomerang is in translational but not rotational equilibrium. Since the net moment is positive, it would tend to rotate in a counterclockwise fashion.

Free body diagrams

The boomerang in Figure 1.7 seems much simpler to understand than the patient's leg in Figure 1.5. This is because the boomerang is shown as a *free body diagram*; that is, it is shown free of all other objects, but with all forces acting on it depicted. Similarly, to simplify the understanding of loading applied to the patient's leg and foot, Figure 1.8 is a free body diagram of the depiction in Figure 1.5. There are five forces shown, two of which are unknown. Solving for two unknown forces requires the construction of at least two equations of equilibrium. Forces that are

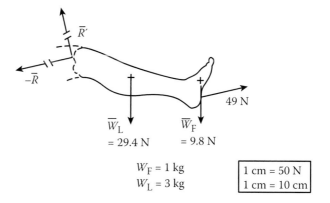

FIGURE 1.8   Free body diagram of leg and foot.

known are those exerted by the foot weight (49 N) and the gravitational force of the foot and the leg. The latter two are directed vertically downward and are shown acting on the *center of mass* of each segment. The center of mass is a point that appears to be exactly in the center of a homogeneous object.

The properties of the center of mass are such that, if the entire mass of the object were transferred to that single point, it would behave the same as the object with a distributed mass.

The two unknown forces are $-\bar{R}$, the joint reaction force produced by the desired tension on the femur, and $\bar{R}'$, the transverse force applied by the joint capsule, which is assumed to be orthogonal to $-\bar{R}$. Since the limb is known to be at rest, both equilibrium conditions apply (Sum $F_x = 0$, Sum $F_y = 0$), and given two conditions, one may solve for both $|\bar{R}|$ and $|\bar{R}'|$. In this case, and often in others, it may be convenient to transfer all forces into mutual orthogonal directions using trigonometric functions presented earlier in this chapter.

Thus, the combination of the use of a free body diagram and the application of the equilibrium conditions permits solutions of quite complex force and moment problems. Such solutions are essential to an understanding of the behavior of materials under load, since the forces within the material are dependent on the forces acting on the outside of the material.

Dynamics

It is necessary to understand statics to perceive the relationship between internal and external forces in the steady state. However, within the human body, there is a relatively constant state of motion, resulting from respiration, blood circulation, locomotion, and so on. The relationship of forces to changes in velocity is the subject of *dynamics*. The field of biomechanics addresses this field primarily at the level of organs, limb segments, and the whole body. Biomechanics and biomaterials merge together when consideration is given to dynamic effects at the tissue or material level. Specific velocity-related issues will be discussed in later chapters, as in consideration of the strain rate dependence of the mechanical properties of articular cartilage (see Chapter 5). For our purposes, it is not necessary to deal completely with dynamics but merely to extract some simple principles.

Force and acceleration

Acceleration is the relationship between force, in the sense of a net resultant force on an object, and a change in velocity of that object. This is embodied in Newton's second law and is, in fact, the origin of the specific derivation of force units from the sets of basic units given in Table 1.1.

Suppose that we return to Figure 1.1 and increase the magnitude of the applied force $\bar{A}$ until the cube begins to move. We have a common-sense idea that we may do this by pushing with increasing effort along the line of action of $\bar{A}$. Further, suppose that the cube has a mass of 100 g (0.1 kg).

A change in either speed or direction of motion is called *acceleration*. The change in acceleration over a period, if constant, can be determined by measuring the velocity of an object at two separate points in time (Figure 1.9). Initially, we locate the cube and measure its speed as 1 m/s in the left direction. Then, 1 s later, we measure its speed as 3 m/s in the same direction. The speed (magnitude of velocity) has increased by 2 m/s. This change in velocity is only possible because of an external force.

Newton's second law states, in a very familiar form:

$$F = m \cdot a$$

That is, a, the acceleration of an object with mass m, is directly related to the force that is applied to that object. Since force is a vector and mass is a scalar, acceleration must also be a vector, pointing along the line of action of the force.

Thus,

$$\bar{F} = m \cdot \bar{a}.$$

In this case, an object with a mass of 0.1 kg experiences acceleration (change in magnitude of velocity) of 2 m/s in 1 s. This can be accounted for by a force of 0.2 N acting in the direction of the velocity for the intervening second. In fact, by knowing the mass and observing the change in velocity, we infer the presence of the force. This is the only way we have of directly perceiving the presence of a net resultant force. Thus, it should come as no surprise that a newton is defined as the force that produces an acceleration of 1 m/s per second (1 m/s²) when applied to an object with a mass of 1 kg and that the intrinsic units of the newton are $kg \cdot m/s^2$.

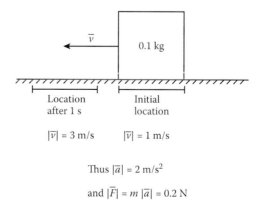

FIGURE 1.9   Newton's second law.

Momentum and impulse

In the same way that forces produce acceleration in the movement of objects with mass, changes in velocity of objects produce reaction forces. Calculation of such forces requires introduction of the second concept, conservation of momentum.

A moving object with a mass m and a velocity $\bar{v}$ is said to have a momentum equal to $m \times v$ (written as $m \cdot v$). This quantity, $m \cdot v$, is also sometimes called the inertia of an object, since it is a reflection of Newton's first law; that is, it remains constant in the absence of an applied force. If no external forces act on a group of objects, then the sum of the momentum of all objects in the group remains a constant, even if the velocities and thus the momentum of the individual objects change. Therefore, we say that momentum is *conserved* in such a group; this principle permits us to calculate the forces that moving objects exert on each other when they collide.

Suppose an osteotome is placed on a piece of bone and struck with a surgical mallet (Figure 1.10). Is it possible to calculate the force that the osteotome exerts on the bone from observing the mallet? (This is a somewhat artificial example since a mallet head swings in an arc rather than moving in a straight line. The actual case may be analyzed with more difficulty, but the conclusions are qualitatively the same as for this simplified case.)

Let us suppose that the mallet ($m = 0.5$ kg) moves with a speed of 0.1 m/s and comes to rest after striking the osteotome. Thus, before striking, the mallet has a momentum of 0.05 kg · m/s or 0.05 N · s, and after striking, it has a momentum of zero. The osteotome must have acquired a momentum of 0.05 N · s. If it were free to move, it would move in the same direction as the mallet, with a greater velocity, since it has a lower mass. However, it is positioned against the bone so that it cannot move to any great degree and must transfer its momentum,

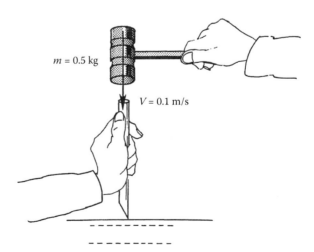

$m = 0.5$ kg

$V = 0.1$ m/s

FIGURE 1.10   Momentum and impulse (Problem 1.5).

in turn, to the bone. The change in momentum is related to the force it applies to the bone:

$$F \cdot t = \Delta m \cdot v$$

The quantity $F \cdot t$, the average force times the time it acts, is called the *impulse*, whereas $\Delta m \cdot v$ is the magnitude of the change of momentum during time t. Thus, if the momentum is transferred in 1 s, it will produce a force of 0.05 N acting during that period; if it is transferred in 0.001 s (1 ms) it will produce a force of 50 N during that period. The impulse is constant for any change in momentum; the resulting force is determined by the time over which the change in momentum takes place.

PROBLEM 1.5

Suppose that the mallet in Figure 1.10, instead of coming to rest, rebounds in the opposite direction with a speed of 0.05 m/s. Assuming that the period of force application to the bone is unchanged, does the force on the bone

    A. Remain unchanged?

    B. Decrease by 50%?

    C. Increase by 50%?

    D. Double?

    E. None of the above

ANSWER:

The answer is C. The change in momentum is now 0.05 + 0.025 or 0.075 N · s. Since the change in momentum and thus the impulse increases by 50%, if all other conditions remain the same (as stated), then the force must increase by 50%.

Coefficient of restitution

The ratio of the final relative speed of the mallet and osteotome to their initial speed is called the *coefficient of restitution* (e). It is a characteristic of any pair of materials and may take on values between one and zero. In the text case of the mallet striking the osteotome, $e = 0$, whereas in Problem 1.5, $e = 0.5$ (with an obvious change in material of one object in the example). Clearly, as e increases, the impulse and possible resultant forces increase. We can easily feel the difference between walking on a hard surface (large e, small t) and a soft surface (small e, large t). A direct conclusion is that objects in contact transmit smaller forces than ones that can rebound and separate, producing larger impulses. The increased force in a rebound situation (compared with that in a full-contact situation) is often called an *inertial force*, reflecting its origin in a change in momentum.

Conservation of energy

The last principle that we must consider related to dynamics is that of *conservation of energy*. A moving object with a mass m and a velocity *v* is said to have a kinetic energy equal to one-half $m \times v \times v$ (written as $m \cdot v^2/2$). Energy content reflects the ability to do work, defined as movement of mass through distance. The total energy of a group of objects is conserved if no external forces act on the objects; however, the total kinetic energy is only conserved if $e = 1$ for all impacts. Impacts for which $e = 1$ are called elastic and do not produce any lasting change of shape in the objects involved. When $e < 1$, the impact is called inelastic; some kinetic energy is converted to other forms (heat, sound, etc.) or stored within the objects as a result of each impact, and these calculations become more difficult. As opposed to kinetic energy, which is possessed by a body in motion, potential energy is possessed by a body due to its position or state. For example, gravitational potential energy is energy due to its elevation relative to a lower elevation. This can be calculated by $m \times g \times h$ (written as $m \cdot g \cdot h$), where g is acceleration due to gravity and h is the height/position of the object. Potential energy can be converted into kinetic energy, but unlike kinetic energy, it cannot be transferred directly from one object to another.

Therefore, we may understand the ability of materials to bear and distribute forces by considering them in a static way, introducing additional forces that arise from changes in velocity or position.

Additional problems

PROBLEM 1.6

In Figure 1.11a, suppose that forces $\bar{A}$, $\bar{C}$, and $\bar{J}$ act at a point P. Find the resultant of these forces $(\bar{R})$ and the vertical component $\bar{R}_v$.

ANSWER:

Graphic. See Figure 1.11b. The line of action of $\bar{R}$ is shown, $R = 210$ N. $\bar{R}'$ is also shown; $R_v = 110$ N.

Numeric. The simplest way is to resolve the three forces into vertical and horizontal components, since R_v will then equal the sum of the vertical components.

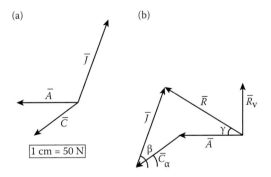

FIGURE 1.11   Resultant force (Problem 1.6).

Sum of horizontal components

$$R_h = A + C\cos\alpha - J\cos\beta$$
$$= 150 + 125\cos 36.9° - 200\cos 70°$$
$$= 150 + 100 - 68.4 = 181.6 \text{ N}$$

Sum of vertical components

$$R_v = (-)C\sin\alpha + J\sin\beta$$
$$= -125\sin 36.9° + 200\sin 70°$$
$$= -75 + 187.9 = 112.9 \text{ N}$$

Length of resultant

$$R = \left(R_v^2 + R_h^2\right)^{1/2} = 213.8 \text{ N}$$

Direction of R

γ = angle whose tangent $(= \tan^{-1}) = R_v / R_h$
$\gamma = 31.9°$

PROBLEM 1.7

For the limb in Russell's split traction (Figures 1.5 and 1.8), find the component of the resultant traction force parallel to the femur (R) (Figure 1.12).

ANSWER:

Graphic. Add $\bar{W}_L$, $\bar{W}_F$, and $\bar{W}_T$ together graphically; the "closing" vector, $-\bar{Y}$, is the sum of $(-\bar{R}$ and $\bar{R}')$ ($Y = 60$ N). Draw a circle with this

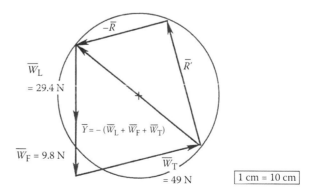

FIGURE 1.12 Component of resultant (split Russell's traction) (Problem 1.7).

vector as its diameter; any two vectors that meet on the circumference of such a circle are orthogonal components of the vector serving as the diameter. Lay out the lines of action of $-\bar{R}$ and $\bar{R}'$ and measure R. R = 35 N.

Numeric. From Figure 1.8:

$$Y_h = 49 \times \cos 15° = 47.3 \text{ N}$$

$$Y_v = 9.8 + 29.4 = 39.2 \text{ N}$$

$$Y = 61.4 \text{ N}$$

$$\tan^{-1}(Y_v/Y_h) = \tan^{-1}(39.2/47.3) = 39.6°$$

Therefore, $R = Y \cos (39.6° + 15°) = 35.6$ N

PROBLEM 1.8

The wheel in Figure 1.13a is mounted in an axle at P and loaded, through two cables, at A by a 3 kg mass and at B by a 5 kg mass. What is the resultant moment at P? If the wheel is free to rotate on its axle, in which direction does it turn?

ANSWER:

Graphic. Construct moment "boxes" on the lines from A to P (3 × 9.8 N × 0.15 m) and from B to P (5 × 9.8 N × 0.1 m) (Figure 1.13b). Partition up into units of 0.25 N·m. Then the force at A contributes about −18 squares and the one at B about +20 squares. Therefore, the net moment is +2 × 0.25 or +0.5 N·m (i.e., counterclockwise rotation).

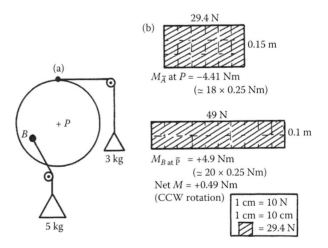

FIGURE 1.13 Wheel and cables (Problem 1.8).

Numeric.

$$M_{\bar{A}} \text{ at } P = -3 \times 9.8 \times 0.15 = -4.41 \text{ Nm}$$
$$M_{\bar{B}} \text{ at } P = +5 \times 9.8 \times 0.1 = +4.9 \text{ Nm}$$
$$M_{\text{net}} = -4.41 + 4.9 = +0.49 \text{ Nm}$$

PROBLEM 1.9

A bone plate is placed in a bending press (Figure 1.14a), and a load of 150 N is applied. What are the magnitudes of the resultant forces at A and B? Assume that the plate has a mass of 0.5 kg (a very heavy plate!) and draw a free body diagram.

ANSWER:

Graphic. Represent the plate by a line (since there are no horizontal components) and construct the appropriate moment "boxes" for moments about point A (Figure 1.14b). Partition into squares of 0.625 N·m each. The 150 N force contributes –18 squares, and the plate contributes about 1 square. Therefore, the force at B must contribute +19 squares. Thus, B must point up and have a magnitude of (19 × 0.625)/0.2 or about 60 N. Constructing 150 + 4.9 = A + B yields $A \approx 95$ N.
Numeric.

$$M_{\text{net at } A} = -150 \times 0.075 - 4.9 \times 0.1 + B \times 0.2$$

Therefore: $B = 58.7$ N
Since: $A + B = 150 + 4.9$, $A = 96.2$ N
Note: If the mass of the plate is neglected, $B = 60$ N and $A = 90$ N; their values are the inverse ratio of their lever arms measured to the point of action of the 150 N force.

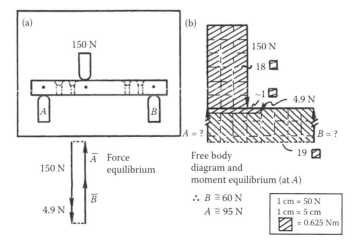

FIGURE 1.14 Bone plate in bending press (Problem 1.9).

PROBLEM 1.10

In Figure 1.15, the force that would tend to cause the screw and proximal fragment (head) to telescope is

    A. 1750 N

    B. 1625 N

    C. 615 N

    D. 40 N·m

    E. 40 N

ANSWER:

Graphic. See Figure 1.16. The best answer is *B*. The device in question is a Richards-type sliding nail–plate. It has an included angle of 145°, its distal portion is positioned 7° from vertical, and the joint reaction force, equal to 2.55 times standard body weight, is inclined at 12° to the vertical (see Ref. 8 for a full discussion of hip mechanics). By construction, as in Problem 1.7, the component parallel to the nail (the telescoping force) is found to have a magnitude $R_T = 1650$ N. Answer C is the magnitude of the cutting out force R_C, which is orthogonal to R_T. Answer D is clearly wrong, since it is a moment rather than a force magnitude.

    Numeric.

$$R_T = 1750 \times \cos(90° - 55° - 12°) = 1610.1 \text{ N}$$
$$R_C = 1750 \times \sin 23° = 683.8 \text{ N}$$

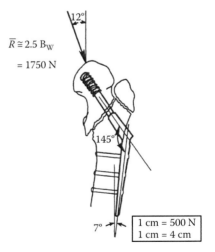

FIGURE 1.15 Nail–plate fixation of intertrochanteric fracture (Problem 1.10).

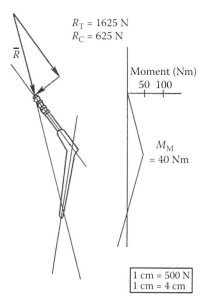

FIGURE 1.16   Moment diagram for nail–plate fixation device (Problem 1.11).

PROBLEM 1.11

In Figure 1.15, where in the device is the maximum moment experienced?

ANSWER:

In Figure 1.16, a moment diagram is constructed by plotting the perpendicular distance from the line of action of the force to the device times the magnitude of the force. It can be seen that the maximum moment, approximately $40\ \text{N} \cdot \text{m}$, occurs at the base of the barrel of the nail–plate. This is the location of the nail–plate junction in one-part devices; most devices are strengthened in this location to withstand this peak moment.

Annotated bibliography

1. ASTM SI10 - 10 IEEE/ASTM SI 10 American National Standard for Metric Practice, *Annual Book of Standards, 2010, Vol. 14.04*, American Society for Testing and Materials, Conshohocken, 2010.
    The standard reference on the SI metric system.
2. ALEXANDER RM: *Animal Mechanics*. University of Washington, Seattle, 1968.
    Biomechanics of swimming, crawling, running, and flying things. Chapter 1 has an elegant illustration of free body analysis in the examination of the mechanics of chewing in several species of fossil reptiles.
3. DEMPSTER WT: Free body diagrams as an approach to the mechanics of human posture and motion. In Evans FG (ed): *Biomechanical Studies of the Musculo-Skeletal System*. Charles C Thomas, Springfield, IL, 1961.

A detailed account of the use of free body diagrams in the analysis of muscle and joint forces.

4. FRANKEL VH, BURSTEIN AH: *Orthopaedic Biomechanics*. Lea & Febiger, Philadelphia, 1970.

    Chapter 1 is a brief introduction to forces, resolution of forces, and free body analysis.

5. FRANKEL VH, NORDIN M (eds): Basic Biomechanics of the Skeletal System. Lea & Febiger, Philadelphia, 1980.

    A good descriptive review of the mechanics of the human musculoskeletal system. Of particular value are the foreword by DR Carter on SI units and the extensive bibliographies at the end of each chapter.

6. GOWITZKE BA, MILNER M: *Understanding the Scientific Bases of Human Movement*. 2nd Ed. Williams & Wilkins, Baltimore, 1980.

    Chapters 2 and 3 deal with the fundamentals of motion and of static and dynamic equilibrium. Of particular note are later chapters that couple neurophysiology and behavior to biomechanics, although in a qualitative manner.

7. LEVEAU B: *Williams and Lissner: Biomechanics of Human Motion*. WB Saunders, Philadelphia, 1977.

    This is a revision of the classic 1962 first edition by M Williams and HR Lissner. Particularly useful are Chapter 3 on resolution of forces, Chapter 4 on static equilibrium, Chapter 5 on applications of static analysis, Chapter 7 on dynamics, and Appendix A, which contains tabulations of the mass and coordinates of the centers of mass of body segments.

8. MATTHEWS LS, SONSTEGARD DA, DUMBLETON JH: Repair of intertrochanteric fractures with a sliding nail. In Black J, Dumbleton JH (eds): *Clinical Biomechanics: A Case History Approach*. Churchill Livingstone, New York, 1981.

    A thorough discussion of the mechanics of reduction and fixation of proximal intertrochanteric femoral fractures, with many useful diagrams.

9. NORTHRIP JW, LOGAN GA, McKINNEY WC: *Introduction to Biomechanic Analysis of Sport*. WC Brown, Dubuque, 1974.

    A largely qualitative introduction to forces and motion in sports activities. Chapter 4 has some good quantitative examples of momentum and energy transfer during impact.

10. WIKTORIN CvH, NORDIN M: *Introduction to Problem Solving in Biomechanics*. Lea & Febiger, Philadelphia, 1985.

    Chapters 1 and 2 are an excellent overview of biomechanical principles. Later chapters offer more than two dozen extended problems involving static or dynamic equilibrium. Assumptions are clearly stated and solutions, in most cases both graphic and mathematical (exact), are provided.

CHAPTER TWO

Deformation

Statics and dynamics describe the motion of objects, such as body segments, surgical instruments, or implants, in response to forces. In solving such problems, one usually assumes that the object is rigid, that is, nondeformable. If that assumption were correct, then static and dynamic analysis would yield a full description of the interaction between forces and materials.

However, the assumption is incorrect. In fact, the opposite assumption is correct: all material objects deform under the action of forces and moments. The resulting deformations may be temporary or permanent and may lead to changes in physical properties and cumulative or sudden loss of integrity. In some cases, either by chance or design, their deformations and cumulative effects are so small that they can be neglected in biomechanical analysis. In the general case, force-induced deformation must be included and the mechanical analysis must be extended from the extrinsic, structural (or biomechanical) level down to the intrinsic, material (or mechanics of materials) level. In this chapter, we shall deal with the principles of deformation of materials.

Elongation

Tensile deformation

Suppose two equal and opposed forces, $F/2$ and $F'/2$ $(= -F/2)$, act on a bar of material with initial length L_0, as shown on the far left in Figure 2.1. We know from experience that if the rod is made of a "soft" material, such as a soft plastic, it will stretch visibly—that is, deform longitudinally under the action of the two forces. Since it is getting longer, we call this type of deformation *elongation*.

In Figure 2.1, we can see this happen as the load increases from a to c. The bar is also becoming narrower; this is because materials tend to conserve their volume when undergoing deformation. If we continue to increase the force, a strange thing begins to happen. A region of the bar begins to narrow, at the expense of the rest, as at d. This is called "necking." At the same time, we find that the bar begins to stretch more easily with a sense of "giving way"; that is, it elongates more rapidly even when

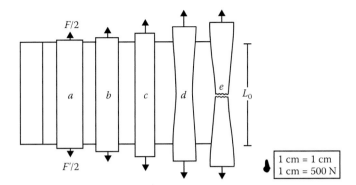

FIGURE 2.1 Tensile deformation of a bar.

we try to stretch it at a constant rate. If we were to do the experiment by stretching the rod at a constant rate and measuring the resultant force, we would find that the force is actually decreasing while elongation continues after necking occurs. Finally, the rod breaks somewhere in the region of the neck.

If we were to start the experiment with a very small force and slowly increase it by stages, using a ruler to measure the new length L after each increase, we would obtain the data in Table 2.1. The applied load and measured length are given in columns 2 and 3, respectively. Column 4 is the difference between the initial length L_0 and the length at each measurement ($L - L_0$). We could also measure the width of the bar, taking care to use the region of necking for measurements later in the experiment. These data are given in column 5; the differences between the initial width W_0 and these measurements are given in column 6.

Load–deformation curves

If we plot force as a function of the difference between the new length and the original length ($L - L_0$), we would obtain the diagram shown in Figure 2.2. Force could be plotted against length directly. However, using the quantity $L - L_0$ produces a graph that conveys the same information but appears to vary more rapidly. In addition, this difference has a special use in the determination of strain. This is called a *load–elongation* or tensile *load–deformation* curve. Similar curves may be

Table 2.1 Elongation of a rod

State	Load (N)	L (cm)	$L - L_0$	w (cm)	$w_0 - w$
	None	4.0	0	1.0	0
a	200	4.2	0.2	0.98	0.02
b	400	4.4	0.4	0.96	0.04
c	700	4.8	0.8	0.92	0.08
d	700	5.2	1.2	0.75	0.25
e	300	5.6	1.6	0.60	0.40

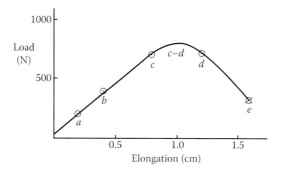

FIGURE 2.2 Load–elongation curve (tensile deformation).

obtained by plotting any force or moment as a function of some measure of the deformation.

If we connect the points a–e with a smooth curve, we find that the force apparently reached a maximum (= 750 N) when the bar had an elongation of 1.0 cm ($L = 5.0$ cm), somewhere between points c and d. This point, c–d, is the point of maximum load and coincides, observationally, with the onset of necking.

Types of load–deformation curves   There are two types of load–deformation curves. The first type is produced by forces alone and records changes in linear dimensions of objects without change in shape. The two types of forces that produce linear dimensional changes are *tension* and *compression*. These can be seen in Figure 2.3. The bar has been ruled with ghost rectangles; after either tensile or compressive deformation, the sides of these rectangles have different lengths but the rectangular shape is retained.

The second type of load–deformation curve is produced by moments and records changes in shape. Since the change in shape is frequently

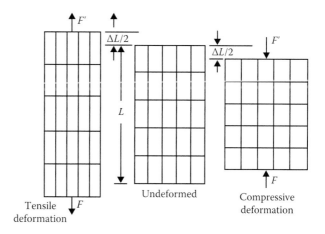

FIGURE 2.3 Tensile and compressive deformation.

determined by measuring the angle between the original and final location of an edge, these curves are sometimes called *moment–angulation* curves. The three types of moments that produce shape changes are *shear*, *torsion*, and *bending*.

Figure 2.4 shows shear deformation of a plate. Ghost rectangles retain the length of their sides, but are transformed into diamonds as the plate is deformed. The deformation is measured as the angle θ between an edge perpendicular to the direction of forces before and after the deformation. In the case of Figure 2.4, the deformation is 30°.

Figure 2.5 shows bending of a bar. The ghost rectangles are distorted, with their upper edges becoming longer and their lower edges shorter. This suggests that bending is a combination of tension and compression, depending on location in the bar. The dashed line is called the *neutral axis*, along which no length change occurs. The vertical edges of the ghost rectangles change slightly, becoming shorter in the tensile portion of the bar (above the neutral axis in this case) and longer in the compressive portion. The angle θ between lines perpendicular to the ends of the

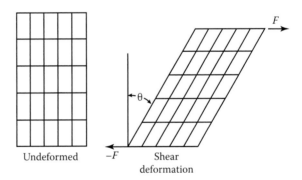

FIGURE 2.4   Shear deformation.

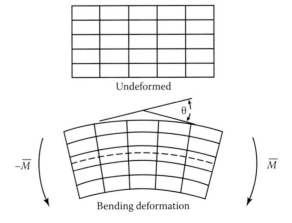

FIGURE 2.5   Bending deformation.

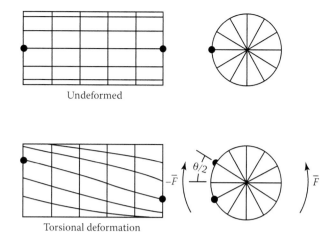

FIGURE 2.6   Torsional deformation.

bar is a measure of the amount of bending deformation. In the case of Figure 2.5, the deformation is 30°.

Figure 2.6 shows torsional deformation of a rod, the result of opposing moments acting around its longitudinal axis. Again, the ghost rectangles are distorted, but even more so than in shear or bending, with the long edges becoming longer, slanting with respect to the rod axis, and taking on a distinct curvature, whereas the short edges are unchanged in length, orientation, or shape. This shape change suggests that torsional deformation includes shear deformation. Marks at the end of a line on the side of the cylinder provide a way of measuring the amount of torsional deformation. In the case of Figure 2.6, the deformation is 60°.

Elastic deformation

Each of these load–deformation curves has two characteristic parts or regions. At low force or moment magnitude, the curve is straight and then begins to curve gently. The deformations recorded are reversible; prompt removal of the force or moment will permit the object to return to its original size and shape. Deformations in this region are called *elastic deformations* and are said to be fully recoverable. There is a point of maximum force or moment that is just enough to produce a permanent deformation after unloading; the level force or moment just below this value is called the *elastic limit*. The word *elastic* comes from a Greek root *elaunein* meaning "to drive," reflecting the power with which such materials "snap back" when released.

The elastic limit is a useful point to identify. It predicts the maximum force or moment that a designer would wish to permit a device, such as an intramedullary (IM) rod, to sustain. On a moment–angulation curve, this point corresponds to the highest value of force attained, the peak of the curve. Unfortunately, this point is difficult to determine experimentally. More importantly, if a bending moment–angulation diagram were to be made for a group of IM rods with different diameters, the elastic limit would occur at different values of moment for each device. This is

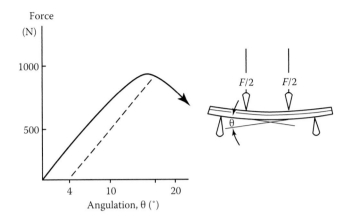

FIGURE 2.7   IM rod in four-point bending (Problem 2.1).

because the elastic limit, as determined in this manner, is an extrinsic property, dependent both on the size and shape of each device, as well as on properties of the material from which it is made.

Load–deformation curves have a valuable use; they may be used to determine general aspects of deformation under loading of devices. Of particular value is the fact that deformation above the elastic limit for a metallic device is unrecoverable, although the relationship between force and deformation is essentially unchanged.

Plastic deformation

Loading beyond the elastic limit results in deformations with increasingly large degrees of unrecoverability after load release. This is called *plastic deformation*.* The Greek root *plassein* means "to shape or mold," nicely reflecting the observation that plastic or unrecoverable deformation changes the dimensions or shape of a material in a permanent way, as already seen in necking during tensile deformation. The amount of plastic deformation can be determined by locating the point of interest on a load–displacement curve and constructing a line parallel to the elastic portion of the curve. The intersection of this line with the displacement/angulation axis gives the quantity of permanent plastic deformation (see Problem 2.1).

PROBLEM 2.1

An IM rod tested *in vitro* has the load–angulation diagram in Figure 2.7. If a removed rod of this size were found to have a 4° bend (although it had been inserted non-pre-bent), what is the maximum angulation that it would have undergone *in vivo*?

---

* The word *plastic* has unfortunately come to describe a class of materials more properly known as polymers (see Chapter 6). The use of the term *plastic* to describe unrecoverable deformation is the more general and appropriate use; polymers have come to be called plastics in common usage because most display plastic deformation at room temperature.

ANSWER:

If a straight edge is laid parallel to the elastic portion of the curve (dashed line), intersecting the angulation scale at 4°, it will intersect the curve at 16.5°.

The answer to Problem 2.1 suggests that any permanent angulation seen in a device *in vivo* is an indication of much greater elastic (recoverable) deformation having taken place. In this case, the total (transient) deformation was 16.5°, of which 12.5° was elastic and 4° was post-elastic or plastic.

Stress and strain

Force–displacement and moment–angulation data are only useful for devices of specific dimensions. To have broader utility, it is necessary to convert this information into intrinsic material properties. Such intrinsic information permits the prediction of the elastic limit, and other properties, for a device of any dimensions made from that material.

In Figure 2.8, we can see the considerations that lead to this conversion. In Figure 2.8a, we see that the effect of the application of a force F to a bar of length L_0 is an elongation $(L - L_0)$. If the initial length is L' $(= 2L_0)$ (Figure 2.8b), then the elongation $(L' - L'_0)$ is also twice as much $(= 2(L - L_0))$. Thus, the effect of the force is to produce an elongation proportional to the initial length. We can remove this proportionality, to be able to express a constant effect of the force on the rod, irrespective of length, by defining a new quantity, *strain*:

$$\varepsilon = \frac{L - L_0}{L_0}$$

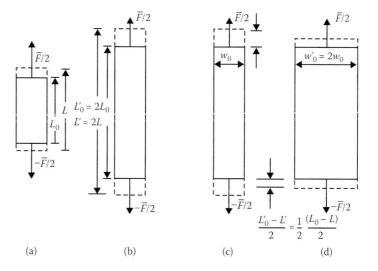

FIGURE 2.8 Derivation of strain and stress.

Table 2.2   Units of stress[a]

System		
British	CGS	SI
Pound/inch^2 (psi)	Dyne/cm^2	Newton/m^2 (Pa)
1	= 6.895 × 10^4 =	6.895 × 10^3
1.45 × 10^{-5}	= 1 =	0.1
1.45 × 10^{-4}	= 10 =	1

[a] 1 kgf/m^2 = 1.422 × 10^{-3} psi = 98.07 dynes/cm^2 = 9.807 Pa.

Since strain is the ratio of two lengths, it has no dimensions. It is either expressed as the ratio or multiplied by 100 and expressed as a percent.

Similarly, if the initial width is $w_0'(= 2w)$ (Figure 2.8c), then the elongation $(L' - L_0')$ is one-half as much (= 0.5*$(L - L_0)$) for a given force. Thus, the effect of the force is to produce an elongation inversely proportional to the initial width in the two-dimensional case. In three dimensions, the force produces an elongation that is inversely proportional to the cross-sectional area. We can remove this proportionality, to be able to express a constant effect of the force on the rod, irrespective of cross-sectional area, by defining a new quantity, *stress*:

$$\sigma = F/A_0$$

where A_0 is the initial cross-sectional area. Stress has the dimensions of force per unit area and may be expressed in several ways as seen in Table 2.2.

Stress is found by multiplying a scalar (1/area) times a vector (force), so it is a vector quantity and is often shown as such, especially to denote stress distributions.

PROBLEM 2.2

Which part experiences the greater internal compressive stress?

A. A stainless steel bar with a rectangular cross section measuring 1.2 cm × 3.0 cm under an axial load of 1.25 kN, or

B. A titanium alloy rod 3.5 cm in diameter under an axial load of 2 kN.

ANSWER:

For A, σ = 1250/(0.012 × 0.03) = 3.47 MPa

For B, σ = 2000/(3.14 × (0.035/2)^2) = 2.08 MPa

Therefore, the correct answer is *A*, even though the load in *A* is less than that in *B*. Note that stress depends only on dimensions, not on the material from which the object is made.

Table 2.3 Conversion of load and deformation of a bar into stress and strain

State	Load (N)	w (cm)	w^2 (cm²)	Stress[a] (MPa) Nominal	True	L (cm)	Strain Nominal	True
	None	1.0	1.0	0.0	0.0	4.0	0.0	0.0
a	200	0.98	0.96	200	210	4.2	0.05	0.049
b	400	0.96	0.92	400	435	4.4	0.1	0.095
c	700	0.92	0.85	700	830	4.8	0.2	0.182
d	700	0.75	0.56	700	1245	5.2	0.3	0.58
e	300	0.6	0.36	300	835	5.6	0.4	1.02

[a] Rounded off to the nearest 5 MPa.

These definitions are for quantities called *nominal* or *engineering* strain and stress. Nominal values are easy to calculate and are correct for small elastic deformations. True values may be defined, which are valid over wide ranges of both elastic and plastic deformation.

True stress and strain

True values for stress and strain can be thought as accounting for the instantaneously changing length and cross-sectional area, respectively. True strain is defined as:

$\varepsilon = \ln(L/L_0)$ (before onset of necking)

$= \ln(A_0/A)*$ (after onset of necking)

where the value of cross-sectional area (A) that corresponds to a particular stress beyond that which produces necking is measured in the neck region and is determined after loading to that stress followed by load release.

True stress is defined as:

$\sigma = F/A$

where A is the instantaneous cross-sectional area (in the neck region, if necking has occurred) rather than the original cross-sectional area.

Let us take the data (Table 2.1) we obtained in the experiment of stretching a bar (Figure 2.1) and convert the load and deformation values into stress and strain (Table 2.3).

For the sets of values below the onset of necking (between c and d), there is a very good correspondence between nominal and true values of both stress and strain. Because of this, and the fact that most devices are designed for very small peak strains, nominal and true values tend to be used interchangeably and the Greek letters sigma (σ) and epsilon (ε) are used conventionally for all values of stress and strain.

Plotting the true values of stress as a function of true strain and connecting them with a smoothly curving line produces a *stress–strain* curve (Figure 2.9). This expresses the intrinsic behavior of the material

---

* This form is correct; the apparent inversion from the prenecking formula occurs since volume (= $L_0 A_0$) is conserved. "ln(x)" is the natural logarithm of x.

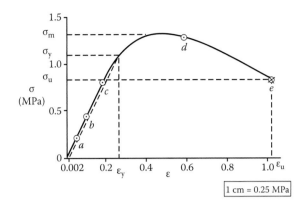

FIGURE 2.9   Stress–strain diagram (tensile).

that was tested in Figure 2.1, without any complications introduced by the dimensions of the specimen or by the onset of necking.

PROBLEM 2.3

The bar shown in Figure 2.1 contracts in width as it extends elastically. This corresponds to a transverse compressive strain. What are the true elastic compressive strains for points a, b, and c in Table 2.3?

ANSWER:

$\varepsilon = \ln(w/w_0)$

$w_0 = 1$ cm

for $w = 0.98$, $\varepsilon = -0.020$

for $w = 0.96$, $\varepsilon = -0.041$

for $w = 0.92$, $\varepsilon = -0.084$

Poisson's ratio

The absolute value ratio of the transverse compressive strain divided by the longitudinal tensile strain is called *Poisson's ratio* (symbol: ν). In the case of point c, $\nu = 0.084/0.182 = 0.46$. Poisson's ratio may take on values from 0 (for a fully compressible material) to 0.5 (for a material that maintains constant volume during deformation). Most materials have Poisson's ratios between 0.2 and 0.5. A Poisson's ratio of 0.5 means that the material is incompressible, such as rubber. A material that has a Poisson's ratio of nearly zero exhibits little lateral expansion when compressed. An example of such a material is cork. It is this property of cork that makes it widely used for serving as a stopper in wine bottles. As the cork is inserted into the bottle, the upper part which is not yet inserted will not expand as the lower part is compressed. Values greater than 0.5 imply expansion of volume during deformation and are unknown for simple materials. Some materials (known as *auxetic* materials) can also have negative Poisson's ratio, such as polymeric foam. This means that they become thicker in the cross-sectional directions when they are stretched.

Primary properties from the stress–strain curve

A stress–strain curve, such as Figure 2.9, has a number of properties that are important in understanding the behavior of materials. They are defined as follows:

Yield stress (σ_y). The stress at which plastic deformation begins.

0.2% offset (or proof) stress ($\sigma_{0.2\%}$). The stress that produces an unrecoverable strain of 0.2%. This is usually used in place of the yield stress to define the limit of elastic behavior, since it, corresponding to the onset of necking, is so difficult to determine accurately.

Maximum stress (σ_m). The maximum value of stress sustained before fracture.

Ultimate (or fracture) stress (σ_u). The value of stress just before fracture.

Elastic modulus (*E*). Ratio of stress divided by strain in the elastic region ($\sigma < \sigma_y$); the slope of the initial (linear) portion of the stress–strain curve. When the experiment is done in tension, this is called Young's modulus (symbol: *Y*). The elastic modulus in tension and compression is usually the same magnitude for simple materials. However, the shear modulus (symbol: *G*) is less, roughly one-third of *E* for metals.

Yield strain (ε_y). The instantaneous strain when the yield stress is applied; the largest value of recoverable strain.

Ultimate strain (ε_u). The strain at which fracture occurs.

PROBLEM 2.4

Find the characteristic values of stress and strain and the elastic modulus for the stress–strain curve in Figure 2.9.

ANSWER:

Construct a line parallel to the linear portion of the curve, intersecting the strain axis at 0.002. Then, construct vertical and horizontal lines from the intersection between this parallel and the stress–strain curve.

$$\sigma_y = \sigma_{0.2\%} = 1.1 \text{ MPa} \qquad\qquad \varepsilon_y = 0.26 \text{ or } 26\%$$
$$E = \sigma_y/\varepsilon_y = 4.23 \text{ MPa*}$$

---

* This is correct for a material whose stress–strain curve is linear all the way up to σ_y. However, some stress–strain curves show a distinct curvature between a lower value of stress and the yield stress. This lower value of stress is called the proportional limit (σ_p), and for materials possessing it, the modulus must be found directly by measuring the slope of the linear portion of the stress–strain curve.

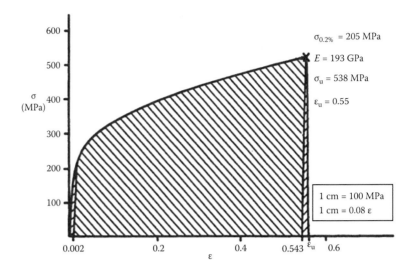

FIGURE 2.10   Stress–strain diagram (strain hardening).

σ_m = 1.33 MPa (by inspection)

σ_u = 0.835 MPa ε_u = 1.02 (by inspection or from Table 2.2)

The value of $\sigma_{0.2\%}$ (= 1.1 MPa) that occurs at ε = 0.26 predicts that the total force at yielding was 850 N. This is somewhat greater than the value we had estimated from the load–deformation curve for the onset of necking (800 N) (Figure 2.2) but is more accurate, since it is based on true strain.

The imaginary material described by Figure 2.9 is of a type that is called *strain softening*. This name comes from the fact that the ultimate stress is lower than the maximum stress; that is, there is a region of the curve for which the stress is decreasing despite an increase in strain. This is characteristic of polymers and some particular metals. The more usual type of behavior is called *strain hardening*, in which stress increases continuously with increasing strain and $\sigma_m = \sigma_u$. Figure 2.10 illustrates this more usual type of material behavior.

Structural aspects of deformation

Deformation in response to tensile or compressive loading is easy to comprehend, since a uniform distribution of stress may be assumed across the loaded faces perpendicular to the line of action of the applied forces. Thus, we can write

$$\sigma = E \cdot \varepsilon$$

This means that if we know the applied forces, we know the stress everywhere in the object and also the strain since it is related to stress by a constant, the elastic modulus. The same is true for shear loading, except that the shear stress is uniformly distributed over the face parallel to the line of action of the force and the proportionality constant is the shear modulus. These relationships are always true at a point; however, if the stress distribution is not uniform, then it must be known in detail to know the local strain and thus to predict the overall deformation from the intrinsic elastic material property, the elastic modulus.

Bending

In bending (Figure 2.5), the stress varies across the depth of a beam. The stress at any point is given by

$$\sigma = M \cdot y/I$$

where M is the bending moment at that point, y is the distance from the neutral axis, and I is areal moment of inertia, an expression of the distribution of material across the cross section of the beam. Values of I for various cross-sectional shapes are given in Table 2.4.

The values of interest, which will predict material failure, are the extreme values of the stress. These occur for $y = \pm d/2$, where d is the depth of the beam. These locations are the so-called *outer fibers*: the upper (maximum tensile stress) and lower (maximum compressive stress) surfaces of the beam shown in Figure 2.5.

Table 2.4   Areal moments of inertia

	Shape	Areal moment of inertia (I)
	Square	$\frac{1}{12}d^4$
	Rectangle	$\frac{1}{12}wd^3$
	I beam	$\frac{1}{12}(wd^3 - w'd'^3)$
	Solid rod	$\frac{1}{4}\pi r^4$
	Thick-walled tube $(r' > r/8)$	$\frac{1}{4}\pi(r^4 - r'^4)$
	Thin-walled tube: $(t \leq r/8)$ Intact Slit	$\pi r^3 t$ $2\pi r^3 t(1 - 3t/2r)$

PROBLEM 2.5

If three beams shown in Figure 2.11 with the same cross-sectional area were subjected to the same bending moment M, which would have the greatest outer fiber tensile stress?

ANSWER:

See Figure 2.11. The answer is A. The maximum stresses in A, B, and C have the ratio of 4:2:1. Another way to say this is that if the moment M were large enough for $\sigma = \sigma_y$, in A, then C could sustain a moment of $4M$ before yielding. However, the stiffness of the beams, the extrinsic resistance to deformation in any type of bending, whether three-point, four-point, or cantilever (one end fixed, the other loaded), is related to the areal moment, I, rather than to the outer fiber stress; thus, A, B, and C, while having the same cross-sectional area, have stiffnesses in the ratio 1:4:16.

Types of bending   Deformation in bending depends on the type of supports and constraints present as well as the distribution of loads. Figure 2.12 shows three common examples of bending geometries with their associated moment diagrams.

Three-point bending. A single load applied at the midpoint of a beam supported freely at each end. The bending moment and the outer fiber stresses are a maximum at the point of load application.

Four-point bending. Two loads, in this case taken as one-half each of the previous load, applied at separate points on a freely supported beam. The geometry used is one common to materials testing, with the end point–load point separation, a, one-fourth the length of the beam, L. The maximum bending moment, while smaller than before, still occurs at a load point but is constant between the load points (if the loads are equal).

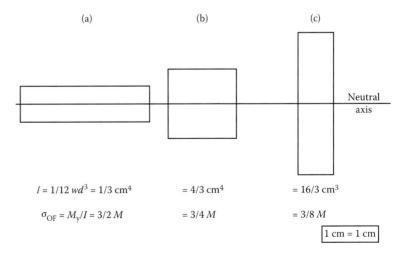

(a)   (b)   (c)

Neutral axis

$I = 1/12\ wd^3 = 1/3\ \text{cm}^4$ $= 4/3\ \text{cm}^4$ $= 16/3\ \text{cm}^3$

$\sigma_{OF} = M_y/I = 3/2\ M$ $= 3/4\ M$ $= 3/8\ M$

1 cm = 1 cm

FIGURE 2.11   Beam cross sections (Problem 2.3).

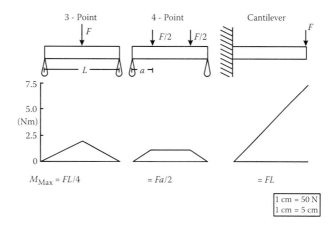

FIGURE 2.12   Bending geometries.

Cantilever. A single load is applied at the end of a beam with the other end fixed. This fixed point produces a maximum moment that decreases to the point of load application.

Each of these loading situations has advantages. Three-point bending concentrates the bending moment at a point away from the ends of the beam and is thus useful for measuring stiffnesses of healing long bone fractures in animal studies. Four-point bending maintains a constant bending moment over a region of the beam and is thus preferred when intrinsic properties of materials are being determined. Cantilever bending produces the greatest bending moment for the applied force; thus, it is helpful in testing very stiff materials and structures.

Structural efficiency

The relationship between areal moment of inertia and resistance to deformation is seen both in engineering practice and in nature. A structure (such as a beam or a bone) that adequately resists deformation while using the minimum amount of material is said to be highly *efficient*.

Let us look at an imaginary biotechnology experiment with the results shown in Figure 2.13. Section *a* is that of a solid, circular bone, with a radius of 1.4 cm. Sections *b* through *d* were constructed by allowing the radius to increase to 2.0 cm and forming a medullary canal so that the area of the cross sections remained constant; that is, the same amount of bone material was present per length of bone. The results are somewhat striking: as the radius increases from 1.4 to 2.0 cm (a 43% increase), the stiffness (as measured by the areal moment of inertia, I) increases by 210%, while the maximum outer fiber stress, for a given applied bending moment, decreases by 54%. Thus, *d* is a very much more efficient structural cross section than *a*.

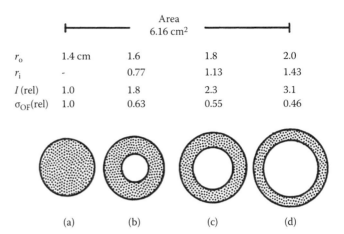

FIGURE 2.13   Structural efficiency of circular cross-sections.

This example may explain why most bones have medullary spaces; their presence is a sign of relative structural efficiency. It also helps to understand why endosteal absorption and periosteal accretion occur in osteoporosis: since stiffness is proportional to the product $E*I$, when E decreases, as in osteoporosis, a response that increases I by remodeling will help restore stiffness without increasing the amount of bone present.

Buckling

There is, however, a limit to which this principle may be extended. A bone is generally considered a thick-walled tube, since its cortical thickness (t) is rarely less than one-eighth its radius (r). Tubes with ratio (t/r) less than one-eighth tend to behave as curved sheets rather than as tubes; thus, different formulas are required to calculate moments of inertia, as seen in Table 2.4. What is different about thin-walled tubes is that they are subject to *buckling*: local, concentrated deformation.

Buckling in bending is difficult to discuss in general because it depends on many factors, including the shape and location of the supports. However, buckling may occur under any type of loading and is usually considered in compressive (end) loading of a cylinder, as in Figure 2.14.

There is a critical force, F_C, that will produce buckling:

$$F_C = \frac{2E \cdot I}{L_e^2}$$

where L_e is an *effective* length, dependent on the degree of constraint at the ends of the column. If the column ends are free, then $L_e = L$; if they are fixed, then $L_e = L/2$.

It is useful to restate this relationship as follows:

$$F_C = \frac{2E \cdot A}{(L_e/k)^2}$$

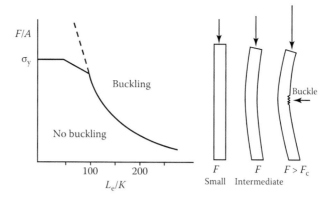

FIGURE 2.14   Conditions for buckling.

where A is the cross-sectional area and k is called the radius of gyration ($= (I/A)^{1/2}$) ($= r/2$ for a column).

It is then possible to make a plot of critical stress (critical force/A) versus the ratio L_e/k. For low values of this ratio (below approximately 50), the critical stress for buckling exceeds the yield stress, so that no buckling occurs. There is a small intermediate range ($50 < L_e/k < 100$) in which buckling also does not occur but in which the yield stress appears to be modestly reduced. Finally, there is a range in which buckling always occurs ($L_e/k > 100$). This region is called the region of elastic buckling, since structural deformation, although resulting in plastic deformation as loads redistribute, begins as an elastic instability.

Buckling may occur easily in a lamellar structure, such as bone, if delamination produces individual portions of material with very high L_e/k ratios. This phenomenon is probably responsible in part for the so-called buckle fracture that is seen in poorly mineralized immature bone. Trabecular buckling may also occur in osteoporotic vertebral bodies as loss of horizontal spicules radically increases L_e in the remaining vertical spicules.

Torsion

In torsion (Figure 2.6), the major stress is a shear stress that increases with radial distance from the center of a rod. The shear stress, τ, at any point is given by

$$\tau = M \cdot r/K$$

where M is the torsional moment at that point, r is the radial distance from the rod axis (the neutral axis in torsion), and K is the polar moment of inertia, an expression of the distribution of material across the cross section of the rod. Values of K for various cross-sectional shapes are given in Table 2.5. As before, the torsional stiffness (resistance to torsional deformation under load) depends on the value of K.

Table 2.5 Polar moments of inertia

Shape	Polar moment of inertia (K)
Square	$0.141a^4$
Triangle	$(\sqrt{3}/80)a^4$
Solid rod	$\frac{1}{2}\pi r^4$
Thick-walled tube	$\frac{1}{2}\pi(r^4 - r'^4)$
Thin-walled tube	$\frac{1}{2}\pi r^3 t$
Thin-walled tube, open	$\frac{2}{3}\pi r t^3$

PROBLEM 2.6

If a 16-mm-diameter thin-walled tube (wall thickness, $t = 1.0$ mm) were to be used as an IM device, how much would its torsional resistance be reduced if it were slit parallel to its axis?

ANSWER:

From Table 2.5:

$$K(\text{intact}) = \frac{1}{2}(3.14)(8)^3(1) = 804 \text{ mm}^4$$

$$K(\text{slit}) = \frac{2}{3}(3.14)(8)(1)^3 = 16.8 \text{ mm}^4$$

Therefore, the slit produces a 98% reduction in torsional stiffness. Fortunately, IM devices function primarily in bending; a similar calculation shows no reduction if the slit is positioned on the level of the neutral axis, and only modest reductions, depending on slit width, if the slit is located at other positions.

Secondary properties from the stress–strain curve

In addition to the relationship between stress and strain, there are other, secondary properties that may be derived from the stress–strain curve. *Strength*

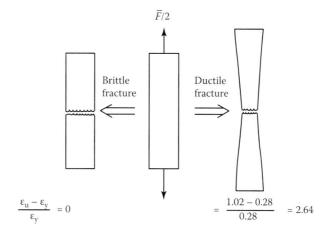

$$\frac{\varepsilon_u - \varepsilon_y}{\varepsilon_y} = 0 \qquad\qquad = \frac{1.02 - 0.28}{0.28} = 2.64$$

FIGURE 2.15 Ductile versus brittle fracture.

is understood as a measure of the ability of a material to sustain stress. Thus, σ_y is called the *yield strength* and σ_m or σ_u, whichever is larger, is called the *ultimate (tensile) strength*. *Ductility* is literally the ability of a material to be drawn out, that is, plastically deformed, before failure. It is defined as ε_u, expressed as a percentage. It is useful to compare the values of ε_y and ε_u. If $\varepsilon_u - \varepsilon_y$ is small compared with ε_y, then the material is called *brittle* and fails with little or no plastic deformation and an absence of necking (Figure 2.15). On the other hand, if $\varepsilon_u - \varepsilon_y$ is large compared with ε_y, then the material is called *ductile* and shows considerable plastic deformation after failure.

Toughness is a measure of the ability of a material to absorb energy before fracture and relates to a commonsense impression of how easily materials may be broken. Toughness is measured by the energy per unit volume required to produce fracture. It is equal to the area under the stress–strain curve to ε_u and has dimensions of force × distance/unit volume. Energy and work have the same units of force × distance; thus, the units in each of the three systems are the same as for moment (see Table 2.5). When used to express energy, these units have special names. The most commonly used is the joule (= 1 Nm). At fracture, a portion of this work, represented by the area in the hatched triangle to the right of Figure 2.10, is released primarily as sound, but the balance has been stored within the matrix. In the case of brittle fracture, in the limit where $\varepsilon_y = \varepsilon_m = \varepsilon_u$, all of the energy is released, which explains why breaking glass produces such a loud sound.

PROBLEM 2.7

What is the ultimate strength, ductility, and work of failure of the material represented by the stress–strain curve in Figure 2.10?

ANSWER:

Ultimate strength = σ_u = 538 MPa

Ductility = 100 × 0.55 = 55%

Work of failure: Rule off the area under the stress–strain curve into 1 cm squares. Using the scales given in the figure, each of these squares is equal to 8 J/m³. There are approximately 26 such squares (fragments added together to make full squares); thus, the answer is $26 \times 8 = 208$ J/m³.

This stress–strain curve is derived from a moderately strong, tough, and highly ductile material frequently used in fracture fixation hardware, 316L stainless steel.

Strain hardening

Strain (or work hardening) alters the properties of materials that have been subject to plastic deformation. Let us return to the example of 316L stainless steel and imagine an experiment that produced the results shown in Figure 2.16. This experiment was performed in three steps.

1. A tensile load was applied to produce a stress of 350 MPa. This is above σ_y (as measured by $\sigma_{0.2\%} = 205$ MPa) so that plastic deformation takes place.

2. The load was released, and a residual (unrecoverable) strain of 0.11 was measured.

3. The load was restored and increased until the stress reached 400 MPa.

Looking at the portion of the stress–strain curve that this experiment generates, we can make the following observations:

1. Loading beyond the yield stress produces a residual deformation; thus, plastic deformation *reduces* ductility.

2. When the initial load is released and then reapplied, the linear portion of the stress–strain curve is parallel to that found initially. Therefore, strain hardening does not change the elastic tensile modulus.

3. However, the yield stress upon reloading is apparently higher than before loading (~300 MPa vs. 205 MPa, an increase of approximately 45%). Thus, strain hardening *increases* the yield strength.

4. Since the ductility has decreased, the work to failure on reloading also decreases. Thus, strain hardening *reduces* toughness.

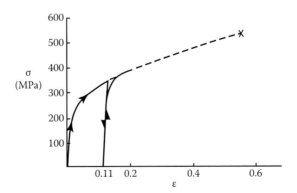

FIGURE 2.16   Work hardening.

Thus, in summary, strain hardening increases yield strength at the expense of lower ductility and toughness, while leaving intrinsic stiffness (modulus) unchanged. This effect is sometimes used deliberately in fabrication of implants and surgical instruments (see Chapter 7) and is a necessary result of any plastic deformation in a metallic device.

PROBLEM 2.8

Suppose that the experiment described in Figure 2.16 was continued until the material failed. Find the ultimate strength, ductility, and work of failure of the material represented by the stress–strain curve from the point of reapplication of load after the initial load–unload cycle and compare the answers with those obtained in Problem 2.5.

ANSWER:

Ultimate strength = σ_u = 538 MPa (unchanged)

Ductility = $100 \times (0.55 - 0.11) = 44\%$ (vs. 55%)

Work of failure: Again, using the method of squares, the answer is $23 \times 8 = 184$ J/m^3 (vs. 208 J/m^3). Thus, prestressing 316L stainless steel to 350 MPa leaves its ultimate strength unchanged, but reduces its ductility by $100 \times (1 - 0.44/0.55)$ or 20% and its toughness by $100 \times (1 - 18.4/20.8)$ or 11.5%.

Initiation of fracture

When materials fracture, it is because the chemical bonds between their atomic constituents have been stretched beyond their cohesive ability. This process may be thought of as either a critical stress (σ_u) being exceeded or an energy storage (work of failure) capacity being surpassed. The former (critical stress) view is instructive in that it predicts the position and orientation of the initial crack.

Fracture will occur when either the maximum tensile or shear strength of a material is exceeded. In either case, the initial crack occurs in the plane of the maximum resolved stress. In Figure 2.15, it would be clear, even without the presence of the force vectors, that the transverse failures were tensile, since they occur in a plane of maximum tensile stress.

Initial crack patterns in simple loading of the other types discussed are more complex (Figure 2.17) and may depend on surface constraints.

In compression, when the ends of a short cylinder are free to move, shear failure occurs. However, if the ends are restrained by friction or other forces, the rod "barrels" and a large circumferential tensile stress, called a *hoop* stress, results, leading to the formation of a vertical tensile failure. This mode of failure is often seen in incomplete burst fractures of vertebral bodies.

In shear, a simple "delamination" failure occurs. This is difficult to distinguish from a tensile failure; careful stress analysis is needed to identify it.

In bending, the initial failure is a tensile failure of the outer fiber under maximum tensile stress, on the convex surface of the beam.

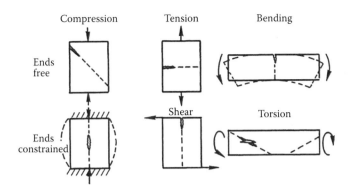

FIGURE 2.17   Fracture initiation patterns.

In torsion, the failure is usually a shear failure that follows a spiral path. Such a spiral pattern is absolutely diagnostic of torsional failure, even in combined loading situations. However, there may be an additional small vertical tensile failure component.

These are ideal patterns. The actual details of crack initiation and propagation are complex, depending on the addition of stresses, on the relationship between ultimate tensile and shear strengths for the material, and on the presence of internal structural features and defects. (These issues will be dealt with at greater length during the discussion of fracture of bone [Chapter 5].)

Practical aspects of material deformation

Ideality

The discussion of deformation so far has dealt in ideal terms. In the real world, a number of complicating factors arise that significantly affect the results obtained, even in apparently simple circumstances. There are three primary sources of these complications.

1. The materials discussed have been assumed to be uniform and homogeneous internally. In fact, real materials contain many structural and compositional inhomogeneities.

2. It was also assumed that the surfaces of materials have the same properties as their interiors. This is also not so, leading to some interesting difficulties.

3. Finally, it was assumed that forces applied to an object lead to uniform internal stress distributions, in the presence of homogeneous material. This is not the case, even for the apparently simple cases of compressive and tensile deformation.

These departures from ideality produce many practical problems in the examination and analysis of the mechanical properties of material. However, one of these problems plagues us in day-to-day life: the concentration of stress by inhomogeneities, leading to premature and unexpected failure.

Stress concentration

One of the puzzles of material behavior is why a relatively strong material such as window glass may be broken easily after it is scratched. Careful studies have revealed that the stress around a defect, such as a surface scratch or an internal pore, is much higher than expected. In fact, it may be shown generally that the true stress near such a defect, σ_T, is given by

$$\sigma_T = k \cdot \sigma$$

where σ is the average stress $(= F/A)$ and k is some multiplier that always exceeds 2. Thus, a scratch on a surface may produce local stresses that exceed σ_u even when the average stress is below σ_y.

For cracks or pores,

$$k = D/r$$

where D is the width of an internal defect or twice the depth of a surface crack perpendicular to the applied force and r is the smallest radius of the defect or crack, usually at a crack root. The minimum value of k is thus 2 for a hemispheric notch and may reach values of 10–12 for scratches made with a sharp knife blade.

PROBLEM 2.9

Which biopsy hole (Figure 2.18) through the lateral cortex of the femur will have the least weakening effect on the femoral shaft?

ANSWER:

The approximate values of K $(= D/r)$, where D is taken as the width of the cortical defect perpendicular to the line of action of the maximum tensile stress (here, the long axis of the bone, since this is the direction of maximum tensile force in both bending and torsion) are as follows:

A. Sharp-edged hole: 4

B. Four small holes, joined by osteotomy cuts: 3

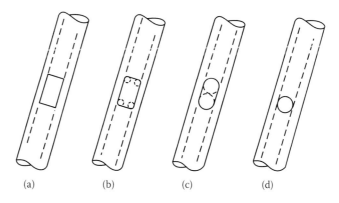

(a)   (b)   (c)   (d)

FIGURE 2.18 Effect of differently shaped biopsy holes.

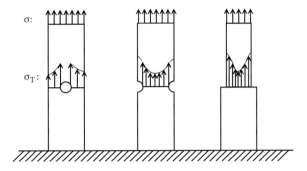

FIGURE 2.19   Stress-concentrating design features.

C. Two large holes, with "saddle" broken out: 2.1

D. Single large hole: 2

Thus, the best answer is *D*; the best way to take a bone biopsy is with a trephine or a Craig needle. Extending the defect proximal–distal as in *C* causes a small secondary structural weakening effect not directly related to stress concentration. This is a small effect, since the bone is a thick-walled tube. The values for *A* and *B* are less than the theoretical calculations would suggest (≈10 and 4, respectively) for homogeneous defect-free material. Cortical bone has such a high density of inherent defects (lacunae, Haversian canals, cement lines, etc.) that the stress concentration factor cannot practically exceed 4, even for holes with sharp corners. Finally, in living bone, the stress concentration effect of a hole may be removed by local remodeling, even if the hole persists, as in a sequestrum. (For discussion, see Clark et al. 1977.)

In addition to obvious cracks and defects in materials or hard tissue, engineering design may contribute to stress concentration by providing internal holes, external retaining notches, or simply by abrupt changes in cross-sectional area (Figure 2.19). One design response to this is the "constant strength" fracture fixation plate, which has a greater thickness at screw hole locations to compensate for stress concentration effects. Acquired defects, such as scratches, nicks, and so on, are also points of stress concentration. For this reason, it is advisable not to use fracture fixation components with obvious surface flaws.

Additional problems

PROBLEM 2.10

For the two materials in Figure 2.20, select the best answer:

A. *b* is equal in strength to *a*.

B. *b* is stronger than *a* since it can undergo more strain before failing.

C. *b*, while having a lower yield stress than *a*, is more ductile and therefore absorbs less energy before failure.

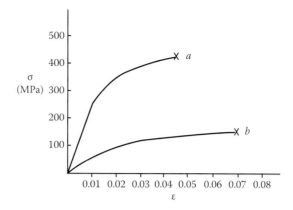

FIGURE 2.20 Stress–strain curves for two materials (Problem 2.10).

  D. *b*, while having a lower yield stress than *a*, is more ductile but absorbs less energy before failure.

  E. *b* is stronger than *a* since it has a higher yield stress and a bigger elastic modulus.

ANSWER:

The best answer is *D*. *b* is weaker than *a*; therefore, answers *A*, *B*, and *E* are false. In addition, *E* is also false, since *b* has the smaller elastic modulus. Although *b* has a lower yield stress than *a* and is more ductile, energy absorption is the area under the stress–strain curve, not the ductility; therefore, *C* is false.

PROBLEM 2.11

For material *a* in Figure 2.20, find the following quantities: yield stress, maximum stress, ultimate stress, ultimate strain, elastic modulus, and work to failure. Use correct symbols in the answer, where applicable.

ANSWER:

  σ_y = 250 MPa

  $\sigma_m = \sigma_u$ = 425 MPa

  ε_u = 0.07 or 7%

  E = 250 MPa/0.01 = 25 GPa

  Work to failure = 14 × (100 MPa × 0.01) = 14 J/m³

PROBLEM 2.12

The two plates shown in Figure 2.21 have identical lengths and are made of the same material, but *A* is twice as thick as *B*. If the plates were to be tested in three-point bending, with a force of 200 N applied, which of the following statements are true?

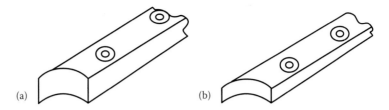

FIGURE 2.21   Fracture fixation plates (Problems 2.12 and 2.13).

A. The elastic modulus of plate *A* is higher than that of *B*.

B. The bending stress of plate *A* is higher than that of *B*.

C. Plate *A* will fail at a lower level than plate *B*.

D. Plate *A* will bend less than plate *B*.

E. Plate *A* will fail in shear while *B* will fail in tension.

ANSWER:

A. False, since modulus is intrinsic. It is proper to say that *A* is stiffer than *B*, although the moduli are the same.

B. False. If "bending stress" means bending moment, these are identical, as they are determined by the test apparatus and the applied force. If "bending stress" means σ_{of}, then $\sigma_{of(A)} = 1/4\sigma_{of(B)}$.

C. False. Whether fail means plastically deform or fracture (if the bending moment applied is high enough), *B* will fail before *A*.

D. True. Deformation is linearly related to M/E^*I; thus, it varies inversely as *I* and $I_A = 8I_B$.

E. False. Both plates will deform if σ_{of} exceeds the tensile yield stress and fracture if it exceeds the ultimate tensile strength. Changing *I* does not change the failure mode.

PROBLEM 2.13

If plate *B* (Figure 2.21) were to be doubled in thickness, which of the following statements would be true?

A. Axial stiffness in tension or compression would increase four times.

B. Axial stiffness in tension or compression would increase eight times.

C. Elastic modulus would increase two times.

D. Bending stiffness would increase four times.

E. Bending stiffness would increase eight times.

ANSWER:

A and B. Both false as axial stiffness depends on cross-sectional area and would increase two times.

C. False. See Figure 2.12, answer *A* above.

D. False. See *E* below.

E. True. Bending stiffness of a beam increases as the cube of its depth. See Table 2.4.

PROBLEM 2.14

Figure 2.22 is a stress–strain diagram. Point *P* is the proportional limit, point *A* is the yield point, and point *U* represents the fracture conditions. Which of the following statements are true?

A. This material is not linearly elastic.

B. Stresses exceeding the yield stress produce large plastic deformations.

C. Young's modulus of the material is 26.7×10^9 N/m.

D. *U* represents brittle failure.

E. This material is not ductile owing to the small difference between the yield stress and the ultimate stress.

ANSWER:

A. True. The proportional limit is less than the yield stress.

B. True.

C. False. At *P*, Y = stress/strain = 400 MPa/0.015 = 26.7 GPa (1 GPa = 10^9 N/m², see Table 2.2). Right number, wrong units!

D. False. Plastic/elastic deformation ≈ 3.5.

E. False. Ductility is related to the difference between yield and ultimate strains, not stresses.

PROBLEM 2.15

Consider the load–unload cycle that passes through points *A*, *B*, and *C* in Figure 2.22. Which of the following statements is true?

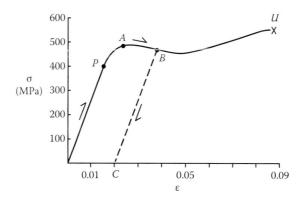

FIGURE 2.22 Stress–strain curve (Problems 2.14 and 2.15).

A. There is always unrecoverable (permanent) plastic deformation after the stress passes point *P*.

B. The permanent deformation is 3.75%.

C. The energy required to produce failure in the material is less than that required to produce a strain of 0.0875.

D. The plastic deformation after unloading is 0.02.

E. The load–unload cycle shown does not result in any net energy loss since the final state of stress (point *C*) is zero.

ANSWER:

A. False. Point *A* (yield stress) must be passed for unrecoverable deformation.

B. False. This is the deformation under load at point *B*.

C. False. The net energy loss is less, but the total energy input is that required for a strain of 0.0875. The difference is elastic energy recovered during rebound after fracture.

D. True.

E. False. The energy loss per unit volume is the area between the load and unload portions of the cycle.

PROBLEM 2.16

A desirable material for an internal fracture fixation device should (select the answer that appropriately completes the sentence)

A. Have a high modulus and a low yield strength

B. Have a low modulus and a high yield strength

C. Have a high modulus and a high yield strength

D. Have a high tensile strength

E. Be flexible

ANSWER:

The best answer is *C*. A fracture fixation device must have minimum volume (high modulus) and a large range of possible elastic loads (high yield stress). A low yield strength does permit plate contouring during insertion but also permits plastic deformation postoperatively, leading to possible failure of prompt bony union. Tensile strength is less important, since most fracture fixation hardware does not fail in single-cycle loading.

Reference

CLARK CR, MORGAN C, SONSTEGARD DA, MATTHEWS LS: The effect of biopsy-hole shape on bone strength. *J Bone Joint Surg* 59A:213–217, 1977.

Annotated bibliography

1. BECHTOL CO, FERGUSON AB, LAING FG: *Metals and Engineering in Bone and Joint Surgery*. Williams & Wilkins, Baltimore, 1959.

    Chapter 6 is a good description of early work on the strength of bone and the effects of stress concentration.

2. DONALD GD, POPE MH: Design of intramedullary nails. In Seligson D (ed): *Concepts in Intramedullary Nailing*. Grune & Stratton, Philadelphia, 1985.

    An excellent discussion of intramedullary nail design features with an emphasis on mechanical requirements.

3. FRANKEL VH, BURSTEIN AH: *Orthopaedic Biomechanics*. Lea & Febiger, Philadelphia, 1970.

    Chapter 2 discusses stress and strain and the deformation of structures. Chapter 3 contains some material on energy of deformation. Chapter 7 covers the design of fixation devices. A useful supplementary source.

4. WEIGHTMAN B: Stress analysis. In Swanson SAy, Freeman MAR (eds): *The Scientific Basis of Joint Replacement*. John Wiley, Chichester, 1977.

    Detail on internal stress distributions as a function of loading conditions. A good brief discussion of experimental methods for determining strain distributions.

5. WILLIAMS DF, ROAF R: *Implants in Surgery*. WB Saunders, London, 1973.

    Plasticity is briefly covered on pp. 80–83. Deformation of structures and performance of devices are well covered in Chapter 7 (pp. 364–375, 394–409). This book contains extremely thorough citations to prior work.

CHAPTER THREE

Mechanical properties

The previous chapter deals with the relationship between external loading and internal elastic–plastic deformation in materials. Relationships are provided to reduce these extrinsic factors to stress and strain, which are associated with the behavior of materials rather than with structural behavior. Stress–strain curves for materials then become the fundamental mechanical data that are used to examine the suitability of a particular material for a given load-bearing application. These data are generally acquired in tension for simplicity, and various calculations, on the basis of a number of assumptions, have to be made to predict the behavior of materials in compression and shear or in more complex situations including bending, torsion, and combined loading.

If this were the totality of considerations necessary, then selection of materials would be relatively easy. However, loading may vary with time, in either an irregular or a repetitive manner. The environment under which the material will operate may be air, if it is an external application, but even this involves wide ranges of temperature, humidity, and possible immersion in water, whereas internal (implant) applications present quite different exposure conditions. These conditions resemble those encountered in other engineering applications but present unique problems, especially since there is a requirement, not usually present in other applications, to maintain almost absolute environmental purity. In addition, these conditions vary from patient to patient.

Furthermore, materials possess a variety of deformational mechanisms not directly predictable from classic elastic–plastic stress–strain relationships. Even taking these into account, actual manufactured materials may show different mechanical behavior from that predicted either theoretically or on the basis of handbook values, which are based on limited testing. These latter differences arise from controlled and uncontrolled variations in manufacturing processes and require proof testing of a portion of each batch of devices to determine the values of critical properties in high mechanical requirement applications, to assure that selection assumptions are correct and safe.

All of these considerations enter into selection of materials for mechanical applications.

Stress–strain characterization

Handbook or reference properties of materials are sometimes limited to six primary values, obtained from moderate strain rate single cycle to failure tensile testing in air of specimens with round or square cross sections. Although the values quoted are the mean of many determinations, uncertainties (confidence interval, standard error of the mean, etc.) and actual composition and source (other than grade) of materials are not usually provided. Thus, these properties, given in the order of frequency of citation, are *nominal* or *handbook* values (Figure 3.1).

1. *Elastic modulus.* The Young's modulus (E or Y) is calculated directly from the slope of the stress–strain curve in the linear region and can be used to predict fully the elastic deformation of the material. Since some materials show distinctly nonlinear but proportional behavior near the yield point, such calculations set a *lower* limit for deformation and are only accurate for small deformations ($\varepsilon \ll \varepsilon_y$). Viscoelastic materials, such as soft tissues and polymers, are not characterizable by a single value of modulus (see Chapter 4).

2. *Yield point (or yield strength).* The most usually cited value is the 0.2% yield or proof stress ($\sigma_{0.2\%}$), since it is easier to obtain accurately than the true yield stress σ_y (see Chapter 2). Thus, this value sets an *upper* limit on the stress necessary to produce unrecoverable deformation. Viscoelastic materials demonstrate a wide range of strain recovery ability; thus, the yield point is not a useful descriptive parameter for them.

3. *Tensile strength.* The value cited is usually the highest stress encountered on the stress–strain curve, but it is frequently based on the initial area (engineering stress) rather than the actual area

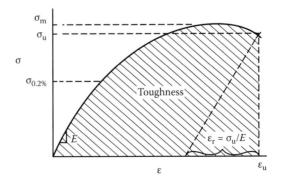

FIGURE 3.1 Engineering properties from the stress–strain diagram.

(true stress), again for easy experimental determination. Modern handbooks and tables cite true values of σ_m. This value is given rather than the stress at failure (σ_u) since σ_m is either equal to or greater than σ_u and it is assumed in actual applications that if external loads are sufficient to produce σ_m, they will be sustained and lead to rapid post-necking fracture.

4. *Elongation at fracture (or elongation to failure).* Again based on laboratory tests, this is the amount of deformation remaining *after* failure and thus is a measure of ductility. Frequently expressed as a percentage, it is then called *percent elongation*. It is usually determined by placing marks 1 to 2 inches apart on the tensile specimen before testing. This dimension is called the *gage length* and may be quoted in the data table. After testing to failure, the two parts of the specimen are reapproximated and the separation between the gage marks is measured. Then, the elongation is calculated as follows:

$$\text{Percent elongation} = \frac{\text{Final length} - \text{Gage length}}{\text{Gage length}} \times 100.$$

This is a strain; thus, it has no dimensions and is equal to $\varepsilon_u - \varepsilon_r$, where ε_r is the elastic strain at failure ($= \sigma_u/E$) (see Figure 3.1).

For highly ductile materials, percent elongation is an excellent, but still slightly *low*, estimate of ε_u (expressed as a percentage). If it is cited as "percent elongation *before* (or *at*) failure," then it is measured intraexperimentally and is explicitly equal to ε_u, without allowance for elastic recovery after fracture.

5. *Reduction in area.* This is another measure of ductility, which is easy to obtain experimentally in highly ductile materials. Frequently expressed as a percentage, it is then called *percent reduction*. No gage length or specimen marking is required. A circular cross-section tensile specimen is used, and its diameter is measured initially and after failure. Then,

$$\text{Percent reduction} = \frac{((\text{original diameter})^2 - (\text{final diameter})^2)}{(\text{original diameter})^2} \times 100.$$

For incompressible materials ($\upsilon = 0.5$), this will be the same as percent elongation but will be less than that if $\upsilon < 0.5$. It may also be measured intraexperimentally, with some difficulty, and then the value is cited as "percent reduction *before* (or *at*) failure" and is related to percent elongation obtained under the same conditions.

6. *Toughness.* This is the ability to absorb energy before failure and is especially important for applications involving impact, such as the striking face of a surgical mallet or impactor. As previously

discussed (see Chapter 2), this is the total area under the stress–strain curve to ε_u and is expressed as an energy per unit volume, typically with units of J/m³.

Material types

It is a usual practice in engineering discussion to generalize the comparative values of these parameters and to use overall descriptive terms for materials. Thus, using the general shape of the stress–strain curves in Figure 3.2, material *A* would be called "strong, brittle," material *B*, "strong, tough," and material *C*, "weak, ductile." We associate type *A* curves with ceramics, type *B* curves with metals, and type *C* curves with polymers (and soft tissues). Composite structures (see Chapter 8) have no single characteristic stress–strain behavior; their utility lies in being able to combine the mechanical properties of different materials, such as a ceramic fiber and a polymer matrix, to produce new, intermediate behavior.

PROBLEM 3.1

In Figure 3.2, which material (*A*, *B*, or *C*) is the

Stiffest?

Strongest?

Most ductile?

Most brittle?

Toughest?

ANSWER:

A, A, C, A, B.

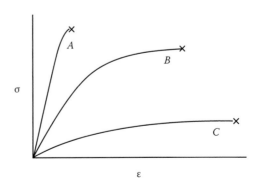

FIGURE 3.2   Typical stress–strain curves.

Atomic origin of mechanical properties

These different types of stress–strain behavior derive from the fundamental physics of interaction between the atoms of the solid involved. It is important to consider these, at least qualitatively, as these interactions provide some insight into the origin of mechanical behavior not predictable from the data presented on stress–strain curves or in their tabular summaries.

Atomic association within solids (and liquids) at body temperature is chemical in nature and depends on the fundamental attraction between electrical charges of opposite sign, expressed in Coulomb's law:

$$F = \frac{k \cdot q_1 \cdot q_2}{d^2}$$

where F is the interactive force (attractive when the charges are of opposite sign), q_1 and q_2 are the magnitudes of the charges, d is their physical separation (1–3 Å in solids), and k is an experimentally derived constant that adjusts the units appropriately. At the extremely short distances between atoms in solids and liquids, coulombic forces are very large and are the origin of the structural cohesion of materials.

Charges are formed on atoms (atoms are converted to ions) by the addition and subtraction of electrons. The "structure" of electrons around the nucleus of any atom produces preferred numbers of electrons, described as constituting a "filled outer electron shell"; thus, ions derived from any atom have one or more favored net charges.

Interatomic bond types

Combination of these two effects in solids produces four types of bonds or interactions between atoms (Figure 3.3):

1. *Metallic.* Atoms that form metallic solids, such as iron, nickel, chromium, cobalt, and so on, are able to lose one or more electrons easily. This is seen in their ability to conduct current (in this

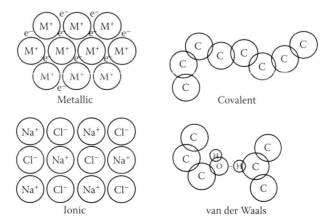

Metallic

Covalent

Ionic

van der Waals

FIGURE 3.3 Types of bonds between atoms in solids.

case, a stream of moving electrons). The resultant positive ions pack together into high-density planes and structures, surrounded by a cloud of delocalized electrons. Metallic bonds are very strong but not particularly oriented in space. Planes of metallic atoms can slide* over each other fairly easily, producing ductile deformation but generally associated with considerable toughness, owing to the strength of the metallic bond and the ease of re-establishing it after adjacent planes of atoms move one atomic diameter.

2. *Ionic.* Some pairs of atoms can easily exchange one or more electrons, producing filled outer shells in each and a resultant pair of positive and negatively charged ions that are strongly attracted. Metal atoms in particular can donate electrons to atoms of gaseous elements such as nitrogen, oxygen, and chlorine. The result is a dense three-dimensional structure with oriented bonds but with a high degree of order imposed by alternation of ionic type. These materials are extremely strong but, at body temperature, tend to fail catastrophically along a plane of symmetry when the ultimate strain is exceeded. Thus, the ionic bond contributes brittle behavior to solids.

If these compounds are stable in the presence of water, they are called *ceramics*, such as aluminum oxide (alumina), zirconium oxide, and silicon nitride. If they are appreciably soluble in water, they are called *salts*, such as sodium chloride.

3. *Covalent.* Some atoms can fill their outer electronic shells on a virtual basis by sharing electrons with an adjacent uncharged atom. This is represented in Figure 3.3 by a slight overlap of the circles representing the atoms. The resulting bond is strong but very directional, owing to the details of electronic structure in the atom. The result can be long chains of covalently bonded atoms, with carbon being the best and most common example. The resultant chains possess relatively fixed angles between bonds on a particular atom but permit easy rotation around single-exchange bonds and are quite strong. Therefore, these solids possess very large molecules (polymers) that can deform easily but break only with difficulty, exhibiting significant plastic behavior.

4. *van der Waals.* Hydrogen in particular can participate in a very weak form of nonexchange bonding with oxygen and a number of other atoms. This is weaker and less directional than the covalent bond, but the very great quantity of hydrogen in *hydrocarbons* (polymers containing carbon, hydrogen, and oxygen, including proteins and other structural molecules in tissues as well as most man-made polymers) produces large contributions to the cohesion of materials. *Polymers* (long-chain molecules made up of identical or repetitive molecular groups) have strong covalently bonded

---

* The process is called "slip" and the motion planes are called "slip planes." Slip requires the application of shear stresses; reference to Chapter 2 will reassure the reader that in all but uniform (hydrostatic) compression, shear stresses result from any external force.

"backbones" linked together with a few covalent bonds ("cross-links") and many van der Waals bonds. Thus, they are generally weak and ductile but may be very tough, especially if the molecules are very long (of high molecular weight) and are tangled together or covalently cross-linked.

Relationship of interatomic bonds to properties of materials

Elastic behavior depends very strongly on the nature of the most common bond in a material. Thus, ionically bonded materials (ceramics) are generally stiffer than metallically bonded ones (metals) and they in turn are stiffer than covalently and van der Waals–bonded ones (polymers). Furthermore, the stiffness of a material is very poorly related to details of its chemical composition. Thus, all types of stainless steels (see Chapter 7) have essentially the same Young's modulus, despite wide variations in the alloying elements.

Ductile behavior is much more difficult to predict. Metals are generally ductile since layers or planes of metallically bonded atoms can move over each other. Polymers are also ductile, resulting from the relative ease with which van der Waals bonds can be broken and remade and covalent bonds may rotate about their axes. Ceramics, on the other hand, are brittle, since one atomic spacing deformation between adjacent planes of atoms produces repulsive rather than attractive forces. However, details of structure, including inhomogeneities in metals and physical arrangement (intertwining) and cross-linking in polymers, can radically affect ductility. (These topics will be discussed at greater length in Chapters 6 through 8.)

However, the problem of strength is more general. Like elasticity, it should depend directly on the nature of the most common interatomic bonds in any solid. However, in the vast majority of cases measured, strengths are one-tenth to one-hundredth those that are expected, on the basis of the properties of the interatomic bonds involved. This disparity between theory and experience has two principal origins.

1. At an atomic level, well-ordered solids, such as metals, may possess "defects" in the planes of atoms. These may be missing atoms, extra atoms, folds, steps, and so on. Although some of these defects interfere with slip, others, such as extra atoms or extra partial planes of atoms, make slip easier than predicted and the materials will fail when the strength of their weakest portion is exceeded. This is a common effect in metals. However, polymers are generally not sufficiently ordered for slip to be an important deformation mechanism.

2. At a molecular level, and on a somewhat larger scale, real materials usually are not ideal, containing cracks, voids, and so on. As discussed in Chapter 2, these discontinuities produce significant stress concentrations, causing apparently premature failure resulting from local stresses far exceeding those determined from external loading and dimensions. At the atomic level, cracks may be extremely "sharp," producing stress concentration factors of as great as 100. This effect is very obvious in brittle materials,

such as window glass, which can be bent significantly but fails at very low external load if scratched, as with a glass cutter. Similar effects exist in ductile materials, but the ability to dissipate energy by local plastic deformation at the tip of the defect tends to produce much less degradation in strength than in brittle materials.

Thus, defects significantly reduce the strength of metals, polymers, and ceramics, but the inherent plasticity of polymers tends to protect them. Composites are, by design, highly defective, owing to the large area of interface between the components involved. Accurate strength predictions are nearly impossible since the nature and strength of bonding across these interfaces are unknown except in a few special cases.

In any case, fracture of a material is caused by the formation and propagation of a crack until material integrity is lost. Any material feature that either produces cracks or reduces the energy needed to produce or propagate them will weaken the material, whereas, conversely, any feature that reduces the number of cracks or increases the energy needed to form or propagate them will strengthen the material.

One may further characterize materials by comparing the ease of defect formation to defect (crack) propagation. If it is difficult to produce a defect but easy to propagate it in a material, then that material is said to be "notch (or crack) sensitive." There is no comparable term for the opposite situation (easy production, difficult propagation), but simple reflection suggests that such a material would be easy to scratch or mar but would be relatively tough. Glasses and brittle materials tend to be notch sensitive, whereas polymers are softer (easier to scratch) and relatively tough (in terms of retention of predicted ultimate strength).

Strengthening mechanisms

The "art" of strengthening materials by changing composition, structure, or processing is sufficiently complex to merit a book in its own right. All such variations involve increasing the difficulty of either crack initiation or crack propagation. Some simple examples are as follows:

Surface hardening. Increasing the hardness of the surface in an otherwise relatively defect-free but notch-sensitive material, such as a glass, can greatly strengthen it. Such surface hardening may be brought about by alloying or, in the case of metals, by cold working. In some cases, heat treatments can produce phase transformations selectively at the material's surface to produce the same effect.

Increased cross-linking. In polymers, strength may be remarkably increased by increasing the volume density of cross-linking (covalent) bonds. This may be restricted to the surface, if it is desired to retain bulk plasticity, or produced throughout to increase overall toughness. Cross-linking may be produced by a variety of means, including heat, ultraviolet illumination, or ionizing radiation. In some cases, gases of unsaturated organic molecules, such as acetylene, may be used to further strengthen the material through incorporation during cross-linking.

Particulate reinforcement. Weak materials, such as polymers, may be strengthened by adding small quantities of very strong particles or fibers. In materials in which the limitation on strength is easy crack propagation, such materials produce increases in strength since cracks must either break through them or "detour" around them to propagate. This effect can be produced in some metal alloys by careful heat treatment producing precipitation of very strong materials, usually metallic carbides, or by the introduction of oxygen to form internal dispersions of metallic oxides. (These latter processes may degrade corrosion resistance; see Chapter 12.)

Other mechanisms of deformation

In addition to elastic (recoverable) and plastic (nonrecoverable) deformation, there are three other principal modes of materials deformation that must be taken into consideration in selection of materials. None of these types of behavior are predictable from standard stress–strain curves but must be characterized by other experimental means.

Creep
Creep is simply plastic deformation at stresses below the yield point. The phenomenon is usually observed as a time-dependent increase in strain when a material is maintained at a constant stress below the yield stress. Most materials exhibit creep, but it is most noticeable in metals at elevated temperatures and in polymers and tissues at body temperatures. It may or may not be recoverable, depending on the nature of the internal deformation process.

There are three distinct stages of the creep process (Figure 3.4), which are often referred to as types of creep:

Primary (type 1) creep. Occurs at an initial high rate, which rapidly decreases.

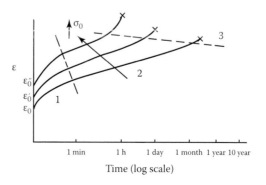

FIGURE 3.4 Creep curves.

Secondary (type 2) creep. Occurs after primary creep and is characterized by a rate that is constant with the logarithm of time until immediately before failure.

Tertiary (type 3) creep. A final, rapid increase in rate to a maximum and failure.

These three stages or types are easily associated with three parts of a creep curve. However, all three stages may not be seen. At low temperatures or low stresses, only types 1 and 2 may occur, whereas elevated temperatures and stresses are needed to cause type 3. Under these latter conditions, the transition between types 1 and 3 may be very rapid, with no type 2, or so-called "steady-state," creep seen. Note that the initial values of strain, such as ε_0, ε_0', and so on, are the elastic responses to the load application (= E/σ_0).

There is no minimum stress below which creep will not occur in materials capable of plastic deformation; however, all three creep rates increase with increasing stress. Temperature also has a profound effect on creep. Many materials will not creep below a minimum temperature, and most exhibit rapidly increasing creep rates as temperature increases. This is a factor in selecting polymers for orthopaedic applications since most engineering data are determined at room temperature.

Determination of creep deformation Creep deformation is quite important in orthopaedic applications of polymers. It is generally referred to in the clinical literature as "cold flow." It is believed that perhaps as much as one-half of the apparent wear in polyethylene acetabular cups and perhaps a greater proportion of that in polyethylene knee components are due to creep deformation rather than material loss.

Information on creep rates is provided in three forms.

1. *Rupture strength.* Failure (fracture) by creep is called "rupture" in engineering usage and is described by the stress needed to produce it in either 100 or 1000 hours.

2. *Creep rate.* Less common, this is the value of type 2 or steady-state creep, at a particular temperature and stress, expressed as a strain rate.

3. *Creep deformation.* This is a measurement of the deformation of a cube of material under a static stress (value given) after 24 hours at room temperature. A related parameter, *residual* creep deformation, is the deformation, usually expressed as a percent strain, after a post-static stress recovery period of 1–3 days.

None of these parameters permit easy prediction of creep in a particular application, since this will be dependent on the complete stress history of the device. However, any of these three parameters is useful for comparative predictions.

Creep processes are quite similar, at the material level, to those producing single-cycle failure (as in the derivation of a stress–strain curve). Thus, any material modification that improves strength has the possibility of improving creep behavior (reducing creep rates or increasing creep rupture strength) and vice versa. However, other factors, including environmental interactions, may also act, and thus it is extremely difficult to predict creep behavior from fundamental considerations.

Stress relaxation   Stress relaxation is, in a sense, the opposite of creep: reduction of internal stress while a constant strain, below ε_y, is maintained. It is characterized by an early rapid release of stress followed by a rate that is constant with the logarithm of time (Figure 3.5). There is no third stage, comparable to tertiary creep, since the final condition is not rupture but simply the loss of all internal stress. As is suggested by the initial strains present in creep experiments, the initial values of stress, such as σ_0, σ'_0, and so on, are the elastic consequences of deformation ($= \varepsilon_0 E$).

As is the case with creep, the rates of stress relaxation increase with increasing initial stress, deformation, σ_0, and increasing temperature. Stress relaxation rates are usually not listed in handbooks directly. However, the interrelationship with creep rates is obvious. The constant (later) stress relaxation rate may be calculated, with some difficulty, from the secondary creep rate. However, the direct comparison between the two behaviors is easy: a higher secondary creep rate is always associated with a higher steady-state stress relaxation rate.

Note that if both creep and stress relaxation data are plotted on a linear time (horizontal) scale, they appear to reach a limit fairly rapidly for many materials. This is apparent but not real; the vast majority of materials under most conditions lack a real limit to either phenomenon.

The primary evidence for stress relaxation effects in orthopaedic applications is the early reduction of internal elastic stress in internal fixation devices, particularly preloaded hardware, as is used in long bone (internal) fracture fixation (Figure 3.6). The loss in stress at the fracture site, which has been demonstrated in experimental models, is due to a combination of creep of bone at screw contact points and internal stress relaxation in bone and other tissues secondary to the external application of the plate with an initial tensile stress. In addition, creep deformation

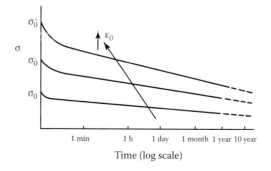

FIGURE 3.5   Stress relaxation curves.

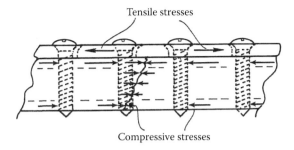

FIGURE 3.6   Stresses in internal (plate) fixation of fractures.

in polymeric components, such as tibial inserts in total knee replacements, can be mistaken for wear (see Chapter 11).

Fatigue

Materials may fail under stresses below the ultimate stress and even below the yield stress if these stresses are applied in a repetitive or cyclic manner. The rhythmic nature of human motion imposes such cyclic stresses on the bones and soft tissues in the limbs and thus on fracture fixation devices and partial and total joint replacement coupled to them.

For instance, if a patient after total hip replacement arthroplasty were to walk a distance of 2 miles per day at an average gait of 30 steps per minute, a relatively modest pace, the femoral stem of the device would experience a total of 1.2 million (1.2×10^6) bending stress cycles, at a frequency of 0.5 Hz, each year. Over a period of years, enormous numbers of cycles can be accumulated on a prosthetic device. To account for the observation that more than one relative stress peak may occur within one gait cycle and to afford a margin of safety, the usual estimate of cyclic load number in orthopaedic applications is 2×10^6 per year.

Such loading may produce brittle fractures, as seen in Figure 3.7. This cast cobalt chrome hip resurfacing component was removed 3 years after

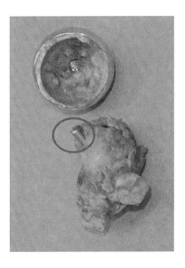

FIGURE 3.7   **(See color insert.)** Fatigue failure in a hip resurfacing stem.

implantation. The failure occurred through the stem of the resurfacing component, owing to contributions from both body weight– and gait-imposed forces. The failure occurred after a loss of bony support due to remodeling,

PROBLEM 3.2

If a runner attempts to run a marathon with a cortical screw securing a medial malleolar fracture, how many cycles will the screw accumulate?

ANSWER:

A marathon is 26 miles and 385 yards. Assume a running stride of 4 feet. Thus, the runner takes 34,609 strides to complete the race. Multiply by 2 to account for forces at heel strike and push off to yield an estimate of 6.92×10^4 cycles.

The S–N curve The general fatigue behavior of materials is shown in Figure 3.8, which is called an *S–N curve* (for stress–number) or *fatigue life curve*. The vertical axis is the peak stress per cycle, on either a logarithmic (as shown here) or a linear scale, whereas the horizontal axis is the number of cycles accumulated, always on a logarithmic scale. The more or less diagonal line on the *S–N* curve divides the regions of failure and nonfailure at a 50% confidence level. Any particular point on that line represents the combination of a number of cycles and a critical stress. After accumulating a certain number of cycles (N), the corresponding value of stress (given by the curve) is the stress that the material can withstand with a 50% probability of failure. Higher stresses are more likely to cause failure, whereas lower stresses may be sustained without reasonable risk of failure.

 S–N curves must be interpreted in such a statistical manner, since the eventual failure is a fracture. In parallel to the term ultimate strength (σ_u), the value of stress at any point on the curve is called the *fatigue strength* (σ_f). The number of cycles required to produce a 50%

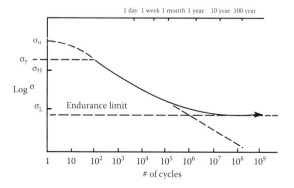

FIGURE 3.8 *S–N* (fatigue life) curve.

probability of failure at a stress (above the endurance limit) is called the *fatigue life*.

As the number of cycles increases, the stress that produces a 50% probability of failure decreases. However, for many materials, including iron-base, cobalt-base, and titanium-base alloys, the curve flattens out in the region of 10^6–10^7 cycles and becomes horizontal. This part of the curve is called the "knee," and the constant stress value is called the *fatigue* or *endurance limit*. Designs for cyclic load applications attempt to keep peak stresses below this value so that an infinite amount of cycles may be sustained without failure. In many metallic alloy systems, it is observed that this endurance limit is an essentially constant proportion of σ_u (as fabricated), typically between 0.5 and 0.3.

Types of fatigue failure Failures occur in two types as a result of cyclic load. The first is the region on the left side of Figure 3.8 and is called *high-stress, low-cycle failure*. The peak cyclic stress required to produce this type of failure is high (designated here as σ_H) and may even exceed the yield stress. The other type of failure occurs to the right of the figure and is called *low-stress, high-cycle failure*. The peak stress that produces this type of failure is low (designated here as σ_L) and may be near the endurance limit.

PROBLEM 3.3

For the material represented by the *S–N* curve in Figure 3.8, what are the fatigue lives for σ_y, σ_H, and σ_L?

ANSWER:

σ_y yields a fatigue life of 100 cycles, and σ_H yields a fatigue life of 300 cycles. Both of these stresses would produce very early failure. σ_L would probably exceed 10^7 cycles in air, since it is so close to the endurance limit. However, in vivo, it might be limited to 5×10^5 cycles or several months of ordinary use.

Fatigue processes may produce modest changes in elastic behavior by an accumulation of work hardening, if local stresses exceed σ_0 owing to stress concentration effects. This is rarely reflected in measurable properties. However, composites often show marked reductions in elastic modulus before fracture, owing to sequential failure of the interfaces between the various phases in those materials. In such cases, a failure criterion, usually a modulus reduction of between 10% and 30%, may be selected, and the *S–N* curve may be plotted to reflect the 50% probability of that reduction occurring.

Each stress–strain cycle has the ability to do a certain amount of work per unit volume of material. In high-stress situations, this work is enough to either initiate or propagate a fatigue crack. However, in low-stress situations, the stress may be inadequate either to form a new crack or to propagate a previously formed crack. Outside of stress magnitude, the difference in response to stress may be affected by other factors, including the following:

1. Introducing surface defects, such as scratches, nicks, changes in section, or other departures from a uniform smooth surface, tends to reduce the endurance limit.

2. Most *S–N* curves are plotted from data obtained in air. If metallic alloys are tested under corrosive conditions, the endurance limit may be reduced or, in some cases, particularly for iron-base alloys, may disappear and σ_f will continue to decline with increasing *N*. This is shown schematically as a dashed line on the right side of Figure 3.8.

Fatigue life in air is not dependent on the frequency of stress application except in polymers in which high frequencies may produce internal heating (and related property changes; see Chapter 6). Fatigue life is dependent on temperature but not in a simple or predictable manner. Metals for which corrosion reduces or eliminates the endurance limit usually have higher fatigue lives at higher frequencies. Thus, accelerated in vitro tests may not adequately predict fatigue life of metals in vivo.

For these reasons, it is usually not possible to design to resist fatigue in a detailed way. The usual engineering practice is to determine the fatigue strength after 10^7 cycles (the most usual value supplied in handbooks) in a suitable environment and design devices so that expected peak tensile stresses do not exceed some proportion, typically 0.5 to 0.7, of this stress.

A further safety factor is provided since most fatigue tests of materials are performed with fully reversible stresses. That is, the test is designed such that during each load–unload cycle, the peak tensile and compressive stresses have the same magnitude. This is expressed in the *stress ratio*:

R = minimum stress/maximum stress

For a fully reversible stress, *R* = −1. Most engineering applications involving fatigue loading have characteristic R_s between 0.9 and 0.1. Under these conditions, fatigue life and endurance limit are usually greater than when stress is fully reversed.

Appearance of fatigue fractures Fatigue fractures have a particular appearance that makes them easy to distinguish from single-cycle failures (Figure 3.9). They display a series of parallel lines or concentric rings, called *fatigue striations*, over a large part of the fracture surface. These rings are also commonly known as river marks because they look like a river on a physical map. If rings, they appear to radiate from or center on one or occasionally several points. This point (or points) is (are) the initiation point(s) of the failure—the place(s) where the combination of overall peak tensile stress and stress concentration features (inclusions, cracks, etc.) combined to produce a local stress that exceeded σ_u. Each line represents the distance that the crack propagated during the peak of the stress cycle. Fatigue failures at higher average peak stresses show wider separations between lines than ones at lower stresses. At the

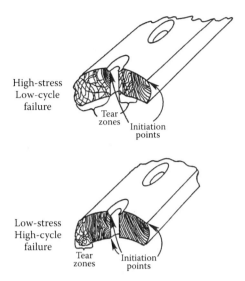

FIGURE 3.9   Types of fatigue failures in fixation plates.

onset of total failure, the cross section is sufficiently reduced that the peak stress on the next cycle is able to completely crack or plastically tear through the remaining material, producing either a granular or a plastic appearance. This is called the *tear zone*. High-stress, low-cycle failures may be accompanied by plastic deformation of the section and have a relatively large tear section (Figure 3.9, left) while low-stress, high-cycle failures appear more brittle, with a large zone of fatigue striations and a small or sometimes absent tear zone (Figure 3.9, right).

Figure 3.10 shows a typical low-stress, high-cycle failure in a pedicle screw. The fracture was initiated on the bottom right corner and grew toward the top left corner until ductile failure of the remaining material.

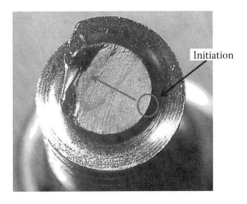

FIGURE 3.10   **(See color insert.)** Low-stress, high-cycle-number fatigue failure in metal component.

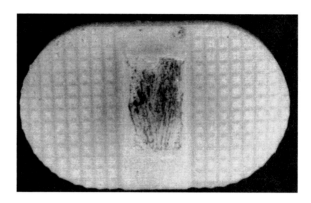

FIGURE 3.11 High-stress, low-cycle fatigue failure in polymeric component.

Figure 3.11 shows a high-stress, low-cycle failure in a polyethylene tibial plateau. Absence of medial support permitted medial–lateral "rocking" of the plateau, leading to a rapid (6 weeks postoperation) fatigue failure of the central stem. Note the wide separation between the major fatigue striations (the fracture surface was shadowed with black spray paint to make these more easily seen) and the ductile tear region in the upper left (anterior).

Temporal aspects of fatigue failure Fatigue failures that occur in the first days to weeks after insertion may be considered, a priori, high-stress, low-cycle failures. However, the more usual orthopaedic device fatigue failure is the brittle-appearing low-stress, high-cycle type.

The knee of the *S–N* curve for most metallic alloys occurs in the predicted 1- to 10-year life period for orthopaedic applications (see upper horizontal scale, Figure 3.8). Thus, late (>2 years) fatigue fractures of metallic components are usually associated with either single peak stress events that exceed the endurance limit or changes in support (bone resorption, fracture, etc.) that change the peak stress. Extreme increases in patient weight or activity level may also produce late fatigue failures.

It is often argued that late device fractures associated with trauma (falls, vehicular accidents, etc.) are "caused" by the traumatic event. Although this is "true," in that the trauma is frequently the proximate cause of the fracture, examination of the fracture surface usually shows it to be a low-stress, high-cycle fatigue failure. Then, the following two points must be taken into consideration.

1. Patients are extremely sensitive to very small changes in joint mechanics and, especially if infirm, may fall as a result of aversion movements associated with small but sudden changes in device configuration. Thus, patients who present after a fall with fatigue fractures of femoral stems or fracture plates frequently report feeling a "shift" or "giving way" or hearing a "crack" before or during such a fall.

2. Even if the forces produced by aversion or impact do produce the fracture, the resultant stresses may be far below σ_u, so that it can more properly be said that the device was essentially "time expired" and that any slight overload would have produced failure. In this case, the overload event should be considered as *contributing* to failure, but the primary cause of failure was the preexisting, ongoing fatigue process.

Static fatigue   All materials are subject to fatigue, with metals and polymers displaying the features discussed here. Ceramics at body temperature do not possess significant ductility and thus do not show fatigue striations. However, when subject to high static or peak dynamic loads, especially in chemically active environments, they may fail suddenly, producing fracture surfaces not distinguishable from those of single-cycle failures. Since ceramics are rarely deliberately designed to sustain high tensile cyclic loads, these failures are often called *static fatigue* fractures. The detailed mechanism is unknown. As mentioned earlier, composites also display fatigue behavior, but the damage appears to be primarily a progressive failure of adhesion between the various components of the material rather than fatigue fracture of any one material.

Clinical observations of fatigue failure   Fatigue fractures of orthopaedic devices usually initiate where expected, in regions of high tensile stress:

On the lateral faces of femoral stems or at the proximal limit of distal support (Figure 3.12)

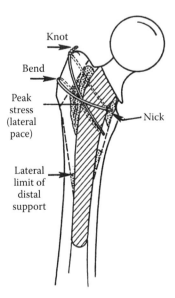

FIGURE 3.12   Points of fatigue failure initiation.

On the superior face or side of internal fixation plates used as tension bands, at a screw hole where the plate cross section is a minimum (Figure 3.9)

At abrupt changes in cross-sectional area or shape (see Figure 3.11)

At scratches or nicks produced in prostheses during installation (Figure 3.12)

At bends or knots in cerclage wire (Figure 3.12)

It may be difficult to determine the point of maximum local stress on a device from the usual external evidence of anteroposterior and lateral radiographs and a general knowledge of anatomic biomechanics. The picture is complicated by the variable stress-concentrating features of cracks (depending on their shape) and by the presence of internal stresses, produced by processes or, in some cases, by deformation during device insertion.

Impact resistance The toughness of a material determines its impact resistance. External devices and implants often undergo impact loading during use owing to patient falls, blows, or other traumatic events.

The toughness is defined as the area under the stress–strain curve to ε_u, as stated earlier. However, since the ability to produce single-cycle failure is dependent on stress concentration factors including inhomogeneities and surface finish, toughness is usually evaluated directly by a specialized test.

In a typical arrangement, a sample of the material is machined to standard fixed dimensions with a carefully prepared notch. It is placed in a clamp, and a swinging hammer is allowed to strike it on one side of the notch. The kinetic energy of the hammer is calculated before and after impact; the difference represents the work of fracture of the specimen. Unfortunately, the results depend to some degree on the shape of the notch and the configuration of the test device, so that the value obtained is best used in a comparative manner than in an absolute manner. The units for impact strength are those of work (N*m or ft*lb), and the most common test arrangement is called the Charpy test, so the result of such a test is frequently reported as a *Charpy (impact) toughness.*

Hardness The hardness of a material is its ability to resist local plastic deformation, especially at its surface. Hardness is an important design parameter in many applications, including impact surfaces, cutting edges, and articulating interfaces. It should be possible to infer it directly from the knowledge of E and σ_y, for any material. However, most materials have different mechanical properties at their surfaces than in their interiors, even if deliberate steps are not taken to alter surface properties. (See Chapter 7 for some examples of surface treatments of metals that affect hardness.)

Hardness is usually measured directly with one or another variation of a basic technique. This consists of pressing an indentor into the surface with a known load and measuring some aspect of the resulting impression. Such tests produce large impressions in soft materials and small ones in hard materials. There are several different eponymic tests that produce scales of relative hardness. All the scales are arranged so that a higher number corresponds to a harder material.

The most common is the Rockwell test, which is based on the measurement of the depth of penetration of the indentor under a fixed load. Different indentors and different loads produce a variety of scales; the Rockwell number reported (R_C, R_M, etc.) is calculated from the reciprocal of the penetration depth. The less common Vickers and Brinell scales express hardness as the mean stress at the point of the indentor (load/area or the impression) and use units of either kgf/mm² or pascals.

The relationship between the different engineering hardness scales is shown in Figure 3.13. An older, geologically oriented scale, the Mohs scale, based on scratch testing, is included for comparison. Orthopaedic alloys are among the harder metals, whereas polymers as a group tend to be fairly soft. Ceramics may be hard or soft depending on their structure and composition, as shown by the Mohs scale. Relative hardness may be important when several materials are used in combination. For instance, softer materials tend to be transferred to harder ones during wear processes. This may be controlled to some degree by altering the hardness of one or the other material.

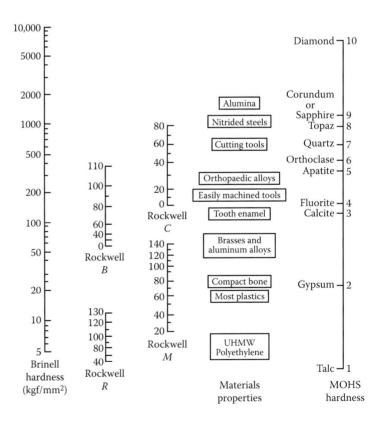

FIGURE 3.13　Hardness of materials.

Additional problems

PROBLEM 3.4

A brittle material

    A. Is stronger in tension

    B. Is stronger in bending

    C. Is fatigue resistant

    D. Is stronger in compression

    E. Is easily shaped

ANSWER:

The correct answer is D since compression will close preexisting cracks and inhibit crack propagation. Brittle materials are weaker under other types of loading. They are hard and not easily shaped.

PROBLEM 3.5

Creep phenomena in materials (true or false)

    1. Are of no concern in orthopaedics

    2. Occur in many materials including metals

    3. Occur only if a material is viscoelastic

    4. Result in fracture

    5. Occur under cyclic load

ANSWER:

F, T, F, F, T. Creep is of concern in orthopaedics as it has been shown to contribute to failure in polyethylene components. Polymers, tissue, and metals (at elevated temperatures) display creep. Viscoelasticity (deformation depending on both load and load rate) is not a precondition for creep. Creep results in fracture (or rupture) only in the tertiary stage. Static loads can produce creep; creep may also occur under cyclic loading conditions and may be greater than expected for the same static average load.

PROBLEM 3.6

The material for a fracture fixation plate should be as hard as possible (true or false).

ANSWER:

False. Surface hardness is desirable to prevent marring or deformation of the plate by the underside of the screw heads. However, since hardness is related directly to σ_y, a fully hard plate would be difficult to deform and be quite brittle. Thus, a better combination of properties would be a soft interior combined with a hard surface; this combination can be obtained by processing.

PROBLEM 3.7

The endurance limit (select the best answer)

    A. Refers to a creep test

    B. Exists for all metals

    C. Is reduced by surface defects

    D. Is increased by a corrosive environment

    E. Is none of the above

ANSWER:

The best answer is *C*. An endurance limit is found during fatigue rather than creep testing and does not exist for all metals. When an endurance limit exists, corrosive conditions tend to remove it, especially for iron-base alloys.

PROBLEM 3.8

Stress relaxation is desirable in internal fixation since it tends to eliminate stresses in the fixation devices (true or false).

ANSWER:

False. Fixation devices remain secure owing to frictional forces generated by stresses produced in them during insertion. Relief of these stresses secondary to either stress relaxation or creep processes may result in loosening of the devices and loss of fixation integrity.

PROBLEM 3.9

A 37-year-old male patient, who works as a mail carrier, sustains a spiral fracture of the right femur that is treated with dynamic compression plates applied to both lateral and anterior sides of the femoral shaft. He is seen on referral 30 months after surgery. He reports pain at the fracture site at the end of his route. Radiographic examination results in a diagnosis of nonunion. Is there any aspect of the fixation one should be concerned with?

ANSWER:

This individual is obviously placing significant cyclic loading on his internal fixation hardware. It may already have one or more partial cracks associated with screw holes. These are usually not seen on radiographs, although stress films may be of some value. The fixation is at risk; whatever therapy is decided for the nonunion, adjunctive measures should be taken to remove or support the hardware or reduce the cyclic loading upon it. Fixation hardware may be expected to fail eventually in the presence of unstable long bone nonunion, owing to the lack of bony support and load sharing.

PROBLEM 3.10

The femoral head resurfacing component shown in Figure 3.7 was removed after a sudden onset of pain and radiographic evidence of fracture 3 years after insertion. Complete the following statements:

The failure is a _____ fracture.

The failure is a _____ stress, _____ cycle fatigue failure.

Modifying the design to _____ the thickness/diameter of the stem or to use a material with a higher _____ might have delayed or prevented this failure.

ANSWERS:

Brittle, low, high, increase, endurance limit. Increasing the thickness/diameter of the device reduces stress; selecting a higher endurance limit tends to compensate for the design. However, material or design changes need to be considered in light of impact on other design factors or implant performance. Generally speaking, design factors interact with one another in terms of trade-offs in different performance measures.

PROBLEM 3.11

The hardness of structural ceramic implants is (select the best answer)

A. Less than that of metals

B. Less than that of polymers

C. Greater than that of metals

D. Less than that of metals but greater than that of polymers

E. None of the above

ANSWER:

The best answer is *C* since ceramics lack any appreciable plasticity their hardness correlates with σ_u rather than σ_y, as is the case of metals. Since useful structural ceramics are stiffer and stronger (in the defect-free state) than most metals, they are also much harder. Polymers are usually softer than all but the softest metals.

Annotated bibliography

1. BLACK J, HASTINGS G: *Handbook of Biomaterial Properties*. Chapman & Hall (Springer), London, 1998.

Useful compilations of reliable mechanical properties of tissues and prosthetic materials.

2. GILLAM E: *Materials Under Stress*. CRC Press, Boca Raton, FL, 1969.

   An insightful but easy-to-read short work that discusses the mechanical properties of materials by classes (metals, polymers, ceramics, and composites). Considerable material on how the different types of bonds produce different internal structures.

3. HAYDEN HW, MOFFATT WG, WULFF J: *The Structure and Properties of Materials*. Vol. III. John Wiley & Sons, New York, 1965.

   This is part of a classic series of four volumes on materials science that is still a standard source. Volume III deals with mechanical properties. See Chapters 1, 4, and 7 especially.

4. NASH WA: *Strength of Materials*, 4th ed. McGraw-Hill, New York, 1998 (Schaum's Outline Series).

   An engineering text, at the undergraduate level, that has an excellent progression of problems with solutions on mechanics of materials. Recommended for the reader who wishes to pursue the analytic aspects of orthopaedic biomaterials.

5. O'KEEFE R, JACOBS JJ, CHU CR, EINHORN RA, Editors. *Orthopaedic Basic Science 4*. American Academy of Orthopaedic Surgeons, Chicago, 2012.

   Chapter 4 is a topical outline of orthopaedic biomaterials. Older editions were accompanied by a slide set useful for teaching purposes.

6. SHACKELFORD JF: *Introduction to Materials Science for Engineers*, 7th ed. MacMillan, New York, 2008.

   Despite the title, this book is highly accessible to those who are not engineers, with a simple orderly approach, solved problems, and excellent illustrations. Chapter 1 deals with structure of materials, Chapter 2 deals with bond types, and Chapter 7 deals with mechanical properties of metals.

Viscoelasticity

Loads applied to materials produce internal elastic and plastic deformations. The stress–strain diagram (see Chapter 2) describes the intrinsic behavior of materials in a general way, such that we speak of stress (vertical axis) as a *function* of strain (horizontal axis). In this conventional manner, strain is taken as an independent variable and a test is performed as follows:

1. A specimen is made to standard dimensions.
2. A suitable apparatus is used to deform the specimen.
3. As the specimen is deformed, the resultant force on a load cell within the apparatus is recorded simultaneously with values of a parameter that measures deformation.
4. The deformation (extrinsic independent variable) and the resultant force (extrinsic dependent variable) are combined with the specimen dimensions to yield the paired values of strain and stress (intrinsic variables) required to plot the stress–strain curve.

The test described above is a standard, repeatable process that can be used to at least partially describe the properties of any solid material. The resulting stress–strain relationship can be referred directly to the nature of the chemical bonds between atoms, with some interpretations based on the presence of structural defects (cracks, etc.).

In a shorthand fashion, we can express the relationship between stress and strain as

$$\sigma = f(\varepsilon)$$

This is a general form of the relationship that we easily recognize in the elastic region:

$$\sigma = E * \varepsilon$$

where the function, f, is given by E, the modulus (a constant).

Unfortunately, the processes of creep and stress relaxation are *not* explainable by reference to the stress–strain curve as obtained this way.

However, the need to show strain and stress, respectively, as functions of time in reporting these behaviors alerts us to the possibility of describing the stress in a material as a function of *both* strain and time. (The choice of stress as the dependent variable is arbitrary here; viscoelasticity is characterized by the involvement of time in any function linking stress and strain.) Materials in which time is a feature of the relationship between stress and strain are called *viscoelastic*. This is a compound word, combining the ideas of viscous flow, such as that of maple syrup straight from the refrigerator, and elastic deformation, such as that of a rubber band, suggesting that both properties are present in such materials.

Similarly, in shorthand fashion, we can write

$$\sigma = f(\varepsilon, t)$$

or more specifically

$$\sigma = E(t)^*\varepsilon$$

This introduces the idea of a modulus (the ratio between stress and strain) depending on time rather than being a constant, as is assumed in the discussion of elastic behavior.

If we take an imaginary material with typical viscoelastic properties and perform a set of load-deformation experiments at increasing rates of loading (and thus at increasing strain rates), we would produce the family of stress–strain curves seen in Figure 4.1.

These curves differ from those for elastic–plastic materials in several ways, including the following:

1. At low strain rates, for the imaginary material selected, there is no observable elastic region.

2. At high strain rates, the material appears elastic and brittle, with no plastic region.

A number of materials behave very much like this imaginary example, including fresh saltwater taffy and the silicone "rubber" used as a hand-exercising material.

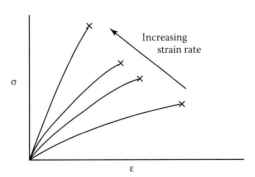

FIGURE 4.1 Stress–strain curves for a viscoelastic material.

Although a broad variety of different viscoelastic behaviors is possible, all such solid materials share these general properties of appearing plastic (or viscous) and ductile at low strain rates and elastic and brittle at high strain rates. Thus, the derivation of the term *viscoelastic* is both obvious and mnemonic.

Models

The variety of viscoelastic behaviors that are observed in real materials do not relate in an easy, generic way to types of materials as do the various shapes of simple stress–strain curves for elastic–plastic materials (see Chapter 3). Additionally, these behaviors are not related simply and directly to the bond types present in the material but are related more closely to details of molecular structure and arrangement and to larger-scale aspects of material organization.

To deal with these problems, it has become the practice to analyze the behavior of viscoelastic materials as if they were composed of arrays of small, simple mechanical elements connected together with pins and tie rods. This is an intellectual exercise; the model elements used in this approach generally have no close correspondence to physical parts of the actual material. However, when taken together, the stress–strain behavior of these model elements mirrors that of the actual material. In addition, when formal mathematical descriptions of stress–strain behavior are required, it is possible to generate them very quickly from these model elements, each of which has a very simple mathematical description.

There are three principal model elements (also called *bodies*) used to construct viscoelastic models.

1. *Spring (or Hooke body)* (Figure 4.2). The simplest element possesses fully elastic behavior and is represented by a spring. The instantaneous application of a stress, by placing a weight on it,

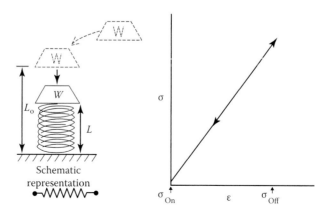

FIGURE 4.2 The spring or Hooke body.

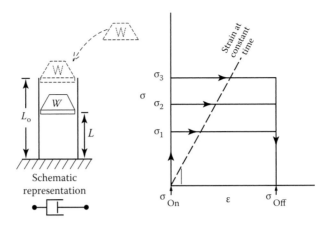

FIGURE 4.3   The dashpot or Newton body.

produces a stress–strain curve that is identical to the behavior of an elastic–plastic material below the yield point, that is, purely elastic. Although produced in an instantaneous experiment, this behavior is presumed to be time independent. Thus, the final strain depends only on the sustained stress. If the stress is released, the strain is fully recoverable.

2. *Dashpot (or Newton body)* (Figure 4.3). The next simplest element possesses fully viscous behavior and is represented by a (perforated) plunger in a closed chamber. The simplest common analogue is a fluid-filled syringe with a small-bore needle. This can be thought of as a dampening device, where the resistance is directly related to the velocity of the applied force. The instantaneous application of a stress produces a constant strain rate dependent on the magnitude of the sustained stress. This behavior is highly time dependent, with strain continuing to change, at a constant rate, so long as the stress is maintained. However, the strain is totally unrecoverable.

In the example of an uncapped fluid-filled hypodermic syringe, the plunger may be made to move at a constant velocity that increases with increasing applied force. The deformation is not recoverable since the plunger will stop moving when the force is removed but will not move back to its initial position. The strain in the fluid at this point is not zero but the strain rate is; thus, there is no restoring force developed to return the plunger.

3. *Frictional (or St. Venant) body* (Figure 4.4). The third simple body resembles the Newton body, but a minimum stress is required to produce strain. For stresses below this value, the body is considered incompressible; for stresses above this value, it behaves like a Newton body. It is best represented by a block sliding on a rough surface: a minimum force is required to move the block, but once in motion, it moves with a constant velocity, dependent on the

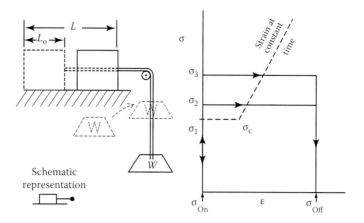

FIGURE 4.4 The frictional or St. Venant body.

force (see Chapter 11). Again, like the Newton body, the strain is unrecoverable when the stress is released.

In these illustrations, the examples are compressive (except for the St. Venant body), whereas the schematic diagrams are tensile. The behavior of these three body types is assumed to be mirrored for tensile and compressive states, and the same schematics are used for tension and compression. Analogous behavior may also be defined in shear and thus extended to torsional loading.

PROBLEM 4.1

How do a Newton body and a fluid-filled hypodermic syringe differ?

ANSWER:

The model Newton body is fully reversible, like a non-spring-loaded automotive shock absorber. The fluid-filled hypodermic is an irreversible body, unless the needle opening is kept immersed in a volume of the same fluid.

Standard test

Figures 4.2 through 4.4 show stress–strain curves for each of the three bodies, respectively, and schematic representations that will be used later in this chapter. These stress–strain curves can be misleading; in fact, the discussion to this point has exchanged the normal roles of stress and strain, making strain the dependent factor and the applied stress the independent one. Figures 4.3 and 4.4 have diagonal dashed lines within the stress–strain curves to show how higher initial stresses produce greater strains after a given (constant) time interval. Even this additional feature leaves these diagrams hard to interpret, so a new approach is needed.

This approach is to define a standard test sequence involving both stress and strain and then to replace the stress–strain diagram with two diagrams showing the variation of stress and strain, respectively, with time.

The *standard test* is defined as follows.

1. At the beginning of the test, $t = t_0$, an external stress is applied instantaneously and then maintained.

2. At a later time, $t = t_1$, the external stress is removed but the strain at that time is *fixed* and not permitted to change.

One simple way to think about the standard test for viscoelasticity is that it consists of a creep test followed immediately (without recovery) by a stress relaxation test. The two subtests, when combined in this way, are sufficient to characterize fully the time-dependent stress–strain behavior of a viscoelastic material.

Figure 4.5 shows the result of the standard test applied to a spring or Hooke body. At $t = t_0$, the strain instantaneously rises to a value ε_0, determined by the stress and the nature of the material. This strain remains constant until it is "fixed" at t_1. At that point, the internal stress must be equal and opposite to the external load (owing to equilibrium considerations). (In this discussion, stresses are set "equal" to loads; stresses describe internal conditions, loads [forces] describe external conditions. It is assumed that equilibrium is produced in the normal manner: the sum of internal stresses times their respective areas must be equal and opposite to the sum of external forces.) However, when the external load is removed and replaced by a constraint on strain, the internal stress remains constant at the same value. For completeness, the modulus $E(t)$, the ratio of stress to strain as a function of time, is also shown. This is constant and it is equal to σ_0/ε_0.

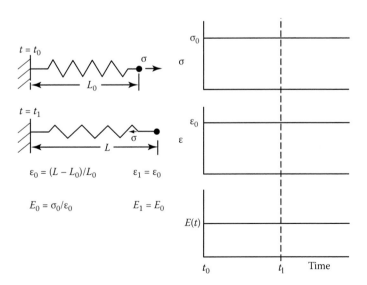

FIGURE 4.5   The standard test for the spring or Hooke body.

PROBLEM 4.2

Doesn't the statement "after removal of the external load, the internal stress remains constant" violate translational equilibrium conditions?

ANSWER:

No. The external load is replaced by a constraint on strain. One can think of it as replacing a weight on a spring with a pin or nail constraining the end of the spring. The internal stress remaining will be balanced by an equal and opposite resultant force exerted by the pin or nail, so that equilibrium is maintained. If there is no internal stress, then there will be no resultant force; this is different from the prior situation in which the external force was fixed at a constant value. So in short, the external force was simply replaced by a reaction force, which balances translational equilibrium conditions.

The utility of the standard test becomes more obvious when it is applied to the Newton body. The results are shown in Figure 4.6. The application of constant stress, σ_0, produces no initial strain ($\varepsilon_0 = 0$), but strain increases at a constant rate. The strain is then fixed at t_1, and the internal stress drops to zero.

In this case, the modulus, $E(t)$, has an interesting behavior. At t_0, it is infinite (since $\varepsilon_0 = 0$), and it decreases asymptotically to σ_0/ε_1 as time approaches t_1. At $t = t_1$, the internal stress becomes zero and so does $E(t)$.

The response of a St. Venant body to the standard test is identical to that of the Newtonian body, so long as $\sigma_0 \geq \sigma_c$. (In Figures 4.6 through 4.9, stress vectors are omitted for simplicity.)

Using these three mechanical elements, it is possible to construct more complex models whose stress and strain behaviors as a function of time begin to resemble those found in real viscoelastic materials. These models contain several of the fundamental bodies and are called *units*.

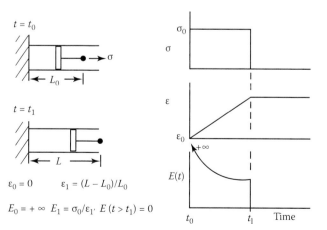

FIGURE 4.6   The standard test for the dashpot or Newton body.

Maxwell unit

The simplest of these units is the Maxwell unit, which consists of a Hooke body and a Newton body attached end to end, that is, in *series*. This is shown schematically, along with the result of the standard test, in Figure 4.7. Note that in such an arrangement, the initial stress must be the same in both bodies, but their strains may be different.

The strain now consists of the sum of two internal strains representing the contributions of the deformations of the two bodies. When the initial load is applied, producing u_0, an elastic strain, ε_0, occurs, which is due only to the elastic deformation of the spring. Then, under the constant stress, the dashpot deforms at a constant rate. At $t = t_1$, the external strain is fixed (made constant) but the stress does not become zero, as in the case of a single dashpot, since there is an internal, recoverable strain in the spring. The spring then acts against the dashpot, producing continuing strain in it, which diminishes in rate with time as the stress (tension) in the spring declines to zero. This is a stress relaxation process and is shown by the way that the overall stress (sum of the stress in the spring and the dashpot) decreases asymptotically to zero.

Kelvin unit

Another way to connect a spring and a dashpot is in *parallel*, as shown in Figure 4.8. In such a figure, it is assumed that the vertical tie bars remain parallel to each other. Note that in this arrangement, the internal strains in each body must be identical and equal to the external strain but the stresses may be different.

The stress now consists of the sum of two internal stresses representing the contributions of the deformations of the two bodies. When the initial load is applied, producing σ_0, there is no initial elastic strain since the elastic deformation of the spring is constrained by the dashpot. Under the initial stress, the dashpot begins to deform. However, as it deforms, the spring is also deformed, since the strain must remain the same in both bodies. This produces a spring stress that subtracts from

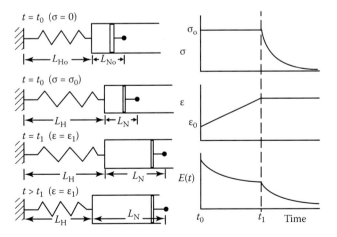

FIGURE 4.7   The Maxwell unit: spring/Hooke body connected to a dashpot/Newton body in series (end to end).

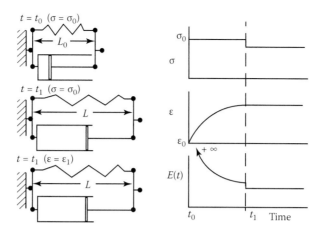

FIGURE 4.8 The Kelvin unit: spring/Hooke body attached in parallel to a dashpot/Newton body.

the externally applied force, reducing the net stress on the dashpot and thus reducing the rate of deformation of the dashpot at a constant rate. At $t = t_1$, the external strain is fixed (made constant), and the stress in the dashpot becomes zero but the stress in the spring does not, since it is strained from its rest position. Thus, there is an instantaneous reduction in stress, but not to zero, as in the case of a single dashpot. In this case, however, the strain is unrecoverable and there are no further changes in stress or strain.

PROBLEM 4.3

In Figure 4.8, what feature regulates the ratio σ_1/σ_0?

ANSWER:

Since σ_1 is the stress in the spring at time t_1, the ratio increases with increasing $t_1 - t_0$, asymptotically approaching a value of 1.

Standard linear (three-body) model

The Maxwell and the Kelvin units combine viscous and elastic behavior but are not sufficiently complex to be able to represent the stress–strain relationships in real solids. The simplest model that can do that is the standard linear (or three-body) model. (There are other three-body models that can represent the properties of real materials. The simplest of these is a Maxwell unit in parallel with a spring. This is equivalent to the standard linear model considered here.) This consists of a Kelvin unit in series with another spring, as shown in Figure 4.9. In this case, the springs are shown as having different stiffnesses.

The results of the standard test are shown in Figure 4.10. There is an initial elastic strain, ε_0, corresponding to a deformation of spring 2, since spring 1 is constrained by the dashpot. The dashpot begins to deform, which produces a restraining stress in spring 1, reducing the stress on the dashpot below σ_0 and thus reducing the strain rate. At $t = t_1$, when

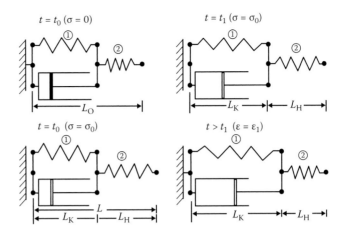

FIGURE 4.9   The linear viscoelastic model: Kelvin unit connected end to end (in series) with a spring/Hooke body.

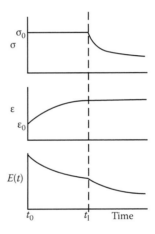

FIGURE 4.10   The standard test of the linear viscoelastic model.

the external strain is set, the stress in the dashpot does not change, since it is stressed by spring 2. However, as it continues to strain, the stress in spring 2 decreases and a restraining stress is produced by additional deformation of spring 1. Eventually, the stress in spring 1 is equal to the stress in spring 2 (but not equal to zero), and internal deformation ceases.

If we compare the behavior of $E(t)$ in Figure 4.10 with that for the Maxwell unit (Figure 4.8) and the Kelvin unit (Figure 4.9), we can see that it is much better behaved, never having either a zero value or an infinite value. Its initial value, immediately after stress is applied but before creep can take place, is called the *unrelaxed modulus*, E_U. Its final value, after all possible internal stress relaxation has taken place, is called the *relaxed modulus*, E_R. In this case, as in the general case for viscoelastic materials, $E_U > E_R$.

The ratio E_R/E_U is often used to compare viscoelastic materials. If it is equal to one, the material is fully elastic. The smaller this ratio is, the more viscous behavior is seen, so the more viscoelastic the material is considered. The ratio has a value of approximately 0.95 for cortical bone but only approximately 0.2 for articular cartilage, for strains within physiologic limits. Thus, we tend to think of cartilage as a viscoelastic material and bone as an essentially elastic material.

Hysteresis

Viscous deformation produces an additional important difference in mechanical behavior between elastic–plastic and viscoelastic materials. If an elastic material is stressed to a point below the proportional limit and then the load is removed, the stress–strain curve will be retraced and the elastic energy, the area below the curve to ε_p, will be fully recovered. However, if the same experiment is performed on a standard linear viscoelastic material by applying an instantaneous stress, the results will be as shown in Figure 4.11. Although the strain can be recovered, in a fully constrained arrangement, the stress–strain curve is not retraced. The area under the curves may be divided into two regions: region 1, the area between the curves, and region 2, the area under the unload portion of the curve. Region 1 represents the portion of the energy of deformation that is lost, whereas region 2 represents the recoverable portion. The unrecoverable energy is dissipated as heat, which can be appreciated by the increase in temperature of clay or bread dough during kneading (repeated deformation).

This phenomenon, the loss of strain energy despite the full recovery of strain, is called *hysteresis*. It will occur in any viscoelastic material in which either internal creep or stress relaxation has been permitted to occur during a load–unload cycle. For a specific model, the area between the load and unload curves will be a function of strain rate.

It is interesting to inquire into the connection between energy dissipation and permanent set (unrecoverable strain). In an elastic–plastic

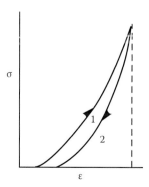

FIGURE 4.11 Hysteresis.

material, such as a metal, energy is dissipated once the plastic region is entered. Elastic deformation occurs at low strains, whereas larger strains are required to produce plastic deformation. Thus, there is some minimum stress, associated with the onset of plastic deformation, required before either unrecoverable strain or energy dissipation occurs. However, in a viscoelastic material, energy is always dissipated if a viscous element (either a Newton or St. Venant body) is required to model the stress–strain behavior. Since this is true for all viscoelastic bodies, then all viscoelastic bodies dissipate energy during deformation, irrespective of either the magnitude of the strain or the degree of recoverability, so long as internal creep or stress relaxation has taken place. Therefore, hysteresis constitutes a considerable problem in the testing of viscoelastic materials, since the intrinsic properties of the materials are temperature dependent. *In vivo*, this effect contributes to muscle heating during exertion, in addition to the heat produced as a by-product of cellular metabolic effort.

Complex materials

Models as discussed here lead to fairly simple stress–strain relationships. However, the relationships in real materials, especially in real structures made of various materials, are far more complex. This complexity in behavior requires much more complex and detailed models.

Repetitive tensile tests of a ligament, performed at increasing strain rates with sufficient intervals in between for "full" recovery, produce a family of stress–strain curves as shown in the left portion of Figure 4.12. These have several features of interest. There is an initial, unrecoverable deformation, called "preconditioning," which occurs during the first cycle (see Chapter 5 for a complete discussion of preconditioning). Each successive cycle shows full recovery, with steeper curves and less hysteresis, as strain rate increases.

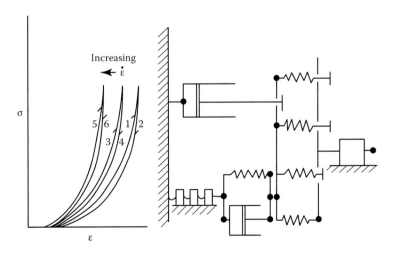

FIGURE 4.12   A model for ligaments.

The model in the right portion of Figure 4.12, with suitable values for the stiffnesses or viscosities for each body, would fully describe this behavior. The large dashpot and the frictional bodies connected with slack ties on the left account for the preconditioning strain. On the right, the spring elements are shown as engaging after discrete strains have taken place. This is necessary to account for the concave-upward shape of the stress–strain curves. This model is very simplified; to account for the detailed shape of the loading curves, a large number of disconnected spring bodies would be required.

Compliance

The reciprocal of a modulus is a *compliance*. The letter J is usually used as a symbol for compliance. The compliance expresses the strain that results from a unit of stress.

Thus, for an elastic–plastic material:

$$J = 1/E = \varepsilon/\sigma$$

and for a viscoelastic material:

$$J(t) = \varepsilon/\sigma$$

If a creep experiment is performed for a linear viscoelastic material and paired (obtained at the same time) values of stress and strain are used to compute $J(t)$, then a plot of $J(t)$ versus the logarithm of time yields some interesting properties. Such an experiment is shown in Figure 4.13. The compliance starts at a low constant value (J_U) and increases to a high constant value (J_R). These are called, respectively, the *unrelaxed* and *relaxed compliances* and are the reciprocals of the unrelaxed and relaxed moduli.

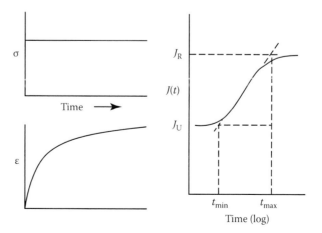

FIGURE 4.13 The compliance curve.

The intersection between the two ends of the compliance curve and the central portion defines two times, t_{min} and t_{max}. The first time, t_{min}, is the time required for viscous flow to begin. For times shorter than this, the material behaves in an elastic manner. The second time, t_{max}, is the time required for viscous flow, at this stress, to be completed. After this time, so long as the stress is below the creep rupture stress, no further deformation will occur, and the material will then appear to be elastic. For articular cartilage in the rabbit, t_{min} is 0.25 s, whereas t_{max} is 20 min.

The slope of the intermediate region is called the *spectrum of retardation times*, $L(t)$, and can be calculated from the four parameters discussed above:

$$L(t) = \frac{J_R - J_U}{\log(t_{max}) - \log(t_{min})} = \frac{J_R - J_U}{\log\left(\dfrac{t_{max}}{t_{min}}\right)}$$

The time-dependent parameter $L(t)$ is essentially a creep rate. It is a constant for a standard linear solid but may not be constant for more complex solids.

The four parameters discussed here (J_U, J_R, t_{min}, and t_{max}) and the function $L(t)$ fully describe the stress–strain behavior of a viscoelastic material and permit predictions to be made for the results of any experiment, including creep and stress relaxation magnitudes, when well away from creep rupture conditions.

Indentation test

Despite the completeness of the standard test, it has been traditional to evaluate the viscoelastic properties of tissues and many engineering materials by the *indentation test*. This test consists of positioning a piton, a round-ended, flat-ended, or hemispherically ended indentor, on the surface of the material to be tested, suddenly applying a load, and measuring the deformation of the surface as a continuous function of time. The test is completed by removing the load at a later time, leaving the very lightweight indentor in place, and measuring the recovery of indentation.

Figure 4.14 shows the results of such a test on rabbit articular cartilage, in place on subchondral bone. The upper curve is the result of a test on normal cartilage; the lower curve is what might occur if the cartilage was degraded for a brief period with a mixture of collagenase and hyaluronidase enzymes. Two parameters have been used to report the results of such tests:

1. The total indentation at "steady state." This is called simply *indentation*.

2. The ratio of the area "below" the unload curve to that "above" the load curve, expressed as a percentage (see areas labeled 2 and 1 in Figure 4.14). This is called *percent recovery*.

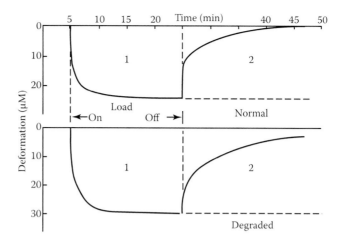

FIGURE 4.14 Indentation tests of articular cartilage.

In the example given, it can be seen that the indentation is greater and the recovery is less in the degraded cartilage than in the normal tissue. However, these measures are extrinsic rather than intrinsic and are difficult to relate to structural details of the tissue. A common problem, avoided in this example, is to unknowingly stop the test before t_{max} is reached. For these reasons, a full characterization, by either a standard test approach or a long-term creep test leading to a compliance curve, is preferred for evaluation of viscoelastic materials.

PROBLEM 4.4

With reference to Figure 4.14, determine whether the sentences below are true or false:

1. The peak strain increases after enzymatic degradation.
2. t_{min} and t_{max} can be determined from these curves.
3. Normal cartilage is more elastic than enzymatically degraded cartilage.
4. Recovery should be 100% for normal tissue.

ANSWER:

T, F, T, F. If the thickness of both specimens is the same, then strain should increase linearly with indentation. It is not possible to determine t_{min} and t_{max} from indentation curves. However, a compliance curve can be plotted if the experiment was continued for a time greater than t_{max}. Elasticity here refers to the amount of immediate elastic recovery after load removal. This appears to be approximately 10 μm for the normal cartilage but only 5 μm for the degraded cartilage. Although for a standard linear viscoelastic solid the recovery would be equal to 100%, details of structure and flow in real materials produce values less than this for all but very small deformations of normal tissue.

Viscoelasticity of fluids

Fluids, as well as solids, exhibit viscoelastic stress–strain behavior. This is easiest to characterize in shear, as in a shear viscometer, as shown in Figure 4.15. In this device, a fluid is placed in the annular space between the inner (rotating) and outer (fixed) cones. A device is provided to measure the torque applied to the outer cone by the fluid, and the inner cone is driven at ever-increasing speeds (producing increasing shear strain rates in the fluid). The force on the outer cone may be expressed, as a function of geometry, as a viscosity, v, expressed in SI units of pascal-seconds (Pa*s). A more common unit is the centipoise with 1000 centipoise = 1 Pa*s. Since energy is continuously dissipated, care must be taken to keep the temperature of the fluid from increasing.

There are three types of behavior of v as a function of shear strain rate (Figure 4.15). If v is *constant* with shear strain rate, the fluid is said to be *Newtonian*. Then we can write:

$$\sigma = v \cdot \dot{\varepsilon}_s$$

where $\dot{\varepsilon}_s$ is the shear strain rate. Many fluids, such as water and blood plasma, are Newtonian.

If v either increases or decreases with shear strain rate, the fluid is said to be non-Newtonian. In particular, if v *decreases* with increasing shear strain rate, the fluid is said to be strain thinning or *thixotropic*. Tomato ketchup, non-drip paint, and normal synovial fluid are all thixotropic. Thixotropy is reversible, but hysteresis heating effects (which generally reduce v, until cooling occurs) may interfere with recovery of viscosity. If v *increases* with increasing strain rate, the fluid is said to be *dilatant*.

Fluids possess modest unrelaxed shear, tensile, and compressive moduli. However, the value of their relaxed shear and tensile moduli is zero; this is an alternative way of defining the fluid state.

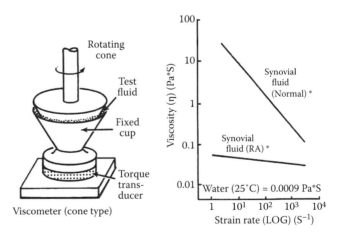

FIGURE 4.15 The viscometer and some results. (Reprinted from *Tribology of Natural and Artificial Joints*, Dumbledon, J.H., Copyright 1981, with permission from Elsevier.)

PROBLEM 4.5

It has been observed that synovial fluid from both normal knees and from those of patients with rheumatoid arthritis (RA) has a low viscosity at high shear rates. However, at low shear rates, normal synovial fluid is extremely viscous, whereas RA synovial fluid is nearly Newtonian (see Figure 4.15). What clinical implication might this observation have?

ANSWER:

Patients with RA complain about difficulty in getting joints to move initially after periods of rest. Perhaps this is associated with the lower viscosity of RA synovial fluid at low strain rates, which might permit it to squeeze out from and permit interference between irregular articular surfaces.

Molecular basis of viscoelasticity

Deformations of elastic–plastic materials were considered at the atomic scale in Chapter 3. Elastic behavior results from the straining of interatomic bonds, whereas plastic deformation requires the rearrangement of bonds, made easier by defects of various types.

Viscoelastic behavior is more difficult to relate directly to movements at an atomic level, since most viscoelastic materials consist of polymers with backbone covalent bonds and van der Waals and occasional covalent intramolecular and intermolecular bonds. The simplest "thought model" is a plate of spaghetti and tomato sauce at room temperature. If one takes hold of the end of a single strand, small forces produce an elastic or rubbery response as the strand stretches. If greater force is used, the strand will begin to pull out of the main mass. Heating the mass makes it more fluid and less elastic, whereas freezing converts it into an elastic, brittle solid.

This is a fair description of the molecular basis of viscoelastic behavior, if the spaghetti represents individual long-chain molecules and the sauce represents the intermolecular bonds and the effect of a fluid phase, as in soft tissue. In general, as temperature rises, viscoelastic materials become more viscous (E_R/E_U decreases) but their "internal" viscosity also decreases ($L(t)$ increases, E_U may decrease). The transition to elastic, brittle behavior takes place fairly abruptly at a specific temperature as temperature is decreased. This is called the *glass transition* (*point* or *temperature*) and represents the temperature at which internal viscosity has increased so much that it is easier to disrupt intramolecular bonds than to cause molecules to move with respect to each other. The molecular basis of mechanical behavior of tissues is more complex since their internal viscosity depends on water content, which may change in response to strain. For example, viscoelasticity of human ligaments is the result of the interaction of ground substance and collagen with water, which typically composes two-thirds the weight of ligamentous tissue. Water is initially trapped inside protoglycan molecules, but will exude under cyclic loading as the internal structure of the tissue changes. As water is lost through the "wringing out effect," the tissue is less relaxed. Similarly, there is a known decrease in relaxation with larger strains, also likely due to a decrease in hydration. Alternatively, the decrease in the rate of creep with increasing load is suspected to be due to more fibers being recruited initially with larger loads, which ultimately decreases the creep response.

In another example, cartilage is a low-friction, avascular, load-bearing tissue, which can also exhibit a highly viscoelastic response and large deformations. It is a triphasic material with a porous matrix made of type II collagen, proteoglycans, and extracellular matrix, along with 70% to 90% without water and ions. Its flow-dependent viscoelasticity is mostly due to its low permeability. Compact bone can be described as a matrix of Haversian sites and hollow osteons embedded in ground substance, which acts as cement lines between the osteons. When subjected to extended periods of stress, there is slippage along the cement lines and the ground substance is understood to behave in a viscous manner. Detailed models have been developed to explain the features of such processes, especially at large deformations, but are too complex to consider here.

Additional problems

PROBLEM 4.6

Figure 4.16 (left curves) shows the stress versus time response for two constrained strain-versus-time experiments (right curves). Answer the following questions (yes or no):

1. Can curves A and B (stress versus time) result from experiments on the same material?
2. Is t_{min} less than t_1 for case A?
3. Does curve A (upper) display stress relaxation?
4. Could a compliance curve derived from case A yield the spectrum of retardation times, $L(t)$?
5. If a strain of 0.025 were applied in a time = $t_1/2$, at a constant rate, as in case A, would the peak stress be 20 MPa?

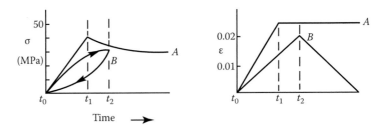

FIGURE 4.16 Stress and strain versus time (Problems 4.5 and 4.6).

ANSWER:

Y, N, Y, Y, N. Cases A and B show the results of constrained constant strain rate experiments on a single material for which $t_1 < t_{min} < t_2$. Case A is a stress relaxation experiment, which yields data equivalent to those of a creep experiment. For strains applied in times less than t_{min}, the material will behave elastically; thus, $\varepsilon = 0.025$ leads to $\sigma = 40$ MPa, irrespective of strain rate.

PROBLEM 4.7

For the material represented in Figure 4.16, find E_U, E_R, and σ_y.

ANSWER:

E_U may be calculated from the end point of unrelaxed deformation (curves A): $E_U = 40/0.025 = 1600$ MPa = **1.6 GPa**. E_R is calculated from the fully relaxed (horizontal) parts of curves A: $E_R = 30/0.025 =$ **1.2 GPa**. Curves A and B display viscoelastic behavior; thus, there is no definable yield stress.

PROBLEM 4.8

How much energy is lost in the hysteresis loop shown in curve B displayed in the left graph of Figure 4.16?

ANSWER:

Since strain is linear in time (constant strain rate), the left curves are equivalent to stress–strain curves (relabeling the time axis as a strain axis). Therefore, the left curves display hysteresis, and the energy loss per strain cycle (estimated by ruling squares under the upper and lower portions of stress vs. time in curve B) is approximately 45%.

PROBLEM 4.9

A viscoelastic material (select best answer)

    A. Behaves like a spring when stressed

    B. Is never found *in vivo*

    C. Degrades mechanically with time

    D. Exhibits deformation that depends on both the load applied and the rate of load application

    E. None of the above

ANSWER:

The best answer is D, which is a good definition of viscoelasticity. Viscoelastic materials only behave elastically (as springs) for stress and strains observed in times less than the minimum relaxation time (t_{min}). Virtually all soft and hard tissues are viscoelastic. Despite their viscous nature, these materials possess a wide range of reversible behavior unaccompanied by permanent damage.

PROBLEM 4.10

The bending of a viscoelastic cantilever-loaded beam (select best answer)

A. Can be calculated from the Young's modulus

B. Is time dependent and can be determined from a creep curve

C. Is determined by the hysteresis of the material

D. Only occurs at low temperatures

ANSWER:

B. A viscoelastic material does not have a Young's modulus, although E_U can be used in the same manner for times less than t_{min}. Hysteresis determines energy loss, not deformation. At low temperatures, many viscoelastic materials become fully elastic, but they undergo deformation in response to load at all temperatures.

PROBLEM 4.11

A model for a viscoelastic material must include at least one spring/Hooke body, one dashpot/Newton body, and one frictional/St. Venant body (true or false).

ANSWER:

False. The combination of *either* a Newton body *or* a St. Venant body with a Hooke body is sufficient to produce the elastic–viscous behavior characteristic of viscoelasticity.

PROBLEM 4.12

Viscoelastic fluids (true or false)

1. Include blood and synovial fluid

2. Display a constant viscosity

3. Are thinned irreversibly by shear strains

4. Are sticky

5. Have no elasticity

ANSWER:

T, F, F, F, F. Viscoelastic fluids, such as blood and synovial fluid, have shear rate–dependent viscosities. They display elastic behavior at very high shear rates and short times, as do viscoelastic solids. Shear thinning is generally reversible unless molecular structure has been damaged by physical or thermal disruption. "Stickiness" or adhesiveness is dependent on fluid–surface interactions and is not related to flow behavior.

PROBLEM 4.13

Considering the viscoelastic material in Figure 4.1, testing the material under a higher strain rate will generally change the appearance of the material behavior according to the following (true or false):

1. Decreasing ductility
2. Decreasing stiffness
3. Increasing amount of recoverable strain
4. Decreasing the elongation to failure

ANSWER:

T, F, T, T. Increasing the strain rate will give the material a response more closely aligned with the curves on the left of Figure 4.1. Because testing at a faster rate will not allow as much time for molecular rearrangement, plastic flow behavior will not develop as sufficiently. As a result, the material response is characterized as having a stiff elastic curve, with more recoverable (elastic) strain, less ductility, and less strain to failure.

PROBLEM 4.14

Viscoelastic properties can be affected by the following (true or false):

1. Temperature
2. Moisture content
3. Load history
4. Atomic bonding type (e.g., ionic vs. covalent)

ANSWER:

T, T, T, T. Because viscoelasticity is associated with larger-scale molecular rearrangement, temperature and moisture content will directly affect this flow potential of the material. Similarly, the atomic bond type will directly affect the ability of a material to rearrange over time. We also know that viscoelastic materials can display significant hysteresis, implicating load history as having a direct effect on current creep and relaxation behavior.

PROBLEM 4.15

Polymers typically have a critical property termed the glass-transition temperature. At temperatures below the T_g, the polymer behavior is characterized as glassy, while above T_g the material behavior is described as more rubbery. High-density polyethylene (HDPE) has a T_g of $-110°C$ and polyetheretherketone (PEEK) has a T_g of $145°C$. Which would we expect to have a greater potential for creep when implanted in the body?

ANSWER:

HDPE—Because body temperature is well above the T_g of HDPE, this material will be characterized by more rubbery behavior and is thus more susceptible to creep under constant loading.

PROBLEM 4.16

Characterize the following viscoelastic phenomena as more indicative of creep or stress relaxation:

1. A polymeric component showing little signs of wear after explantation has been significantly deformed from its original state
2. A decrease in tension in the rotator cuff ligaments as a result of overuse
3. Skin wrinkles during the aging process
4. Straightening of teeth using orthodontic bracing
5. Stretching of the rotator cuff ligaments as a result of aging

ANSWER:

Creep, stress relaxation, stress relaxation, creep, creep.

Annotated bibliography

1. BURSTEIN AH, FRANKEL VH: The viscoelastic properties of some biological materials. *Ann NY Acad Sci* 146:158–165, 1968.
   An early but useful introduction to the viscoelastic properties of hard and soft musculoskeletal tissue. Easy to read.
2. COLETTI JM, AKESON WH, WOO SL-Y: A comparison of the physical behavior of normal articular cartilage and the arthroplasty surface. *J Bone Joint Surg* 54A:147–160, 1972.
   Illustrates the indentation test and discusses the behavior of normal and abnormal cartilage. An appendix shows how the viscoelastic behavior of these tissues may be represented by a model.
3. DUMBLETON JH: *Tribology of Natural and Artificial Joints*. Elsevier, Amsterdam, 1981.
   Tribology is the combined science of friction, lubrication, and wear. This is a good source on the orthopaedic aspects of these topics. Chapters 2 and 3 discuss viscosity.
4. FLUGGE V: *Viscoelasticity*. Blaisdell, Waltham, UK, 1967.
   An intermediate level book on viscosity. Chapter 1 covers the standard test (this is the apparent source of this approach) and may be followed with an elementary knowledge of differential equations.
5. FRANKEL VH, BURSTEIN AH: *Orthopaedic Biomechanics*. Lea & Febiger, Philadelphia, 1970.
   Chapter 4 discusses viscoelasticity, using the body and model approach, without mathematics.
6. FRISEN M, MAGI M, SONNERUP L, VIIDIK A: Rheological analysis of soft collageneous tissue. Part 1: Theoretical considerations. Part 2: Experimental evaluations and verifications. *J Biomech* 2:12–20, 21–28, 1969.

A classic paper developing a "body" model for ligamentous tissue and then comparing it with some of Viidik's results.

7. PARSONS JR, BLACK J: Viscoelastic shear moduli of normal rabbit articular cartilage. *J Biomech* 10:21–29, 1977.

Building on earlier theoretical work by others, shows how the indentation test may be adapted to produce a compliance curve and intrinsic parameters.

8. PROVENZANO PP, LAKES RS, KEENAN T, VANDERBY R: Nonlinear ligament viscoelasticity. *Ann Biomed Eng* 29: 908–914, 2001.

A discussion of the constituents of ligaments and their contribution to ligament viscoelasticity.

CHAPTER FIVE

Properties of natural materials

There is a school of thought that attempts to restrict the field of biomaterials to the study of manufactured materials derived entirely or in part from nonliving or synthetic sources. This is an inadequate concept. In the same way that we recognize that biomechanics includes the application of the principles of classical mechanics to the study of the function of living systems, we must recognize that the discipline of biomaterials includes the application of the principles of materials science to the study of the "stuff" from which living systems are made. Thus, tissue mechanics, often considered a subdiscipline of biomechanics, is in fact at the border where biomechanics and biomaterials meet: the former discipline considering tissues as materials with definable deformational properties and the latter considering how these properties arise from composition and structure.

This latter approach is the classical process of materials science: relating the measurable physical properties of materials to their chemical composition and the internal arrangement of their constituents and phases. The final goal is the derivation of a constitutive equation: one that predicts mechanical behavior on the basis of quantitative measurements of composition and structure.

Biomaterials applies this approach to two classes of materials: manufactured or modified materials for prosthetic applications on the one hand and tissues, both normal and diseased, on the other hand. Both classes of materials are "made"; that is, they arise by the action of living systems. A third class of materials bridges across these two: "engineered" tissues which may or may not retain prosthetic elements. Prosthetic materials and devices are artifacts of the life of man; soft and hard tissues are artifacts of the life of cells.

Thus, this chapter is devoted to a combined discussion of the mechanical properties of tissues and their constituents and how these properties arise.

In vitro versus *in vivo* properties

There is a general problem involved in understanding the mechanical behavior of tissues. By and large, mechanical properties have been determined in the laboratory, on "dead" tissue. A frequent observation is that the stress–strain relationship observed on an initial test is not reproducible on subsequent tests that are immediately repeated. However, the subsequent tests tend to closely reproduce each other, so long as physical conditions are not changed and tissue autolysis has not begun. This phenomenon, of initial mechanical irreproducibility, is called the "preconditioning effect," and it is the practice, rather than the exception, in studies of tissue mechanics to "cycle" or exercise the tissue specimens until reproducibility is assured. This misdemeanor is compounded, again in the vast majority of cases, by failure to report the initial results.

The origins of the preconditioning effect are unclear but they are related to the differences between the stable *in vivo* situation and the artificial and often poorly controlled *in vitro* test conditions. Release of stresses, owing to failure to maintain original resting length of the tissue as a starting point or to removal of tissue from a supporting structure, is a major contributing factor, as is the inability to restore mechanically expressed fluid owing to the loss of microcirculation. Furthermore, there are continuing property changes in the immediate postexcision period, up to 5–6 h after specimen preparation at room temperature, paralleling the macroscopically observable events of rigor mortis. These occur in all tissues, but are more prominent in soft tissues. Similarly, the storage conditions of the tissue, for example, if they are stored in formalin or some other solution, can also affect the properties.

The property values cited in this chapter are *in vitro* post preconditioning values. In general, overlooking the obvious fact that tissues are viscoelastic rather than elastic–plastic, *in vitro* (post preconditioning) behavior is more elastic and brittle than that *in vivo*.*

Tissue constituents

Poverty of structural elements

The atomic composition of the human body is surprisingly simple. Essentially all of the vast intricacy of the structure is composed of combinations of four elements: carbon, oxygen, hydrogen, and nitrogen. A number of additional elements contribute to creation and preservation of structure: calcium, sulfur, and phosphorus. Once past these seven elements, which together constitute more than 99% of body weight, those remaining are present in amounts treated in general engineering as "trace elements" or "impurities": perhaps possessing chemical activity

---

* For a more complete discussion, the reader is referred to Black J: Tissue properties: Relationship of *in vitro* studies to *in vitro* properties. pp. 5–26. In Hastings GW, Ducheyne P (eds): *Natural and Living Biomaterials*. CRC Press, Boca Raton, FL, 1984. The reader is also referred to Part 1 of Black J, Hastings, G (eds): *Handbook of Biomaterial Properties*, Chapman & Hall, London, 1998.

but not contributing to structural integrity or mechanical properties. Even an element with such a key physiological role as iron represents a contribution of 6 g to the weight of a 70 kg person or less than 0.01% of the total. Disregarding its role as an oxygen ligand, iron dictates the structure of the porphyrins and hemoglobin but is not even able to influence markedly the shape and mechanical properties of the red blood cell. Sickle cell anemia, which is associated with reversible shape changes of the red blood cell, is more directly related to changes in the internal structure of the hemoglobin molecule than to its atomic composition.

Again, at the molecular level, a similar sparsity of structural elements persists. The most common structural molecule is collagen. It constitutes 25% of the organic content of the human body, and despite the presence of perhaps 10 related structural types, more than 90% of it consists of types I and II. Several other proteins have structural roles, and a number of other molecules promote tissue component adhesion and water retention. The inorganic structural composition is even more limited, with a single mineral, calcium hydroxyapatite, making up almost all of it.

Thus, the great variety of structure and mechanical properties present in the human body arise in a traditional engineering fashion: by combining simple elements into complex assemblages designed to provide the desired performance. Whatever one's view concerning the role of creational or evolutionary processes, one must wonder at the richness of results obtained with such poverty of resources.

Collagen

It is not necessary to recite the structure of collagen in detail here. It is sufficient to remember that both type I and type II consist of three individual molecular chains assembled into a right-hand helical spiral fibril. Each molecule contains perhaps 1000 amino acids, made up of one-third glycine, one-third proline and hydroxyproline, and one-third other amino acids. The periodicity and the ability to assemble extracellularly into a spiral are apparently a consequence of the presence of a regular repeating triad (glycine plus proline or hydroxyproline plus another amino acid residue) along the covalently bonded backbone of each chain. These fibrils are stabilized by internal intermolecular van der Waals bonds with occasional covalent cross-links. The resulting structures are 300 nm in length and 1.5 nm in diameter with a screw pitch (distance between "turns") of 0.27 nm. The fibrils, in turn, are assembled into larger bundles or fibers with a longitudinal quarter stagger that results in the familiar 64–68 nm banded structure that is the hallmark of collagen when seen in the electron microscope.

Thus, a collagen fibril may be considered as a long coiled spring, like the one formerly used to close screen doors, and a fiber as an assemblage of springs connected together by a great number of less stiff spring-like cross-links. This model clearly predicts the stress–strain behavior of a single fiber, as seen in Figure 5.1. Small stresses tend to uncoil the springs and to rotate the cross-links, whereas larger stresses begin to stretch the covalent backbone and to break and remake the interfibril cross-links. Thus, the curve has two relatively distinct regions, with the

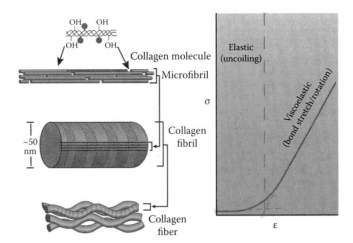

FIGURE 5.1   (See color insert.) Structure and mechanics of collagen.

transition representing the transition between these two load regimes—from elastic to viscoelastic behavior. Collagen fibrils are capable of reversible deformation, with a resilience of approximately 90%.

Collagen is mostly found in fibrous tissues such as tendon, ligament, and skin, but is also found in other tissues such as cartilage, bone, and intervertebral disc. Collagen is the primary tensile fiber in tissues. Its relatively high aspect ratio (length/diameter approximately 200) renders it ineffective in compression. It is viscoelastic under relatively small strains so that it appears in combination with a more elastic fiber, elastin, in structures such as tendons and ligaments that must bear high stresses without significant deformation. It is also a nonexcitable or passive structure; the active (physiochemically mediated) length changes in muscles are produced by myofibrils containing an interacting complex of two other long-chain molecules, myosin and actin.

Table 5.1 lists some estimated values for the mechanical properties of these fibers. Such data are extremely difficult to obtain in the absence of structural effects imposed by tissue organization.

Elastin

This molecule is sometimes called the "biologic rubber." Its composition is highly variable, consisting of approximately 55%–70% of the triad glycine + alanine + serine intermingled with 8%–10% of other amino acids. It possesses a spiral form, as does collagen, but lacks the repetitive

Table 5.1   Properties of biological fibers

Fiber	Elastic modulus (MPa)	Elastic limit (%)	Ultimate strength (MPa)	Ultimate strain (%)	Contractile stress (MPa)
Collagen	1000	1–2	60	10	—
Elastin	0.6	60	>0.35	>60	—
Myosin–actin	0.4	—	>0.35	75–85	0.2–0.4

periodicity of collagen and thus does not form large-scale fibers. Highly hydrophobic, it is usually seen as 5–7 μm fibers in a matrix of other fibers, such as collagen.

The elasticity of elastin is thought to be related to its high hydrophobicity and its random, crumpled structure. As it is extended, elastin will uncoil into an ordered configuration, decreasing the entropy of the system. Entropy changes are due to an increase or decrease of order in the atomic structure owing to a change in strain. Because the tendency of a closed system is to experience an increase in entropy, upon removal of the extension force, a restoring resultant force will return elastin to its random, crumpled structure.

Tendon and ligament

The properties of collagen and elastin lead directly to those of tendons and ligaments. Collagen and elastin primarily provide resistance to tension and shear, while proteoglycans resist compression. Tendon is relatively inextensible, to permit muscle extension–contraction to act directly through bony attachments. Figure 5.2 shows the resulting stress–strain curve for a typical tendon, with failure near 10% strain. Ultimate stress varies, depending on the nature of the tendon involved. The peculiar upward curve results from the interaction between the low-modulus elastic elastin fibers and the higher-modulus but viscoelastic collagen fibers. At low strains, elastin dominates, but at higher strains, collagen fibers, which possess a zigzag crimp, begin to take an increasing portion of the load, resulting in an upward curvature of the stress–strain curve and hysteresis upon unloading. At low strains, otherwise known as the toe region, the macroscopic crimps in the collagen fibrils are removed. Then as the strain increases beyond 2% to 3%, the heel region develops where there is a straightening of the kinks in the collagen—first at the fibrillar level and then at the molecular level. At higher strains, the collagen triple helices or the cross-links between the helices are stretched, which produce a linear response. If there is cross-link-deficient collagen, slippage within the fibrils occur, which causes a

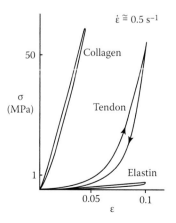

FIGURE 5.2 Stress–strain properties of tendon and its components.

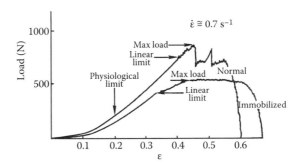

FIGURE 5.3 Load–strain properties of bone–ligament–bone unit. (Adapted from Noyes, F.R. et al., *J Bone Joint Surg* 56A:236–253, 1974.)

creep behavior or a plateau in the stress as the strain increases. Beyond 8% to 10% strain, macroscopic failure occurs and further stretching causes tendon rupture.

Ligaments, on the other hand, tend to have a somewhat different collagen composition and a greater elastin content as well as generally straighter fibers with a greater density of cross-links, leading to load–strain behavior as shown in Figure 5.3. This tissue is generally tested as a bone–ligament–bone complex; thus, cross-sectional area (and stress) determinations are difficult to perform. This figure shows two important features of soft tissue mechanics:

1. The physiological strain range is frequently only a small portion of the total possible range.

2. Disease states, in this case prolonged disuse, may produce radical changes in properties.

Ligaments (and tendons) have strongly strain rate–dependent mechanical behavior. This is seen not only in the usual increase in apparent stiffness and decrease in ultimate elongation with increasing strain rate but also in their mode of failure. At low strain rates, those appropriate to normal movements, failures tend to occur within the body of the tissue. However, as strain rates increase, to those of high-speed vehicular or missile impact, failure is increasingly likely to occur by avulsion at bony attachments.

Myosin and actin   The molecular structure of muscle is extremely complex. At the center is the association of two proteins, myosin and actin. Myosin is a relatively rigid molecule containing six smaller subunits and having an overall length of 300 nm with a variable diameter between 2 and 7 nm. It represents the active molecule that when combined with actin, a rigid double helix, produces the characteristic interdigitating structure of the sarcomere, the fundamental motion unit of muscle.

Although there have been extensive investigations of mechanical behavior of muscle at the molecular level, it is sufficient for our purposes to consider how the basic fiber, perhaps 1 μm in diameter, behaves. Figure 5.4 shows a frequently used model, as originally proposed by

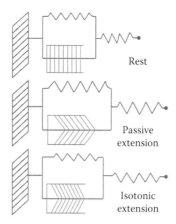

FIGURE 5.4 **(See color insert.)** Model representation of muscle.

A. V. Hill, that expresses this. There are both series and parallel spring elements that account for the elastic behavior of muscle. There is also an active contractile element. This sometimes includes a small parallel dashpot (not shown here) to reflect the velocity-dependent aspects of contraction. This viscous property makes the muscle forces decrease if the muscle is shortened with a certain velocity. The model is, unfortunately, a generalization as none of the elements are linear, as was assumed in the discussion of viscoelasticity in Chapter 4.

However, this model explains the relative load-deformation properties of muscle, as seen in Figure 5.5. This is typical of a pennate or multipennate muscle, such as the tibialis anterior. Fully parallel muscles, such as the rectus abdominis, have a higher passive stiffness and thus have a smaller "dip" in developed force at intermediate elongations.

Muscle develops its maximum stress at lengths slightly longer than its rest length. This stress is somewhat velocity dependent and is between 20 and 40 N/cm² (0.2–0.4 MPa), when the area is the cross-sectional area of the muscle midbelly at its resting length. This is commonly known as the physiological cross-sectional area or PCSA. This feature may be used to estimate the maximum forces that muscles can develop, based

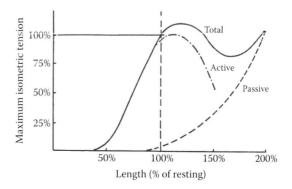

FIGURE 5.5 Passive and active properties of muscle (Blix curve).

on anatomic studies in cadavers, and has proven to be a great aid in bio-mechanical analyses of forces during various motions of limb segments.

PROBLEM 5.1

Suppose that a muscle with a belly cross section of 10 cm² contracts by 20%.

1. What is the maximum external force that the muscle can resist at this contraction?

2. If the attached tendon is assumed to have a cross-sectional area of 1.0 cm², what strain will it experience?

ANSWER:

1. 260 N. This is obtained by determining that the maximum force at 20% contraction (80% of resting length) is (from Figure 5.5) 65% of peak (= 40 N/cm²). Thus:

   $$0.65 \times 40 \times 10 = 260 \text{ N}$$

2. 0.03 (3%). The stress in the tendon is $260/10^{-4}$ or 2.6 MPa. From Figure 5.2, this stress corresponds to 3% strain, near the physio-logic limit for tendon. Training would increase the cross-sectional area (hypertrophy) and reduce both the stress and the resulting strain.

Articular cartilage This extraordinary tissue is responsible for the easy rotational and trans-lational movement of synovial joints. It is very well hydrated, contain-ing 70%–85% water by weight. Its solid components are approximately 50% type II collagen and 50% glycosaminoglycans (GAGs). The GAGs consist of a protein backbone with highly charged polysaccharide side chains. The collagen forms a network, in tension under unloaded physi-ologic conditions, to contain the highly hydrophilic GAGs and its associ-ated water. The result is a markedly viscoelastic tissue.

Complex theories have been proposed to explain the stress–strain and associated stress–electrical potential behavior of articular cartilage at a local level, depending on the properties of its components and their relative presence. These theories arise from the recognition that articu-lar cartilage has a variable composition from the high-collagen-content superficial layer (lamina splendens) to the more cellular regions near the bone–cartilage junction. Moreover, the collagen in the surface layer tends to be elongated along it and to be oriented parallel to the direction of normal movement of the joint from which the cartilage is taken. This superficial layer represents 10% to 20% of the total thickness of articu-lar cartilage. In contrast, the collagen fibrils in the middle zone, which comprises approximately 40% to 60% of the total thickness, are more randomly oriented. This transitions to the deep zone of the cartilage, which forms approximately 30% of the cartilage thickness, where the fibers are woven together and oriented perpendicular to the surface. The collagen content by dry weight varies from approximately 86% in the superficial layer to approximately 67% in the deep zone.

However, examination of intact healthy cartilage, in place on its subchondral support, suggests that within physiologic strain limits (<12%–15%, fully relaxed), it behaves as though it is a homogeneous, isotropic, linear viscoelastic solid. This tissue is linear in the sense that its moduli are independent of stress within this physiologic strain limit. However, this linearity is rapidly lost in a variety of disease states.

Like all materials, articular cartilage has definable tensile, compressive, and shear moduli. However, it has a very low coefficient of friction that results in force application across joints being borne largely as shear stresses near regions of cartilage–cartilage contact. When it is degraded, as in osteoarthritis, the resulting mechanical failures, including delamination of separation of the lamina splendens and deep cracks perpendicular to the surface, closely resemble shear-induced cracks in inorganic materials. Thus, the shear moduli dominate cartilage's behavior *in vivo*.

The shear moduli have been determined extensively in tissues from rabbits and other animals and are in the range of 0.1 MPa (G_R) to 0.5 MPa (G_u). Shear moduli in human material is similar, but elastic moduli, when directly measured parallel to the principal fiber direction in the superficial layer, may be as much as 10 times higher, reflecting the stiffness of collagen in tension. The tensile modulus may range from less than 1 MPa to over 30 MPa, depending on the joint, anatomic location within the joint (weight-bearing vs. non-weight-bearing portions), depth within the cartilage, and degree of degeneration. For example, the tensile modulus of human femoral groove cartilage can vary by more than 10 times, decreasing from 13.9 MPa at the surface to 1.0 MPa in the deep zone. Joint disease, such as osteoarthritis, has been shown to cause a reduction in tensile modulus by approximately 6-fold. The degenerative changes during osteoarthritis, which result in a loss of proteoglycans, can also produce a 10-fold decrease in the tissue compressive modulus.

Studies of rabbit articular cartilage have shown the relative roles that collagen and GAG play in production of mechanical properties. In Figure 5.6, hexosamine is used as a measure of the GAG content of normal and extracted (hyaluronidase-treated) articular cartilage. The shear moduli depend slightly on GAG content, with G_u rising and G_R falling modestly as GAG content decreases. This reflects the water-binding ability of GAG: as GAG content falls, the water content of articular cartilage falls and the remaining water is less strongly bound. The spectrum of retardation times ($L(t)$) rises strongly with decreasing GAG content in normal cartilage, reflecting easier flow of less well-bound water. However, after enzymatic degradation of the GAGs, the relationship changes, indicating that both water and GAG fragments are free to move as a response to pressure. This may lead to loss of GAG fragments from the tissue and may be a contributing mechanism to tissue degradation in arthritic conditions. Similar studies have been done with collagenolytic enzymes but are much harder to interpret since disruption of the collagen network produces GAG loss, even in the absence of GAG degradation. During the progression of osteoarthritis, there is a loss of matrix

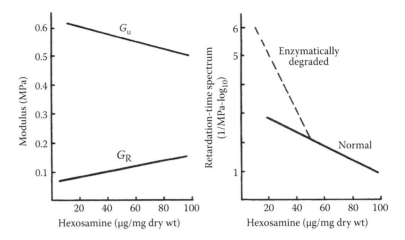

FIGURE 5.6   Dependence of mechanical properties of articular cartilage on GAG content (as measured by hexosamine content). (Adapted
from Parsons, J.R., *The viscoelastic properties of rabbit articular cartilage*. PhD Thesis, University of Pennsylvania, Philadelphia, PA, 1977.)

proteoglycans, fibrillation of the cartilage surface, wearing away of the
collagen fibrils, and eventual exposure of the underlying bone.

Extensive studies of articular cartilage in other modes of deformation
have been made, and there is a large resulting literature. It seems clear that
the properties of articular cartilage are matrix related and are not dependent on the small number of indwelling cells (chondrocytes), despite their
relatively large size. Perhaps the most important finding from these studies
is the observation that articular cartilage is mildly subject to fatigue, with
failure lines propagating parallel to the superficial collagen fiber direction.
It is unknown whether this occurs *in vivo* and, if it does occur, whether it
represents a source of cumulative damage or it is repaired by remodeling.

Other soft tissues   There have been extensive studies of mechanical behavior of other soft
tissues, including skin, fascia, peripheral nerve, and so on, and a wide
literature exists. However, in the vast majority of cases, these tissues
possess sufficiently low effective moduli at the strain rates that they
experience and sufficient ductility that they simply follow movements
of the major elements of the musculoskeletal system without playing a
major role in determining either kinetics or mechanics.

Bone

Material aspects   Bone is the term used to describe both the primary mineralized tissue
in mammalian bodies and the structures that are composed of it. As a
material, it consists of a framework of collagen fibers, essentially all
type I; a mineral matrix, primarily calcium hydroxyapatite; and a small
quantity of mucopolysaccharides and protein polysaccharides, collectively referred to as ground substance or cement.

At a fundamental, structure-free level, all bone has the same properties, with these being dependent on the relative proportions of three phases: organic, mineral, and void. *In vivo*, the void phase is filled with cells, cell processes, and fluid. These have not been shown to contribute to either the static or dynamic properties of fully wet bone. Dry bone, of course, has considerably different properties, but these are not relevant to either tissue mechanics or to the selection of materials to augment or replace bone. A further simplification is the observation that healthy cortical bone possesses a fixed amount of organic tissue per unit volume, approximately 0.6 g/cm^3, and that its density then varies directly as its mineral content up to a peak near 2 g/cm^3. Osteoporotic bone is apparently "normal" at this level of structure; its inferior mechanical properties derive from an absence of bone material per unit volume. Other diseases, such as the osteomalacias, may result in deficiencies of organic material, whereas osteopetrotic bone is essentially hypermineralized "normal" bone.

Cortical bone is a modestly viscoelastic tissue with $E_R/E_U = 0.95$–0.98. Over a wide range of strain rates over several orders of magnitudes, the modulus only increases by a factor of approximately 2. It is highly anisotropic, displaying a fiber pattern or grain that is nearly parallel to the long axes of long bones, with the ratios of tensile moduli in the radial:transverse:longitudinal direction being approximately 1:1:2. Long bones are thus better able to resist stresses *along* the long axis than *across* the long axis. In tension, it displays apparently elastic–plastic behavior, with a "yield" strain of 0.5%–0.6% and an ultimate strain near 3% (Figure 5.7). There is some doubt about this latter value since *in vivo* studies and observations are consistent with considerable ductility, perhaps as high as 5%–6%, whereas *in vitro* studies, even of tissues that are fully wet, frequently show much more brittle behavior, with ε_u, as low as 0.9%–1%. Although these values are higher than those for dry bone, which is quite brittle and fails at ultimate strains of 0.4%–0.5%, the uncertainty reflects a previously discussed problem common to tissue mechanics: the failure to consider postmortem property changes.

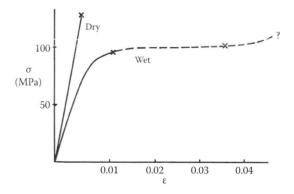

FIGURE 5.7   Stress–strain curves for wet and dry cortical bone.

Hard tissue is relatively immune to post-excision mechanical property changes, if properly handled and maintained, owing to its relative low cell density, especially in cortical bone, but inappropriate storage solutions may produce "softening," reduction in modulus, and increase in ductility resulting from partial demineralization. Older data in the literature were often obtained from formalin-fixed tissues. In general, fixed tissues, although stable in properties, are stiffer and more brittle than unfixed tissues, in direct proportion to the amount of collagen present.

The issue of qualitative changes is much more controversial, because of the difficulty in making reliable physical property measurements *in vivo*. The uncertainty in the relative plasticity of bone as reflected in the uncertainty in the ultimate strain is an example. A more important problem is the question of the fatigue properties of cortical bone.

Figure 5.8 is a compilation of fatigue data obtained from a variety of studies. Stress is plotted on the vertical axis normalized by dividing by σ_u to account for variations in material source test technique, and so on. The logarithm of the number of cycles is plotted on the horizontal axis, in the usual manner for *S–N* fatigue curves. The diagonal line represents the middle of the range of data from various sources using traditional excision and preservation (but not fixation) techniques for fully moist bone. A great deal of data exist for the solid part of the line and less data exist for the high-stress, low-cycle region, which is shown as a dashed line. A single *in vivo* experiment has been done on the tibiae of live immobilized rats (Seireg and Kempke 1969). The results of this are shown in the upper line of Figure 5.8. The qualitative difference is graphic: *in vitro* testing shows no endurance limit whereas *in vivo* results suggest an endurance limit of 42% of σ_u, reached after 5×10^3 cycles. Although the actual biologic situation is far more complex than this short-term experiment, with remodeling processes competing with fatigue processes, the comparison of the two groups of data should give one pause to consider the general problem of extrapolating *in vitro* tissue mechanical results to *in vivo* performance.

More recent data have shown that cortical bone tissue has significantly higher fatigue resistance than cancellous bone tissue. Bending

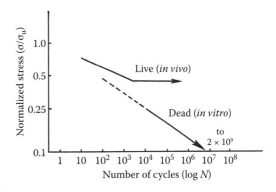

FIGURE 5.8   *S–N* (fatigue) curves for live and dead bone.

tests of human tibial bone has shown cancellous bone fatigue strength of approximately 160 MPa at 10 cycles to approximately 100 MPa at 1 million cycles. On the other hand, cortical bone fatigue strength is approximately 190 MPa at 10 cycles to approximately 160 MPa at 1 million cycles. The loading mode also has an effect on the fatigue lifetimes in bone. For cortical bone, compression loading produces approximately 10%–15% higher lifetimes than tensile loading. Animal studies have also shown that the fatigue strength in torsion is less than half the fatigue compressive strength.

Microstructural aspects

Cortical bone Cortical bone is the best organized mineralized tissue in the body and carries the majority of the load in major bones. It is characterized by lamellar sheets of tissue, 3–4 μm thick. Within each lamella, collagen fibers run more or less parallel in the plane of the sheet. Adjacent lamellae are separated from each other by a relatively nonmineralized layer of ground substance and disorganized collagen called the cementum or cement line, which is approximately 0.1 μm thick.

In the purely cortical diaphyseal portions of long bones, these cortical lamellae are arranged in several microstructures. Parallel circumferential lamellae encircle the outer cortex below the periosteum.

A variety of cylindrical structures exist, with their long axes roughly parallel to the long axis of the bone, as seen in the transverse sections of Figure 5.9. The most common of these is the *Haversian* osteon, with its closed concentric structure centered on a Haversian canal. The central canal contains a circulatory process and, frequently, a nerve fiber. Osteocytes occupy lacunae within the cement lines between lamellae, and fine channels or canaliculi connect the osteocytes with each other

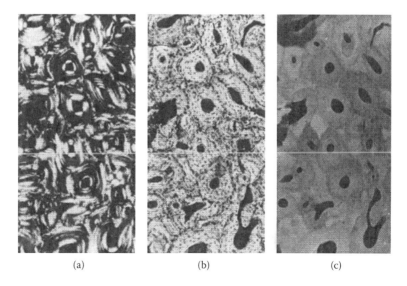

(a)   (b)   (c)

FIGURE 5.9 Structure of cortical bone (human anterior tibial cortex, transverse [100 μm]) section. (a) Crossed polarizers. (b) Transmitted light. (c) Microradiograph (1 inch = 1000 μm).

and the Haversian canal. Occasional vascular processes, in Volkmann's canals, lie across the grain, joining adjacent Haversian canals.

The axis of the Haversian osteon lies generally along the long axis of a long bone, such as a femur or tibia, but tends to pass from exterior to interior surface as it passes in a distal-to-proximal direction, with a slight spiral track. Osteons of this type may extend over several centimeters in length and have diameters (or major axes) of no more than 300–450 μm, apparently limited by the necessity for the osteocytes to be within a diffusion-limited distance from the central vascular process. The Haversian osteon is separated from the surrounding bone matrix by a heavier cement line.

Within the Haversian osteon, adjacent lamellae have different preferential collagen fiber directions. This produces the light and dark bands seen when cortical bone sections are viewed between crossed polarizers (Figure 5.9a). The classic structure has a 90° angulation between fibers in adjacent lamellae, resulting in alternating light and dark bands. Several other orientation patterns are possible, and it appears that any particular osteon shows different collagen fiber orientations along its length.

Haversian osteons also show a wide range of degrees of calcification (Figure 5.9c). Younger osteons are generally less well mineralized, whereas old ones may become infarcted and actually have the canal closed by hypermineralization before remodeling. Thus, the concept of bone density must be taken as an average, even at this level of structural organization.

Intermediate in structure between circumferential and Haversian osteons is the incomplete or *involute* osteon. In some cases, it is an incomplete Haversian osteon, formed by radial growth of the bone with encirclement of periosteal capillaries. In section, it shows a characteristic omega shape, with a portion resembling a Haversian osteon, but with the lamella turning about and streaming away from the open side.

Finally, groups of nearly parallel lamellae are seen in the spaces between Haversian and involute osteons. These are termed *interstitial* osteons and may, in some cases, be fragments of older osteons left behind during remodeling.

The mechanical properties of excised segments of Haversian osteons have been studied extensively. They appear to be more ductile (ε_u = 7%–9%) and somewhat less stiff than cortical bone overall. From this finding and from theoretical considerations, it is believed that Haversian osteons confer resistance to failure in bending on cortical bone.

Other bony microstructures   In addition to cortical bone, there are several other types of material structure within bones in mammals. Each appears to play a different role in load carriage and stress transmission.

Fiber bone Fiber bone is found in the fetus and neonate before functional reorganization takes place. It is a loose, tangled web of collagen fibers, with more ground substance than mature cortical bone and a good degree of amorphous mineralization, primarily octa-calcium phosphate, in addition to the normally expected calcium hydroxyapatite. It is weak, is quite ductile, and does not persist long in normal development.

Because of this immature structure, it is essentially an isotropic material, with equal properties in all directions.

Callus Callus, the mineralized tissue that forms in healing fractures and produces a natural "splinting" or reinforcing effect to the broken bone ends, is similar in organization, composition, and properties to primitive fiber bone (Figure 5.10). It is very poorly bonded to preexisting bone and, thus, its contribution to fracture stiffness and strength is difficult to determine, even in *in vitro* testing. To add to the complexity of quantifying the mechanical properties of callus tissue, there is variability due to its heterogeneous nature. Multiple tissue types exist within the callus, namely, granulation tissue, chondroid tissue, and woven bone. Animal studies, such as from rat fracture healing experiments, suggest that the variability can range by over three orders of magnitude, from approximately 0.6 MPa to 1000 MPa. The nature of the callus tissue will depend on the phase of fracture healing. During the first phase, the inflammatory response leads to the formation of a hematoma and granulation tissue. Then, a soft callus consisting of cartilaginous or chondroid tissue is formed in the second phase, typically starting 2 weeks after the fracture begins to heal. In the third phase (between 6 and 12 weeks), the soft callus ossifies to form a hard or bony callus consisting primarily of woven bone tissue. Finally, the woven bone is remodeled into lamellar bone tissue (between 12 and 16 weeks). At any given time, a heterogeneous mixture of these tissues can be found within the fracture callus.

Cancellous bone Next in order of strength and organization is *cancellous* or spongy bone. This is found in the endochondral areas of long bones, supporting the subchondral cortical plates, in the central areas of smaller bones loaded in complex fashion, such as the metacarpals, and as the diploe between the tables of the calvarium. It consists of spicules or trabeculae of fairly acellular bone surrounded by a highly cellular

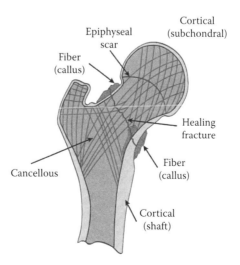

FIGURE 5.10 **(See color insert.)** Microstructural elements of bone.

periosteal membrane. The bone is well organized with a preferred direction for collagen fibers lying roughly along the axis of each spicule. The spicules are organized into a spongy network, which in places condenses into plates connected by spicular struts, as in the patella, or into a closed-cell sponge, as in the diploe.

Cancellous bone, unlike fiber bone and callus, is an organized load-bearing material that appears to follow Wolff's law. Its presence is associated with the following structural requirements:

1. The need to provide a transition of direction of stress (*example*: the transition between the neck and the diaphyseal cortices of the proximal femur)

2. The need to distribute concentrated loads, such as associated with tendon and ligament insertion (*example*: the greater trochanter of the femur)

3. The need to resist impulsive loads (*example*: the calcaneus)

Cancellous bone is anisotropic in terms of both mechanical properties and morphometry. It is stiffer (has higher tensile and compressive moduli) but fails at a lower strain when loaded parallel to the predominant spicular direction than when loaded in other directions. On first examination of sections of cancellous bone, there does not appear to be such defined axes, but they are revealed by closer study. Figure 5.10 shows typical directions or trajectories in the proximal femur, in a plane passing distal–proximal and bisecting the shaft and neck.

Both the degree of anisotropy and the relation between the elastic properties and the density of bone vary substantially with skeletal site and function. Trabecular bone from the pelvis and lumbar spine are relatively isotropic compared to sites such as the calcaneus and proximal tibia (Figure 5.11).

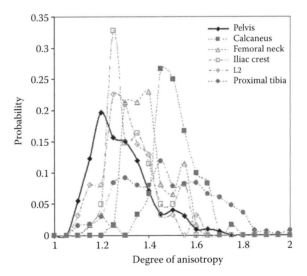

FIGURE 5.11 Degree of anisotropy of bone at various anatomic sites. (Adapted from Day, J.S., PhD Dissertation, Erasmus University, Rotterdam, The Netherlands, 2005.)

The question of ductility of cancellous bone is difficult to resolve. The stresses placed on it, for instance, in compression, are not carried uniformly by all spicules, and the soft tissue and marrow in between cannot adequately redistribute the stress if one spicule buckles or fractures. The deformation limit in the laboratory is defined as the point at which this first collapse occurs. However, *in vivo*, it has been suggested that such spicular collapse produces healing and remodeling processes leading to a stiffer, less ductile structure.

Comparison of mechanical properties of bony microstructures Overall, at typical physiologic densities, compared with cortical bone, cancellous bone is:

1/3 to 1/4 as dense

1/10 to 1/20 as stiff

Five times as ductile

However, the mechanical properties of cortical and cancellous bone represent a continuum, reflecting the behavior of a relatively uniform material modified by differences in density and organization. These findings are summarized in Figure 5.12, which shows σ_u and E (compressive) as a function of density. These curves were created from a broad body of data by a fitting process, assuming the following relationships:

Ultimate strength varies as the *square* of density. Modulus varies as the *cube* of density.

These relationships are derived from theoretical consideration of the relationship of structural and mechanical properties of inorganic porous structures. The experimental data appear to support them except that stiffness rises more rapidly than expected at densities above 1 g/cm^3, as

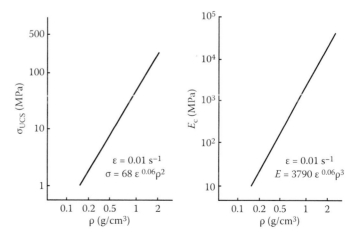

FIGURE 5.12 Dependence of σ_{ucs} and E_c of bone on density. (Adapted from Carter, D.R., Hayes, W.C., *J Bone Joint Surg* 59A:954–962, 1977.)

found in vertebral bodies, owing to a transition of cancellous bone from an open or network sponge to a closed cell sponge structure.

Effects of anatomic location

The mechanical properties of bone are highly localized, in terms of their dependence on the anatomic location. This reflects the evolutionary changes to support the magnitudes and directionality of forces that are experienced at the respective locations. The classic understanding of the modulus of cortical bone is based on femoral diaphyseal bone. However, the mineral content of cortical bone can vary by anatomic location and from the effects of aging or disease. The relevant mechanical properties can also vary on the basis of the type of loading that is typically observed at the site of interest. For example, in a region where flexural bending is commonly experienced, flexural modulus would be the relevant property.

The flexural modulus of the human cortical tibia bone is approximately 5.4–6.8 GPa and decreases to approximately 4.9 GPa in the human iliac crest and 2.5 GPa in the human vertebra. While the longitudinal modulus of femoral and tibia diaphyseal cortical bone is approximately 17 to 20 GPa, it decreases to approximately 5 to 15 GPa for the vertebra endplates and to approximately 0.1 to 0.4 GPa in the subchondral bone of the glenoid. Similarly, the mechanical properties of cancellous bone vary between anatomic locations, as well as within different regions of the same anatomic site. The tissue modulus of cancellous bone has been reported to range from 0.76 to 10 GPa in tension and from 3.2 to 5.4 GPa in bending.

PROBLEM 5.2

What is the resulting local strain in the bone at the insertion of the tendon in Problem 5.1?

ANSWER:

186 $\mu\varepsilon$. From Figure 5.7, estimate the modulus of cortical bone *in vivo* to be 100/0.07 = 14 GPa. Thus, a stress of 2.6 MPa produces a strain of 1.86×10^{-4} or 186 $\mu\varepsilon$. Activities of everyday life produce strains in cortical bone between 100 and 1000 $\mu\varepsilon$.

Fracture of bone

Since bone is viscoelastic, its work of failure may be expected to increase with strain rate. This is the case for both cancellous and cortical bone with the increase being approximately 10% per decade (10-fold) increase in strain rate. At physiologic strain rates, failure is of a "delamination" type, with the fracture line following previous defects, such as cement lines, lacunae, Haversian canals, and so on. However, at very high strain rates, such as encountered in high-velocity-missile impacts, the work of fracture is greatly reduced, and the fracture surfaces propagate at random, producing considerable comminution.

Cortical bone, when tested in compression parallel to the fiber axis of the long bone from which it is taken, frequently shows a buckling or delamination failure, reminiscent of the buckle fracture seen in immature bones in children (Figure 5.13). When tested in tension, the fracture is transverse and brittle, with some minor pullout of lamellae and

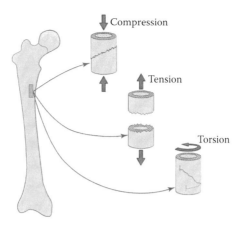

FIGURE 5.13   **(See color insert.)** Fracture of cortical bone.

osteonal segments. Finally, cortical bone tested in torsion around its longitudinal fiber axis produces the expected spiral failure. However, there are frequently vertical splits at the ends of the fracture plane, and the angle of the plane to the axis is nearer to 30°–35° than the expected value of 45°, again reflecting the fibrous nature of bone.

Defects such as screw holes produce significant stress concentration in bone, as in other materials, with the minimum concentration factor K approximately equal to 2. However, unlike inorganic materials, bone shows a considerable ability to remodel. This can remove the stress concentration effect of a screw hole in 6–8 weeks *in vivo* (in dogs) if, for instance, the hole is plugged with silicone rubber. The same effect can be produced if a rigid screw is used and left in place during mechanical testing; however, removing the screw just before testing reintroduces the stress concentration.

Screws anchored in bone may be pulled out directly, producing a shear failure at the points of the screw threads. The strength of screw retention varies somewhat, depending on screw design and diameter, but is 350–400 N/mm of bone thickness in cortical bone and 10–25 N/mm of bone thickness in healthy cancellous bone.

Orthopaedic surgery is sometimes likened to carpentry, since many of the tools of the two disciplines are the same: chisels, rasps, twist drills, saws, and so on. This similarity arises from the "machining" properties of bone, which greatly resemble those of a partly seasoned (dried), moderately strong hard wood, such as yellow birch or elm. Bone can be made to form a "chip" and can be split, sometimes inadvertently. However, bone is different from wood in two significant respects.

1. The production of heat during machining must be actively avoided. Temperature rises of as little as 4°C can produce cell death, whereas larger rises (>10°C) can produce irreversible mechanical property changes.

2. The calcium hydroxyapatite content of bone is highly abrasive and rapidly dulls cutting edges of surgical tools.

There have been a number of studies done to determine the optimum design and use of cutting edges for tools for bone surgery. There is no general agreement, perhaps reflecting the differences in behavior of bone *in vitro* and *in vivo*, but some principles have emerged.

1. Cutting performance varies with edge design.
2. Sharp tools produce less heat than dull ones.
3. Increasing bearing pressure on tools increases heat production.

Thus, good surgical practice suggests selecting tools that work well for the individual surgeon and maintaining them as sharp as possible to diminish required bearing forces and heat production.

Comparative properties of tissues

It is useful to provide a brief overview of the comparison of the mechanical properties of soft and hard tissues with some common prosthetic materials. This is shown in Table 5.2.

Table 5.2 makes the problem of prosthetic replacement of tissues quite clear. No prosthetic materials provide the unique combinations of even these selected mechanical properties that are seen in tissues. Thus, increasing interest is being shown in prosthetic materials that are composites of two or more materials. These show promise of producing properties closer to those of tissues, mimicking the way the mechanical properties of tendon arise from those of two of its components, collagen and elastin. Further consideration also needs to be given to the site specificity of the mechanical properties of tissue. For example, cortical bone modulus is conventionally based on properties for long bone cortical bone. However, the properties can diminish as the cortical bony tissue transitions to a thin layer at the end of the long bone or at the cortical rim of vertebra.

Table 5.2 Mechanical properties of tissue and prosthetic materials

	Tensile modulus (GPa)	Tensile strength (MPa)	Strain to failure (%)
Typical tissues			
Articular cartilage (unrelaxed)	0.001–0.03	5–25	80–120
Tendon	1	55	8–10
Cancellous bone (ρ = 0.1 to 1.0 g/cm^3)	0.2–10	10–20	5–7
Cortical bone (ρ = 2.0 g/cm^3)	10–20	100–200	1–3
Typical prosthetic materials			
Ultrahigh-molecular-weight polyethylene	0.012	40	420–525
316L stainless steel	193	480	40
Aluminum oxide ceramic (compression)	350	4000	0.5–1

Effects of aging

As individuals age, the mechanical properties of their tissues change. This is a variable process with physiologic age, even in normal individuals lagging or leading chronologic age by up to 20%. Although all material properties change, with tissues becoming less stiff, less ductile, and weaker, the most pronounced effect is that of loss of strength. Strength properties in general reach a peak near the age of 20 years in humans and then decrease thereafter. An overall or composite "aging rate" has been calculated at 0.5% strength loss per year (Yamada 1970). Mean effects for various tissues are given in Table 5.3. Another way of thinking about the effects of aging is that ultimate stress, ultimate strain, and energy absorption decrease by 5%, 9%, and 12% per decade, respectively, from the age 20 to 100 years. In terms of trabecular bone architecture, after 60 years of age, there is significant decline in bone volume fraction and trabecular thinning, with a change in the microarchitecture of cancellous bone from plate-like to rod-like structures. As a result, the degree of anisotropy increases with age. Cortical bone also becomes more brittle and fractures with less energy with aging.

Effects of disease

Joint disease may set in as individuals age, from overuse, or progressive wear and tear. Rheumatoid arthritis is an immune-mediated chronic, inflammatory disease that can damage and destroy the joint and is manifested through inflammatory synovitis. Animal studies have shown that the mechanical properties of arthritic femurs are impaired, having lower modulus, yield stress, and ultimate stress, and resultantly making bone more prone to fracture. The deregulation of the immune system disturbs the balance of biochemical bone markers and the arrangement of collagen, therefore affecting bone metabolism and possibly

Table 5.3 Age effects on strength of tissues (as proportion of values for age 20–29)

	Age (years)		
Tissue	30–39	50–59	70–79
Costal cartilage			
Tension	0.93	0.56	0.29
Compression	0.97	0.73	0.73
Tendon—tension	1.0	1.0	0.80
Cancellous bone (vertebral body—compression)	1.0	0.78	0.55
Cortical bone			
Tension	0.98	0.76	0.70
Compression	0.95	0.95	—
Musculoskeletal system (average)	0.97	0.85	0.77

Source: Adapted from Yamada, H., Ratios for age changes in the mechanical properties of human organs and tissues. In Evans, F.G. (ed), *Strength of Biological Materials*, Williams & Wilkins, Baltimore, pp. 255–271, 1970.

indicating rheumatoid arthritis as an independent risk factor for fractures. Significant microarchitectural changes in cancellous bone can be observed after osteoarthritis, leading to a very heterogeneous architecture. Osteoarthritic trabecular bone is thicker and denser, as well as more plate-like, but has lower mechanical strength.

Effects of antiresorptives

Antiresorptive therapy includes bisphosphonates and estrogen replacement. Over the past two decades, bisphosphonates have been used to help arrest bone loss and to treat osteoporosis, by limiting the dissolution of the principal bone mineral, that is, hydroxyapatite. The mechanism is achieved through encouraging osteoclasts, which destroy bone, to undergo cell death and thereby preventing bone turnover. This improves bony microarchitecture by preventing loss of trabecular volume and suppressing activation of remodeling, thereby adding mass to trabecular bone and halting cortical bone erosion on the corticoendosteal surfaces. However, bone formation does not appear to continue beyond filling remodeling sites previously created. Thus, bisphosphonates do not add bone mass or change the macroarchitecture or shape of bone, outside of limiting the effect of increasing resorption. Bisphosphonate drugs include alendronate, etidronate, ibandronate, risedronate, zoledronate, and pamidronate. In contrast, other drugs function anabolically instead by stimulating osteoblasts, which build new bone.

Estimates of human bone strength after the use of bisphosphonates suggest that vertebral strength may be increased by up to 10% after 3 months. Similar changes have also been observed for femoral bone, with 3.6% and 4.8% improvement after 1 and 2 years of treatment, respectively. Consequently, bisphosphonates are also highly effective in decreasing the incidence of hip and spine fractures by up to 30% to 50%. Increased bone strength can be explained almost entirely by increases in bone mineral density, but the increased mechanical properties are partly offset by reduced bone toughness. Differences occur, depending on drug, dosage, and duration of use.

Sex hormones, such as estrogen for women and testosterone for men, have a protective effect on bone. If hormone production is altered because of surgery, illness, or early menopause in women, hormone replacement can be used to replace hormones that the body should be making or used to make. Such therapy can include replacing calcitonin, which acts on the skeleton to regulate the amount of calcium in the blood. Supplements of estrogen or estrogen with progesterone may also be taken.

PROBLEM 5.3

What is the primary mechanism for bisphosphonates on bone remodeling?

A. Creating bone throughout, including beyond remodeling sites

B. Arresting osteoclasts to prevent bone turnover

C. Changing the macroarchitecture of bone

D. Activating osteoblasts

ANSWER:

B. Bisphosphonates do not add bone mass, but instead encourage osteo-clasts, which destroy bone, to undergo cell death and thereby preventing bone turnover.

Electrical properties of tissues

In addition to mechanical properties, tissues possess thermal and electrical properties that arise from their composition and structural arrangement. Thermal properties are not of great interest in orthopaedic applications since, as yet, prosthetic devices intended for implantation by orthopaedic surgeons are not sources of heat. The exception is the role of heat release by polymethyl methacrylate–type bone cements during curing. However, electrical properties have become of great interest, both in the process of understanding naturally occurring processes of growth, remodeling, and repair and in the application of exogenous signals to aid these processes. Thus, a brief discussion of electrical behavior of tissues is in order.

Passive electrical properties

Electricity, or the flow of current, is simply the transfer of charge from one point to another. Solids, liquids, and gases conduct electricity according to Ohm's law:

$$E = I \cdot R$$

where E is the electrical potential difference (in volts), I is the current (in amperes), and R is the resistance (in ohms). This is the relationship used in electrical circuits with direct current (net current flowing in one direction without reversal). It may be converted to an intrinsic expression, suitable for consideration of tissue properties, and written thus:

$$\Delta V = i \cdot \rho$$

where ΔV is the voltage gradient at a point (in $V \cdot m$), i is the current density (in A/m^2), and ρ is the resistivity (in $ohm \cdot m$). Thus, ρ is the intrinsic electrical conduction parameter of the material, describing the density of current that will pass a point in response to an applied voltage gradient.

Current flows in tissue primarily by the movement of ions. If two electrodes are inserted in a portion of tissue and a voltage is placed across them, positive ions (such as H^+, Na^+, K^+, and Ca^{2+}) will move toward the cathode and be reduced, whereas negative ions (such as OH^- and Cl^-) will move toward the anode and be oxidized. The net effect, in the external circuit, is that a current of electrons obtained by oxidation at the anode will flow to the cathode. This current will be equal in magnitude to the current, produced by these ion movements, flowing between the electrodes in the tissue.

If this experiment is done with a battery (which is a nearly constant voltage source at low current) and the current is measured, it will be seen to diminish with time. This is due to a process called *polarization*: the accumulation of charges in the vicinity of the electrodes and the separation of tissue-bound charges of opposite signs. If nonpolarizable electrodes are used, such as pressed silver–silver chloride pellets, the current will still decline with time because of tissue polarization.

This polarization ability, which is seen as an *apparent* increase in resistivity with time in response to a fixed voltage, is governed by the following equation:

$$\Delta V = q/K$$

where q is the density of charge (coulombs/m^2) and K is the dielectric constant (farad/m).

This effect produces a lower initial resistivity (and thus a higher current); the final steady value is called a *resistive* current, whereas the initial contribution by polarization is called a *displacement* current, since a fixed charge is displaced rather than mobile charges being moved.

If the direct current is replaced by an alternating current, then the contribution of the (dielectric) polarization is greater. Thus, in general, apparent tissue resistivity *decreases* with increasing frequency of applied voltage. The dielectric constant of water decreases with increasing frequency, which tends to diminish the decrease of resistivity with frequency above 100 kHz.

The resistivity and the dielectric constant thus completely characterize the passive electrical properties of tissues. Unless current is driven through a cell or tissue membrane, both resistivity and dielectric constants tend to reflect the water content of tissue. For resistivity, the lowest values obtained are perhaps 0.6 (ohm·m) for blood and 1 for muscle, and they range up to 30–40 for cortical bone (fully wet). The dielectric constant of water is nearly 90 (air = 1), and the various tissues are fractions of this value.

Thus, imposed currents, either injected by electrodes or produced internally by various processes, tend to flow through fluid-filled spaces and high-water-content tissues such as articular cartilage, whereas potential gradients are larger in tissue with lower water contents, such as bone.

Active electrical properties

In addition to these passive materials properties, musculoskeletal tissues are themselves the source of a number of electrical signals. Those that arise in nerve tissue resulting from membrane depolarization and repolarization, secondary to ion flows, need not be recited here as they are well known.

However, nonexcitable tissues are the source of two types of electrical potential difference whose significance is now just being appreciated. The first of these is seen in a pattern of constant polarization throughout the bodies of living mammals. They are called *bioelectric potentials* or more simply *biopotentials* and have been shown to be dependent on the presence and magnitude of coupled oxidative phosphorylation. They produce potential gradients on the order of 0.1–1 mV/cm and are oriented such that sites distal from the center of the trunk are relatively electropositive with respect to more central sites. Open epiphyseal growth plates and other areas of growth, including tumors, are electronegative with respect to surrounding tissues. Tissue injury, such as skin abrasion or bone fracture, produces a short-term (<1 h) local positive polarization, ascribed to an "injury current," followed by a strong negative polarization that diminishes but persists until healing and remodeling activity have stopped.

The second of these electrical effects is a group of polarizations called variously *piezoelectric, stress-generated* (SGP), or *strain-related* (SRP) *potentials*. These potentials exist in tissue, whether living or dead, and are produced by deformation in shear of the tissue. Thus, a popular way to elicit them is by bending a slab of cortical bone or a whole bone.

Figure 5.14 shows the results of such an experiment. When a bending stress is applied and shortly thereafter released, the following sequence of events is observed. As the strain develops, an initial or forward polarization develops, oriented such that the concave or compression side of the specimen is electronegative with respect to the convex side. If the strain is maintained constant for several seconds, the forward potential rapidly decays. When the strain is released, the polarization rapidly disappears and a small reverse polarization is seen, which decays to zero in a short time. If the initial strain is maintained, suitable measurement instruments reveal that the forward polarization decays to a very low value (but not to zero), which is called the *offset potential*.

The forward potential is typically 10–20 mV in wet cortical bone for surface strains of 500–1000 μɛ. It increases linearly with strain at a constant strain rate (Figure 5.14, upper right). For a given peak strain, it increases with an increasing strain rate to a plateau value (Figure 5.14, lower right). The offset potential is linearly related to the peak strain but is not dependent on the initial strain rate.

There is some debate as to the origin of SRPs but the consensus is that *in vivo*, they are related to the forced flow of fluid (secondary to strain) over surfaces with net fixed charge densities.

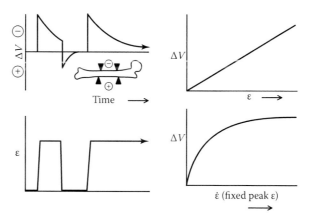

FIGURE 5.14 Production of strain-related potentials (SRPs).

What is more arguable but of great present interest is the role that these two types of potential play in directing growth, healing, and remodeling of musculoskeletal tissues. The temporal association of the biopotentials with growth processes, especially with healing fractures, was certainly a factor in early investigations of the effects of faradic (net current injected with electrodes) stimulation on healing of bony defects in animals and its application in the late 1970s to clinical treatment of nonunions. More recent considerations of SRPs, particularly in relation to the success in the use of inductive and capacitive stimulation in both animal models and in clinical studies and practice, have led to suggestions that these signals represent the necessary translation of stress (or strain) into signals perceivable by cells that are responsible for Wolff's law adaptive remodeling effects. However, the critical experiments remain to be done to demonstrate this hypothesis.*

Additional problems

PROBLEM 5.4

Articular cartilage (select the correct answer[s])

    A. Is elastic in behavior

    B. Is uniform in structure

    C. Is viscoelastic in behavior

    D. Has a high mineral content

    E. Has a high shear modulus

ANSWER:

C is the best answer, since articular cartilage is highly viscoelastic. It shows some elastic behavior, at very short times, so *A* is true, but this answer does not emphasize the time dependence of the response. Articular cartilage has a relatively low shear modulus and has a layered structure with a low mineral content (relative to bone), so the other answers are incorrect.

PROBLEM 5.5

A muscle can exert a maximum force

    A. At its resting length

    B. At slightly longer than its resting length

    C. At slightly shorter than its resting length

    D. After being surgically shortened

    E. Of 40 N

---

* Space is too limited for a full discussion of electrical effects and their consequences *in vivo*. Interested readers may consult Black, J: *Electrical Stimulation: Its Role in Growth, Repair and Remodeling of the Musculoskeletal System*. Praeger, New York, 1987.

ANSWER:

B. Surgical shortening, by movement of tendon insertions, reduces maximum possible muscle forces. *E* is wrong since the maximum force depends on the type of muscle and its midbelly cross-sectional area.

PROBLEM 5.6

Rank (1) articular cartilage, (2) cancellous bone, (3) ligament, and (4) tendon in *increasing* magnitude of

    A. Elastic (tensile) modulus

    B. Strain to failure

ANSWER:

    A. 1, 2, 3, 4

    B. 4, 1, 2, 3

PROBLEM 5.7

Living bone (select the incorrect answer[s])

    A. Remodels to reduce abnormal stresses placed upon it

    B. Requires no energy for maintenance

    C. Is viscoelastic

ANSWER:

B. Living bone requires energy for maintenance as does all living tissue. *A* is a restatement of Wolff's law, and *C* is correct since all tissues are viscoelastic to some degree.

PROBLEM 5.8

Match possible phrases to complete true definitions:

1. SRPs	A. can be predicted from Ohm's law
2. Voltage	B. depend upon life processes
3. Wolff's law	C. depend upon ion movement
4. Biopotentials	D. may depend upon electrical effects

ANSWER:

1, C; 2, A; 3, D; 4, B.

PROBLEM 5.9

Increasing strain rate in bone (select the correct answer[s])

    A. Changes the microscopic nature of fractures

    B. Causes fatigue failure

    C. Causes creep

D. Produces increasing ε_u

E. Produces increased tensile modulus

ANSWER:

A and *E*. Fatigue failure and creep in bone are essentially independent of strain rate. Increasing strain rate decreases ε_u.

PROBLEM 5.10

Select the choices for each material comparison:

A. Bone is generally (stronger or weaker) than plastics.

B. Bone is generally (stronger or weaker) than metals.

C. Bone is generally (more brittle or more ductile) than ceramics.

ANSWER:

A, stronger; *B*, weaker; *C*, more ductile.

References

SEIREG A, KEMPKE W: Behavior of *in vivo* bone under cyclic loading. *J Biomechanics* 2:455–462, 1969.

YAMADA H: Ratios for age changes in the mechanical properties of human organs and tissues. pp. 255–271. In Evans FG (ed): *Strength of Biological Materials*. Williams & Wilkins, Baltimore, 1970.

Annotated bibliography

1. ABDULGHANI S, CAETANO-LOPES J, CANHAO H, FONSECA JE: Biomechanical effects of inflammatory diseases on bone-rheumatoid arthritis as a paradigm. *Autoimmunity Rev* 8:668–671, 2009.

    Discusses the effects of rheumatoid arthritis on bone changes.

2. ASCENZI A, BELL GH: Bone as a mechanical engineering problem. In Bourne GH (ed): *The Biochemistry and Physiology of Bone*, Vol. 1. Academic Press, Orlando, FL, 1972.

    A historical overview of the materials aspects of bone. Includes extensive references to the studies of Ascenzi and coworkers on the structure and mechanical properties of osteons.

3. BASSETT CAL: Biologic significance of piezoelectricity. *Calcif Tissue Res* 1:252–272, 1968.

    A review of the descriptive information on strain-related potentials in tissue up to 1968, with the principal ideas concerning their origin and some interesting suggestions as to their biologic roles.

4. BLACK J: Tissue properties: Relationship of *in vitro* studies to *in vivo* behavior. p. 5. In Hastings GW, Ducheyne P (eds): *Natural and Living Biomaterials*. CRC Press, Boca Raton, FL, 1984.

    Examination of the evidence for differences between properties measured *in vitro* and those actually existing *in vivo*.

5. BLACK J: *Electrical Stimulation: Its Role in Growth, Repair and Remodeling in the Musculoskeletal System.* Praeger Publishers, New York, 1987.

    Covers a variety of subjects, including results of *in vitro*, animal, and clinical studies of electrical stimulation of soft and hard tissue.

6. BURSTEIN AH, REILLY DT, MARTENS M: Aging of bone tissue: Mechanical properties. *J Bone Joint Surg* 58A:82–86, 1976.

    A study of the effects of donor age on bone mechanical properties.

7. CARTER DR, HAYES WC: The compressive behavior of bone as a two-phase porous structure. *J Bone Joint Surg* 59A:954–962, 1977.

    An often cited paper that, for the first time, united the mechanical behavior of cortical and cancellous bone with a single analytical approach.

8. COWIN SC: *Bone Mechanics Handbook*, 2nd ed. CRC Press, Boca Raton, FL, 2001.

    Review of many aspects of cortical and cancellous bone, including their mechanical and architectural properties (see Chapters 10 and 33).

9. DING M: Microarchitectural adaptions in aging and osteoarthrotic sub-chondral bone tissues. *Acta Orthopaedica*, Suppl 340(81), 2010.

    Discusses the effects of aging and osteoarthritis on the mechanical properties and architecture of bone.

10. FRANK C, AMIEL D, WOO SL-Y, AKESON W: Normal ligament properties and ligament healing. *Clin Orthop Rel Res* 196:15–25, 1985.

    Not strictly about tissue mechanics, this relates physiology, composition, structure, and mechanical properties of ligaments with special reference to changes produced by injury and subsequent healing.

11. FREEMAN MAR (ed): *Adult Articular Cartilage*, 2nd ed. Pitman Medical, Bath, UK, 1979.

    The standard work on articular cartilage. Chapters 5 and 6 deal with mechanical behavior.

12. FRICH LH, JENSEN NC, ODGAARD A, PEDERSEN CM, SOJBJERG JO, DALSTRA M: Bone strength and material properties of the glenoid. *J Shoulder and Elbow Surgery* 6:97–104, 1997.

    Provides materials properties for the shoulder joint.

13. GIBSON U: The mechanical behavior of cancellous bone. *J Biomech* 18:317–328, 1985.

    A historical discussion of mechanics of cancellous bone and the role of porosity in the mechanical behavior of cortical bone. Quite accessible discussion in terms of structural types; includes a review of Carter's and Hayes' (1977) results on cortical bone.

14. GOZNA ER, HARRINGTON IJ (ed): *Biomechanics of Musculoskeletal Injury.* Williams & Wilkins, Baltimore, 1982.

    A qualitative treatment of how physical injuries occur to soft and hard tissues in the musculoskeletal system. Chapter 3 has some useful comments on the mechanics of internal fixation.

15. GRODZINSKY AJ: Electromechanical and physiochemical properties of connective tissue. *CRC Crit Rev Biomed Eng* 9(2):133–199, 1983.

    An exposition of the inter-relationships of structural features and composition on one hand and mechanical and electrical behavior of soft tissues on the other hand. Extensive bibliography.

16. JOHNSON TP, SOCRATE S, BOYCE MC: A viscoelastic, viscoplastic model of cortical bone valid at low and high strain rates. *Acta Biomater* 6(10):4073–4080, 2010.

    An extremely useful summary and critique of modeling efforts to describe bone as a viscoelastic material.

17. MOW VC, HUISKES R: *Basic Orthopaedic Biomechanics and Mechano-Biology*, 3rd ed. Lippincott Williams & Wilkins, 2004.

Collection of information on biomechanics of biological tissues and biomaterials, as well as total joint replacements.

18. NOYES FR, DELUCAS JL, TORVIK PJ: Biomechanics of anterior cruciate ligament failure: An analysis of strain-rate sensitivity and mechanisms of failure in primates. *J Bone Joint Surg* 56A:236–253, 1974.

Title speaks for itself—an early work from a prolific laboratory studying ligament mechanics.

19. NOYES FR, TOVIK PJ, HYDE WB, DELUCAS JL: Biomechanics of ligament failure. II. An analysis of immobilization, exercise and reconditioning effects in primates. *J Bone Joint Surg* 56A:1406–1418, 1974.

This and the previous report established the modern understanding of the biomechanics of the bone–ligament–bone unit with the primate anterior cruciate as the model. Large bibliographies.

20. RECKER RR, ARMAS L: The effect of antiresorptives on bone quality. *Clin Orthop Relat Res* 469:2207–2214, 2011.

Provides overview of antiresorptive therapy in treating and preventing osteoporosis.

21. WAINWRIGHT SA, BIGGS WD, CURREY JD, GOSLINE JM: *Mechanical Design in Organisms*. John Wiley & Sons, New York, 1976.

A detailed account of how materials properties arise in tissues and how they are used in the "design" of bones, joints, wings, and so on.

22. WILKES GL, BROWN IA, WILDNAUER RH: The biomechanical properties of skin. *CRC Crit Rev Bioeng* 1(3):453–462, 1973.

Covers the structure and mechanical properties of skin with examples of the effect of test environment on properties.

23. YAMADA H: *Strength of Biological Materials*. Evans FG (ed). Williams & Wilkins, Baltimore, 1970.

An exhaustive collection of the mechanical properties of a broad range of animal and human tissues. A particularly good source of information on the change of properties with patient age and on bone-to-bone variation.

CHAPTER SIX

Polymers

The selection and use of implant materials involve important prospective decisions. Each material has specific combinations and ranges of chemical, mechanical, electrical, thermal, and biologic performance characteristics. Design requirements dictate materials choices; however, once materials choices are made, they strongly affect the design process in both positive and negative ways. If there were a single "best implant material," then all devices would be made from it. There is no such thing; to make all devices from the same material would be like asking a painter to work with only one color of paint. There are classes and groups of materials with similar properties, and within each group different choices may be made of composition and of processing techniques, to yield different combinations of final properties.

Design is a creative process of compromise. Suppose a designer begins to reduce an idea for a new configuration of cemented femoral total hip replacement component to an engineering design so that trial parts may be made. Key or critical design features are identified, such as the desire for the femoral stem to be able to sustain large reversing loads without fatigue failure. However, having done this, the designer cannot reach for his materials handbooks and specifications and select the material with the highest endurance limit. The same material must meet other requirements, such as single-cycle fracture strength, smoothness, corrosion resistance, and so on, and it must be able to be fabricated into the desired shape (Figure 6.1).

Thus, the design is refined by developing the shape of the stem in detail. This leads to calculation of the peak magnitude of the reversing stress that might be expected in the "average" 70 kg patient with an average lifestyle and in turn to specification of a minimum endurance limit, with a suitable safety factor, which is permissible if the stem material is to survive the expected fatigue stresses. All materials that meet this minimum are then candidates for use, and further steps in the design process result in choices being made between them on the basis of other criteria, until a clear final choice of material composition and processing emerges for the fabrication of the femoral stem.

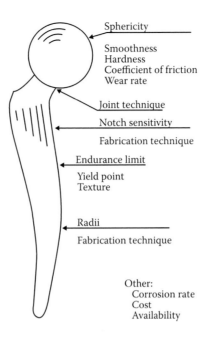

Sphericity

Smoothness
Hardness
Coefficient of friction
Wear rate

Joint technique

Notch sensitivity

Fabrication technique

Endurance limit

Yield point
Texture

Radii

Fabrication technique

Other:
Corrosion rate
Cost
Availability

FIGURE 6.1   Design requirements—proximal femoral component.

Design *is* a creative process and *is not* purely analytic. It is influenced by temporal, cultural, historical, ethical, aesthetic, and practical factors as well as by strict engineering considerations. Even in these engineering considerations, a great deal of uncertainty persists. Patients' anatomy and lifestyles are highly variable and, to a significant extent, unpredictable. Even for "standard" conditions, only the overall outlines of the mechanical, chemical, and biologic challenges are known. Designs must therefore be forgiving during both insertion and use. They have to provide wide ranges of component sizes, each with safety factors in the calculation of critical requirements, to assure acceptable results in a series of patients with defined indications treated with a relatively uniform surgical technique. (The design process, especially as it applies to development of new materials, is considered more fully in Chapter 15.)

For these reasons, enormous variety persists in the choice of materials and designs incorporating them. In femoral endoprosthetic components alone, more than a dozen materials and over a few hundred designs have been used, with many still in use, even without allowance for the complexity of modern modular designs. This is how it should be, since surgeons and designers together constantly strive for improvement in outcome and duration of good to excellent results. However, changes should not be made at random. The progress in total joint replacement over the last 50+ years is striking, with good to excellent 10+ year outcomes to be expected in 90%–95% of "typical" patients with total joint replacement arthroplasty who received proven designs. However, what is considered the expected outcome for patients has changed as well owing to the changing patient demographics, the obesity epidemic, and increase in activity levels of patients and their expectations. The drive to improve this record must be much more cautious than John Charnley's pioneering efforts were. Now, there is a solid foundation of experience and expectation, which is placed in hazard when material and design changes are made in pursuit of further improvement.

In particular, it must be emphasized that selection of materials is *not* analogous to choices among ice cream flavors. A proven design may acquire improved performance through a superior value of a key property of a new material. However, this material possesses a different combination of properties than the one previously used, and a simple change of materials will not produce an optimized design. A change of materials should be accompanied by a complete re-evaluation of the overall design and may result in a different final configuration. Therefore, changes of materials should always be regarded as significant and not be undertaken lightly.

We can place materials on a generic basis into four classes: metals, polymers, ceramics, and composites. These class distinctions are based both on external appearances and on related internal chemical composition and molecular structure differences. This chapter is the first of three that discuss the properties of present and emerging orthopaedic biomaterials with these classes as a central organizing feature.

Comparative properties

It is difficult to make many generalizations about the properties of each class of materials since exceptions may be cited to any such broad conclusion. This is particularly true of composite materials that, ab initio, are intended to have properties adjustable over wide ranges by control of internal details of design.

Table 6.1 Comparison of properties of materials by classes

Property	Highest[a]	Intermediate	Lowest
Tensile modulus (Y)	C	M	P
Yield strength (σ_y)	M	—	P[b]
Ultimate strength (σ_u)	C[c]	M	P
Strain to failure (ε_u)	P	M	C
Toughness	M	C	P
Hardness[d]	C	M	P
Resistance to *in vivo* attack	C	P	M
Local host response (bulk)	M	P	C
Systemic/remote response (degradation products)	M	P	C

[a] C, ceramics; M, metals; P, polymers.
[b] Ceramics do not have appreciable plastic properties at 37°C.
[c] Theoretical; practically metals, as a class, are superior.
[d] Strongly dependent on processing.

However, some general relations are a useful guide in thinking about choices between metals, polymers, and ceramics (including glasses, carbons, and other amorphous inorganic materials). These are summarized in Table 6.1.

Other engineering properties that affect the selection of materials by classes include wear rate, creep and stress relaxation rates, coefficient of friction, endurance limit, nature and biologic effects of degradation products, fabricability, appearance, availability, and cost.

General considerations concerning polymers

It is easy to picture a generic polymer: we think of polymers as "plastics." In this general view, polymers are relatively weak solid materials that soften as temperature increases. They are all around us, more and more so as new and improved polymers begin to displace metals (and ceramics, especially glasses) from traditional applications. Thus, the chrome steel automobile bumper is replaced by high-strength polymer body components, and the glass quart milk bottle gave way to the plastic gallon jug. Polymers also result in new products: compact audio discs, clear food wrap, Frisbees, and so on.

Polymers and polymer-based composites represent one of the most exciting areas of modern materials sciences. They combine moderate strength, low cost, and easy raw material availability with the ability to regulate physical properties by design of composition, internal structural arrangement, and processing. Furthermore, the ease with which they may be colored and joined, by adhesive and other processes, gives them an aesthetic flexibility lacking in more traditional materials.

Nowhere has the impact of modern polymeric materials been greater than in medicine, with the resulting wide use of polymeric disposable supplies, dressings, and sutures and the incorporation of polymers into medical devices and surgical instruments and implants. Many polymers are used in orthopaedics, and the use of just two materials, ultrahigh-molecular-weight poly(ethylene) (UHMWPE) and poly(methyl methacrylate) (PMMA), has radically transformed clinical practice by ushering in the era of successful long-term joint replacement.

Structure

Polymers are distinguished from metals and ceramics in that their structures (and therefore physical properties) are derived more directly from primary molecular features than from interatomic bonds. This molecular structure is characterized, in solid polymers, by high-molecular-weight linear chains or networks formed of identical or similar smaller repeating units.

The repeating structural unit within a polymer is called a *mer*. Polymers (literally "many mers") result from the combination of molecules called *monomers*. A monomer is a molecule containing one or more atoms that can each participate in *two* or more covalent bonds. The most familiar such atom is carbon; having four electrons in its outer shell, it can participate in *four* covalent bonds. Other candidate atoms include nitrogen, silicon, and sulfur.

The most common polymers, which are called *organic* polymers, are based on carbon. These polymers, containing primarily carbon, oxygen, hydrogen, and nitrogen, are so named because they were originally thought to be produced only by cells or organs, that is, by life processes. However, today, the vast majority of commercial organic polymers are produced synthetically from very simple starting compounds, primarily methane derived from mineral stores of hydrocarbons (compounds containing carbon, hydrogen, and oxygen such as petroleum oil, wax, natural gas, tar, etc.).

The monomers are assembled by formation of covalent bonds between these central atoms to form polymer chains. The nature of the single covalent bond is that it has a nearly fixed length (at any given temperature) but permits rotation of adjacent atoms about its axis. In addition, when an atom such as carbon forms multiple covalent bonds, the sizes of the angles between the bonds involving a particular atom are also fixed.

This combination of structural rules (fixed bond length, rotation about bond axes, and fixed interbond angles) has a major effect in determining the molecular structure of polymers. The generic polymer may be thought of as a very long string of beads, in which each bead represents a mer, but with the additional feature that the central string is rigid, jointed, and angulated instead of being limp. Interaction between the strings that is due to either mechanical interference or weak (van der Waals) and strong (covalent) bonding accounts for the rest of the structural features observed in polymers.

PROBLEM 6.1

How many mers does a poly(ethylene) (PE) molecule with a molecular weight of 2,000,000 contain and how long is it?

ANSWER:

The individual mer is derived from ethylene, containing two carbon atoms and four hydrogen atoms for a total molecular weight of 28. Thus, there are 2,000,000/28 or 71,429 mers in a molecule. The carbon-to-carbon distance is 1.54 Å (with two such bonds per mer); therefore, the molecule is $2 \times 1.54 \times 10^{-10} \times 71,428.5$ or 22 μm long. However, it tends to curl up into a sphere with a diameter between 0.015 and 0.8 μm, depending on the local physical conditions.

Polymerization

Polymer molecules obtain both their names and their structures from their monomeric components. Figure 6.2 gives the names and schematic structures of some common monomers and the resulting medical polymers containing them. Most monomers are gases or low-viscosity liquids. They must be polymerized to produce fluids and solid materials with useful engineering properties. As the number of mers increases, the chains become longer and the polymers generally have greater viscosities, strengths, and stiffnesses.

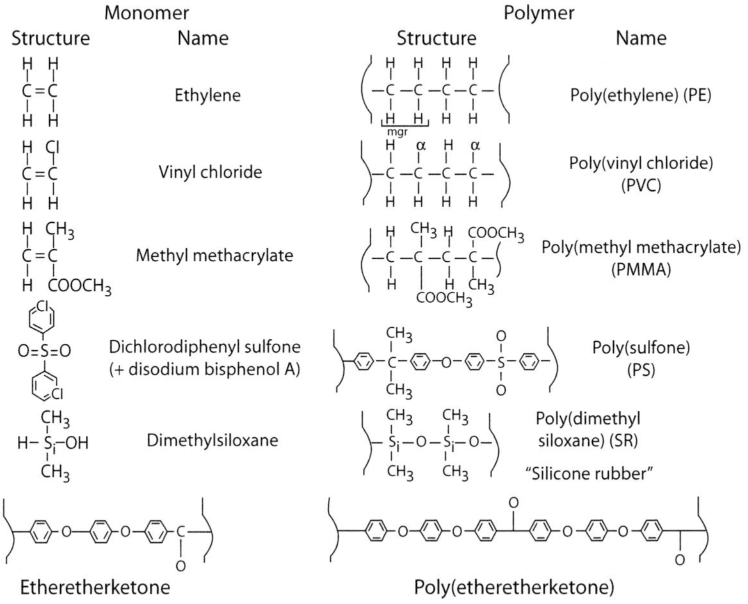

FIGURE 6.2 Monomers and polymers.

The polymers shown in Figure 6.2 all have applications in orthopaedics. PE at very high molecular weight is used in total joint replacements, whereas PMMA is the generic form of the major polymer in the familiar "bone cement." Poly(methyl siloxane) (SR) is used in the fabrication of one-piece proximal interphalangeal (PIP) and metacarpophalangeal (MCP) joint prostheses. Poly(sulfone) (PS) is a very stiff polymer that is an important candidate for fabrication of composites. Poly(vinyl chloride) (PVC) is commonly used in tubing for blood and fluid infusion sets.

Polymer fabrication

There are two distinct mechanisms of polymerization: chain growth (addition polymerization) and step growth (condensation polymerization). The choice of processes, and of variations within each process, depends on both the selection of monomers used and the final desired polymer properties.

Addition polymerization   Addition polymerization is usually used to produce molecules that are linear or simply branched. These polymers have physical properties that are strongly temperature dependent and are referred to as *thermoplastic* polymers or *thermoplastics*. (The distinction between thermoplastic and thermoset polymers is actually based on differences in mechanical properties, rather than on differences in formation processes.) As a rule, thermoplastics become more compliant and weaker with increasing temperature. Examples are PE, PMMA, PS, and PVC.

Formation of addition polymers begins with the interaction of an activator, such as the hydroxyl free radical (from hydrogen peroxide), with a monomer with an unsaturated bond, such as ethylene (Figure 6.3). This forms a new free radical that in turn can interact with another ethylene molecule, extending the chain. The process may be started by physically adding the activator to the monomer or by ionization in situ, by exposure to ultraviolet light, or by other energy input, and its rate may be increased by increasing the temperature of the reactants. This will happen naturally since polymerization, once initiated, is a spontaneous chemical reaction that liberates energy as heat. Polymerization continues until it is terminated by interaction with another free radical. Careful control of reaction conditions permits the formation of linear molecules with molecular weights exceeding 10^6.

Condensation polymerization   Condensation polymerization usually forms interlocking networks. After the initial reaction, which is often accelerated by a temperature increase, the physical properties of condensation polymers are relatively insensitive to temperature. Thus, they are referred to as *thermoset* polymers or *thermosets.* Examples include SR and epoxies.

Condensation is the reaction of dissimilar molecules with each other, resulting in the formation of a larger molecule (polymer) and an elimination product, frequently water. A typical reaction is the formation of poly(ethylene terephthalate), the familiar Dacron (DuPont, Wilmington, Delaware). Thus, in this case (Figure 6.3), an alcohol and a carboxylic acid combine to form a polyester and an eliminated water molecule. Reaction with additional alcohol and acid molecules can extend the chain, in each case with the production of a molecule of water for each ester mer added to the polymer chain. Initiation is usually caused by physically combining and heating the reactants, sometimes in the presence of inorganic catalysts, such as Grignard reagents. No chain termination is required; the reaction ceases when one of the reagents is consumed. As in the case of addition polymerization, a considerable amount of heat may be released.

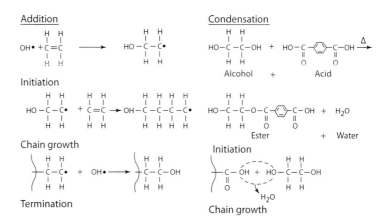

FIGURE 6.3   Polymerization processes.

Polymer structural terms

If a polymer is made from a single monomer, it is said to be *homogeneous* and referred to simply as a polymer. It is possible for there to be differences in structure in a homogeneous polymer. These may arise from branching and from asymmetry in the mer.

If the polymer has a single chain, with no branches, then it is called a *linear* polymer. If, however, there are side chains or branches, as is common in polymers formed by condensation, then it is called a *branched* or *nonlinear* polymer. In general, linear polymers possess higher density than nonlinear ones since the chains can pack more closely together.

If the mer is asymmetric and can be present in two different orientations, then there are three other possibilities for chain structure. Suppose we call the monomer "B" and the two possible orientations of the mer in the chain "b" and "p." Then, the three arrangements and their names are as follows (Figure 6.4):

-bbbbb- (or -ppppp-): *isotactic* (single orientation)

-bpbpbpb-: *syndiotactic* (alternating)

-bbpbpppbp-: *atactic* (random)

As expected, isotactic and syndiotactic molecules can pack more closely than atactic ones, thus forming higher-density solids.

Chain symmetry and the presence or absence of branching are very important in determining the macroscopic structure of polymers. Unbranched isotactic or syndiotactic polymers can form highly crystalline materials with properties that reflect their high density and internal regularity. More irregular polymers tend to form amorphous, lower-density materials with poorer mechanical properties. Most polymers are a mixture, with crystalline regions in an amorphous matrix (Figure 6.5). This aspect is described by the *degree of* or *percent crystallinity*: the proportion of the volume that is crystalline. Higher degrees of crystallinity are associated with increased strength, stiffness, and light transmission, but these are obtained at the expense of reduced toughness.

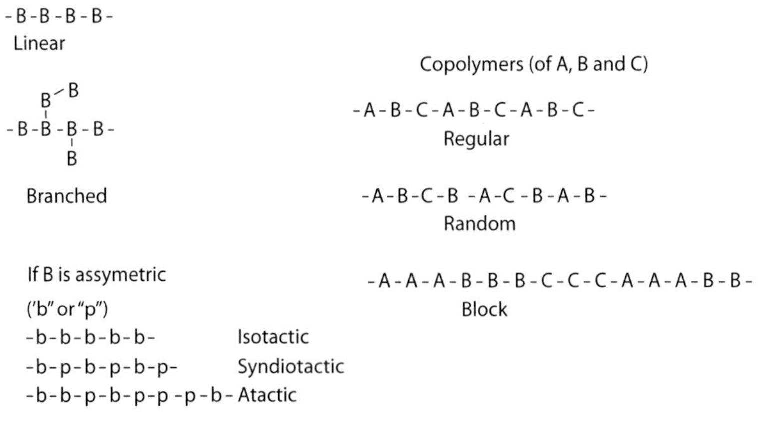

FIGURE 6.4 Polymer structures.

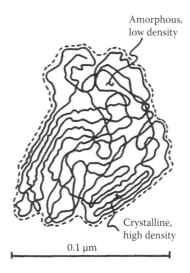

Amorphous,
low density

Crystalline,
high density

0.1 μm

FIGURE 6.5   Amorphous and crystalline regions in a polymer.

Thus, in a general sense, crystalline polymers are more brittle than amorphous ones.

Additionally, if two or more different monomers, let us call them "A," "B," and "C," are combined, the resulting material is called a *copolymer*. Coploymers in which the individual mers repeat in a fixed pattern, such as -ABCABCABCABC-, are called *regular* copolymers (Figure 6.4). Copolymers in which the repetition is irregular, such as -ABCBACBABCAB-, are called *random* copolymers. Another possibility is that the individual monomers are combined into homogeneous polymers that are themselves then polymerized, to produce a pattern such as -AAABBCCCAAABBCCC-. This is called a *block* copolymer and may itself be either regular or random. Copolymers also have the linearity and symmetry features of polymers but with a greater possible complexity.

PROBLEM 6.2

Show the structures of the following linear polymeric chains:

   A. Regular block copolymer with 40% AA, balance B

   B. Random copolymer with 40% A, balance B

   C. Regular block copolymer with 50% AAA, balance B

Which would have the higher crystallinity (assume symmetric A and B mers of the same weight)?

ANSWER:

   A. -AABBBAABBBAABBB-

   B. -AABABBBABBAAABBABBBB-

   C. -AAABBBAAABBBAAA-

If the structure in *C* is actually achieved, then it is easy to see how several of these chains might "fit together" better than those of *A* or *B*:

-AAABBBAAABBBAAA-

-BBBAAABBBAAABBB-

-AAABBBAAABBBAAA-

Thus, *C* would probably have a higher degree of crystallinity than the other two polymers.

Additional aspects of polymer composition and structure

These structural features of polymer molecules, by themselves, produce a great variety of possible materials. However, additional aspects further complicate the production and resultant properties of real polymeric materials. I will briefly summarize some of these topics here; a full treatment is beyond the scope of this work.

Molecular weight distribution. Either addition or condensation polymerization produces molecules with a wide distribution of molecular weights (reflecting different numbers of mers per molecule). It is possible to tailor these distributions, to make them broader or narrower, to assure a minimum or maximum molecular weight, and so on. Each of these choices affects both density and mechanical properties. In particular, low-molecular-weight molecules may act as plasticizers (see below).

Plasticization. Plasticizers are low-molecular-weight compounds that are added to polymers and act as internal lubricants, making relative molecular motion easier. These materials tend to increase elongation and toughness at the expense of reduced melting point, hardness, and ultimate tensile strength. Residual low-molecular-weight species may act as "self"-plasticizers. In implant applications, absorbed water and low-molecular-weight lipids also serve as plasticizers, particularly in hydrophilic and lipophilic low-density materials such as polyamides (Nylon; DuPont).

Other additives. Numerous agents are added to polymers to produce changes in color (colorants), increases in strength (reinforcing materials), resistance to attack by oxygen (antioxidants), easy removal from molds (mold release agents), and so on. These materials, added either deliberately or inadvertently, may be a source of adverse local tissue response. Manufacturers of polymers intended for medical applications routinely screen new compositions and individual production batches by *in vitro* techniques, usually cell culture, to prevent such problems from arising.

In general, polymers that have proven useful as biomaterials have few or no low-molecular-weight additives. The leaching of such additives may promote significant adverse local host responses. However, some additives have proven to be very beneficial. Of particular interest in orthopaedics, the antioxidant vitamin E may be added to UHMWPE, which in turn, reduces the effects of oxidative degradation after gamma irradiation for sterilization or cross-linking. Vitamin E can provide oxidation and wear resistance to UHMWPE by reacting with trapped free radicals in cell membranes and protecting polyunsaturated fatty acids from degradation owing to oxidation. There are currently two methods utilized to mix Vitamin E with UHWMPE. Vitamin E can be either blended with UHMWPE powder prior to consolidation and irradiation (with a side effect of impeding some cross-linking) or diffused into the UHMWPE after irradiation cross-linking.

Alloying. Different thermoplastics may be combined to produce materials with intermediate properties. This is a direct analogy to alloying of metals (see Chapter 7), but the mixture is mechanical and reflects a random mixture of molecules or of regions of fixed composition rather than the atomic mixtures found in metal alloys. Polymer alloys are frequently called composite polymers, but this term is better reserved for true composites in which a defined solid phase or phases (reinforcing materials) and a continuous matrix are combined.

Polymer processing

The first step in the preparation of polymeric materials is the production of the fundamental polymer compound. Initial chemical processing is usually called *compounding* and results in a material called a *resin* (Figure 6.6). It may be manufactured in a powdered or pellet form, or in the case of thermoset polymers, in blocks, sheets, rods, and, that may be additionally formed by conventional machining processes. Most solid polymers can be shaped and formed in the same way as metals, using lathes, grinders, shapers, and so on. However, care must be taken to keep the materials cool, and in general, amorphous materials are more difficult to machine than crystalline ones.

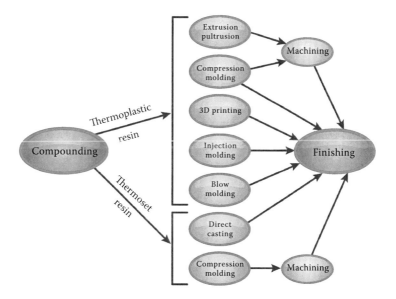

FIGURE 6.6   (See color insert.) Processing of polymers.

There are a variety of special processes used to fabricate polymeric parts and devices that take advantage of basic resin properties.

Molding. Polymers may be machined, as indicated above, but there is a general difficulty in maintaining tolerances and producing smooth surfaces. Thus, molding is a very popular way of producing either partially or fully finished parts. There are several variations of the generic process.

Injection molding (also called *die casting*). Thermoplastic resins are melted and heated to slightly higher temperatures (to reduce their viscosity) and then forced into closed water-cooled molds. Molds are usually made from metal alloys, but the low melting point of some resins permits them to be cast in molds made from high-melting-point polymers. The resin must possess a reasonably low viscosity to permit mold filling, so this technique is not easily applicable to high-molecular-weight polymers. A version of this method, called *reaction in mold* or *RIM* molding, uses components of thermoset resins combined and immediately injected into molds. This technique is especially well suited for making porous polymers, such as sponges, with the pores produced by the addition of a volatile material called a blowing agent.

Compression molding. Precise amounts of finely powdered thermoplastic (or some thermoset) resins are introduced into a split heated mold. The mold is closed, and a combination of heat and pressure produces the finished part.

Blow molding. Preformed sheets of thermoplastic resin are placed in a closed heated mold and formed to shape by air pressure. This technique is well adapted to making bottles and other containers. The material may be drawn into the mold by a vacuum on the other side; then, the process is called *vacuum forming*.

3D printing. During prototyping, it is often desirable to quickly create a 3D form of an object in either very small batches or on its own. 3D printing can create a solid part of any object from just a digital model, and without the traditional sourcing and design effort required of other fabrication techniques. Printing is typically carried out using an additive manufacturing process that will deposit liquid or powder material onto a substrate in successive layers, until a full object is hardened and rendered. The use of 3D printing has continued to accelerate as the equipment continues to become less expensive. Beyond traditional prototyping utility, there is some interest in utilizing 3D printing for custom implants, potentially on site at the point of care.

Other fabrication techniques include the following:

Direct casting. Parts are fabricated in open molds from either molten thermoplastic resin or freshly compounded and unreacted thermoset resin. A variant of this process is to dissolve the polymer resin in a suitable solvent, pour it into the mold, and then drive the solvent off in a vacuum or by heating.

Extrusion. Thermoplastic resins are heated to just above their melting point and then forced through small apertures. This aligns the molecules in high-molecular-weight resins and produces rods with good tensile and bending properties. The rod or bar may be forcibly stretched as it exits from the aperture. This further orients long-chain molecules and is called *pultrusion.* A variant of this process is used to form thermoset fibers when one primary chemical reactant (of a thermoset polymer) is sufficiently viscous to permit extrusion. Then, this reactant is extruded into a bath containing other reactants, and a continuous fiber may be formed and reeled up.

Cross-linking. After fabrication of a part, it may be necessary to change its surface properties, especially to provide increased wear resistance. This can be done by exposing the part to ionizing radiation in the presence of a cross-linking agent, such as acetylene. The radiation disrupts covalent bonds and forms free radicals which will may react and form a crosslink. The net result is to produce an increased density of covalent intermolecular bonds. This process may be applied to both thermoplastic and thermoset polymers. Cross-linking in polyethylene is discussed in detail in the sections below. This should not be confused with radiation sterilization, in which doses, although high enough to kill microorganisms and disrupt viruses, are not high enough to produce significant cross-linking.

Each of these fabrication processes directly affects the orientation and local arrangement of the polymer molecules. In addition, for some polymers, molecular weight distributions may be altered by processing. Thus, the *composition, molecular weight distribution, additives,* and *processing* must be known if the behavior of a fabricated polymer is to be predicted accurately.

Finishing

After completion of the physical shape of a polymer part, there are additional finishing steps that may be required for functional and cosmetic reasons. These include polishing, cleaning, sterilization, and packaging. These steps are required for polymers particularly because of their relative fragility and ability to "pick up" (adsorb or absorb) foreign materials combined with the known degradative consequences of autoclaving. Polymer parts and implants should *never* be autoclaved unless package instructions specifically permit this practice. Most such parts are radiation sterilized (cobalt gamma) after hermetic packaging. Many polymeric materials may be gas (ethylene oxide) or solution (formalin, etc.) sterilized; however, this should also only be done if specifically permitted by package instructions since some polymers are damaged by one or the other or both treatments.

Mechanical properties of polymers

All polymers are viscoelastic to some degree, resulting from the combination of strong covalent "backbone" bonds and relatively weak intermolecular bonds. However, the engineering literature is relatively poor in describing these properties, probably because the general inferiority of mechanical behavior (with respect to metals) generally relegates polymers to low-stress, low-strain-rate applications. Thus, it should be understood that, in this discussion, "modulus" means the modulus obtained by engineering tests at a typical laboratory strain rate, say between 0.1 and 1.0 mm s⁻¹, at 25°C. Thus, these moduli are typically between the true relaxed and unrelaxed values.

Figure 6.7 shows the family of stress–strain curves for a typical polymer of low crystallinity. As for other viscoelastic materials, the initial slope of the stress–strain curve ("modulus") increases with increasing strain rate. Note also the effect of temperature.

Small deformations of polymers produce deformation and failure of weak intermolecular bonds and are frequently recoverable. Larger deformations produce uncoiling of the polymer chains, elongation, and failure of covalent cross-link and backbone bonds and thus are more likely to be irreversible. Thus, it is also possible, at any given temperature, to define an engineering value of "yield" stress. This has the same difficulty as the previously described "modulus," since it is both strain rate and temperature dependent. Most such values are determined under the conditions previously cited for "modulus."

The mechanical behavior of polymers has a very strong dependence on temperature. In Figure 6.8 we can see this, again for a generic polymer with a variety of crystallinities. The middle curve, which is the most characteristic, is for a material with 50% crystallinity, such as that previously seen represented by the stress–strain curves in Figure 6.7.

There are four regions in the "modulus" versus temperature curves shown in Figure 6.8:

Glassy. Below a specific temperature, T_G, called the *glass transition temperature* (or *point*), both crystalline and amorphous polymers are rigid and brittle, much like metals and ceramics.

Leathery. As the temperature rises above T_G, the "modulus" drops very significantly (note that the vertical scale is a logarithmic one) and deformations are slowly recoverable.

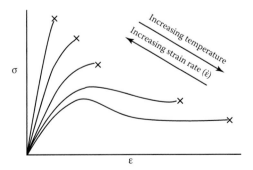

FIGURE 6.7   Typical stress–strain curves for a polymer.

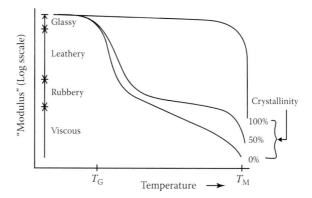

FIGURE 6.8 Temperature dependence of polymer "modulus."

Rubbery. At slightly higher temperatures, there is a transition to a more elastic or rubbery behavior, with rapid recovery of deformation. Polymers that have a long rubbery range with little temperature dependence of modulus in this region (horizontal rubbery "plateau") are called "elastomers" and are commonly known as "rubbers."

Viscous. Finally, near the melting point, T_M, the modulus again drops very rapidly and the polymer behaves like a very viscous fluid. Unlike ionic compounds and metals, polymers do not have an abrupt melting point; T_M is defined as the temperature at which the polymer flows (creeps irreversibly) under the force of gravity (as determined in a defined test procedure).

Note that as crystallinity increases, the rubbery region increases and the leathery region decreases until finally, at full crystallinity, the polymer behaves as an elastic, brittle solid up to temperatures near the T_M.

Cross-linking produces effects parallel to those of increasing crystallinity, except that the values of mechanical constants may be different, since large elongations of cross-linked materials may produce bond failure. The addition of reinforcing agents (fillers, etc.) also simulates the effect of increasing crystallinity. However, plasticizers produce a more amorphous behavior for a given degree of crystallinity.

Strength is much more difficult to predict, but in general, it decreases with increasing temperature in much the same way as modulus, whereas elongation increases.

Engineering properties of polymers

Primary properties   Table 6.2 provides some engineering properties of typical biomedical polymers used in orthopaedic applications. Unlike metals and ceramics, the composition and structure of polymers are poorly controlled. That is, a high-molecular-weight PE (molecular weight 5×10^5) from

Table 6.2   Primary engineering properties of polymers

Polymer	Density (g/cm^3)	Tensile "modulus" (GPa)	Tensile "ultimate strength" (MPa)	Maximum tensile elongation (%)	Glass transition temperature (°C)	Melting temperature (°C)
PE[a]°						
HD	0.94–0.97	1.05–1.09	22–31	10–120	−110	135
UHMW	0.93–0.95	0.94–1.05	39	420–525		
PMMA (in situ)	1.17–1.20	1.6–2.6	25–48 70[b]	5–10	105	Amorphous
PS	0.92	2.0–2.5	100	50–100	90–100	Amorphous
PVC						
Flexible	1.19–1.28	0.02–0.05	16–28	170–400	−40	Amorphous
Rigid	1.35–1.55	0.015	15–40	2–30	80–90	Amorphous
SR	1.34	0.004	10–12	700–800	−105	Amorphous
PEEK	1.23–1.84	2.70–138	51.0–2070	0.3–150	145	335
PLLA	1.2–1.4	8.50	900	25	56	170

[a] HD, high density; UHMW = 2×10^6 molecular weight.
[b] Minimum compressive strength.

one manufacturer may have values of mechanical properties significantly different from that from another manufacturer. Specifications for these materials tend to be methods to describe their composition and properties rather than discrete compositions that will lead to specific properties. Thus, the bioengineering literature refers routinely to these materials by their specific manufacturer's grade and composition designation. Even this is no assurance of uniformity of properties: resin compounders routinely make minor changes in their grade compositions and processing from time to time, without changing the grade designation. In addition, there are no medical grades of most polymers, since the rate of use in medical devices is almost always below the minimum required for commercial production of a specific grade: 5,000,000 lb/year. For this reason, many medical device manufacturers compound their own primary resins, especially of low-volume polymers.

PROBLEM 6.3

Rank UHMWPE, PMMA, cortical bone (CRB), and cancellous bone (CNB) in *increasing* order of

A. Stiffness (modulus)

B. Strength (ultimate)

ANSWER:

(Refer to Figure 5.12, and assume that CRB has a density of 2 g/cm^3 and CNB has a density of 0.3 g/cm^3)

Stiffness: CNB, UHMWPE, PMMA, CRB

Strength: CNB, PMMA, UHMWPE, CRB

Other mechanical properties

Polymers, as a group, have relatively low strength and low hardness are soft so that some specialized tests have been developed to permit accurate characterization. Some of these tests are related to intermediate properties during production, such as characterization of the original resin after compounding. Several of these tests and their resulting parameters are briefly described below.

Creep. Creep is clearly an important parameter, and creep tests are routinely reported for engineering polymers. The most important parameter is the creep modulus, which is the ratio of stress to strain (in compression) after 1000 h under a standard load (usually 1000 psi). The creep rupture strength is also frequently reported as a measure of resistance to creep failure and is the maximum tensile stress that can be sustained without fracture for a fixed time, usually 1000 h. Both the creep modulus and the creep rupture strength are temperature dependent; unfortunately, values at 37°C are rarely available.

Tear strength. Polymers are quite notch sensitive, since notches involve breaks in the covalent backbones of their constituent molecules. Some are sufficiently brittle that they may be broken and the area under the stress–strain curve is integrated to produce a work or energy of fracture as a measure of toughness. However, most are sufficiently ductile that this is not possible. For these materials, a tear test is utilized: a standard tensile specimen is produced with a sharp-rooted slit perpendicular to the direction of tensile test. It is then loaded until the crack propagates and a catastrophic failure occurs. The peak stress is reported as a tear strength and is typically between one-tenth and one-half of the tensile strength.

Shore durometer. Polymers are generally soft and, being viscoelastic, have time-dependent moduli. A quick way to determine an effective modulus is with the Shore durometer. This is a device analogous to the Rockwell or Brinell hardness tester but operating under a different principle. The durometer is a small portable instrument with a spring-loaded piton and an indicator dial. The piton is pressed against the surface of the polymer, and the dial indicates the penetration resistance, which is proportional to some short-time, near to unrelaxed, modulus. The value is reported on the Shore scale as a Shore durometer (number); increasing numbers represent higher values of modulus.

Small Punch Test. It is often necessary to characterize materials when only a small amount of material is available for testing. Examples where this scenario may arise are during the evaluation of retrieved implant components, or when localized differences are of interest in inhomogeneous materials. The small punch test is a useful technique that can address this problem when determining the ductility and fracture resistance of a material. Small punch testing uses a die and guide system to constrain small disc-shaped samples before subjecting the samples to a bending-by-indentation load (constant displacement) until the failure of the material. Typically, a load–displacement curve is determined during the test, from which the modulus of elasticity, ultimate load, ultimate displacement, and work-to-failure can be derived. Although this method is actually a shear test, tensile properties can be obtained by calculation.

Bone cements

The so-called bone cements (BCs) are derived from PMMA materials that had long been used in dental applications, primarily for construction and repair of dentures. Sir John Charnley is generally credited with the first significant use of this material for the support of medullary portions of total hip replacements, beginning in 1958, although there is a long history of applications in general surgery and, dating back into the 1940s, in orthopaedic surgery. Despite many small changes in the material itself and in its use, it remains essentially the same as that used by Charnley, except for the introduction of barium sulfate ($BaSO_4$) to render it radiopaque.

The original role intended for BCs was as a "lute": as a space-filling material that could be interposed between a metal prosthetic stem and bone to distribute the stress, thus preventing the local stress concentration and bony necrosis attendant to early, noncemented device designs. A second goal was to reduce pain by stabilizing, that is, by "fixing," the prosthesis relative to bone. PMMA was not intended to be adhesive and is not; thus, the continued shorthand term *bone cement* is a misnomer. Other, truly adhesive materials have been used experimentally in this application; they are discussed elsewhere in the consideration of fixation (see Chapter 11).

There are a number of commercial BCs, all based on PMMA. Although they differ slightly in composition and properties, it is possible to speak of them in a generic way. There is no convincing evidence that these differences, although in some cases requiring alterations of surgical technique, produce differences in surgical outcome. The resultant material is a dull, opaque pink or white mass. Although (except for fillers) it is chemically identical to the familiar clear Plexiglas (Rohm & Haas, Philadelphia, Pennsylvania) or Lucite (DuPont Co, Wilmington, Delaware), its opacity is due to filler and air inclusions and to a relatively low crystallinity. Typical molecular weights are 1×10^5 to 5×10^5.

The typical PMMA BC is supplied in a sterilized two-part kit, generally containing a 40 g container of a dry component and a 20 ml vial of a liquid component. The dry component is usually 10 weight percent (w/o) $BaSO_4$ with the balance consisting of a fully polymerized microspheric (10–30 μm) powder of PMMA or PMMA-poly(styrene) copolymer. This component also contains a very small quantity of a free-radical source (to be acted on by the initiator in the liquid component); the most common is benzoyl peroxide. The liquid is methyl methacrylate monomer (MMA) (≥97 w/o) with an initiator (typically *N,N*-dimethyl-*p*-toluidine) and one or more stabilizers to prevent premature polymerization. The powder is usually sterilized by cobalt gamma irradiation, whereas the liquid is sterilized by ultrafiltration. Some BCs contain an antibiotic, in dry form. This is most typically gentamicin, supplied at 5–10 w/o in the dry component. In some BCs, the size distribution of the dry component is carefully controlled to produce a lower viscosity during the early stages of polymerization.

When the components are combined, an addition polymerization process ("curing") is initiated that produces long-chain polymers that interpenetrate the previously polymerized microspheres and bind them together into a single mass. There is also a significant amount of dissolution of low-molecular-weight species (from the dry microspheric powder) and incorporation of them by polymerization. Nonetheless, the interface between the microspheres and their new matrix remains and is relatively weak; breaking BC after full curing shows microspheres and their impressions on the resultant fracture surface. It is also of interest to note that the newly formed polymer chains are essentially linear. In addition, there is an almost total absence of cross-linking, either in the initial powder or in the final compact.

BCs are designed to cure with essentially no change in volume, so that prosthetic stems may be bedded in them without subsequent loosening owing to dimension changes. In fact, BCs shrink modestly, perhaps 0.5–1.0 volume percent (v/o) during curing, and then gradually expand by perhaps 1–2 v/o over the first 30 days *in vivo* owing to water and lipid absorption. The shrinkage is partially offset by transient thermal expansion owing to heating during curing but is increased by the presence of internal porosity.

Internal porosity in BCs has been a subject of some interest. When the material is mixed traditionally, with a spatula in an open mixing bowl in the operating room, the result will be 1–10 v/o porosity, depending on technique and experience. Moderate mixing speeds with care taken not to stir air into the cement mass seem to produce the lowest porosity. Various treatments have been suggested, including centrifugation during the early stages of curing and vacuum degassing of the dry component before mixing, to improve this situation. These methods greatly reduce resultant porosity and produce modest increases in ultimate tensile strength and possibly in fatigue life of BCs. However, there is also laboratory evidence that these treatments increase initial shrinkage by 1–3 v/o. Although porosity reduction seems a "good thing" on theoretical grounds, there is as yet no clear evidence of a clinical benefit. Furthermore, with the addition of antibiotic powders in the BC, questions have also been raised about the porosity of the BC after drug elution, as well as changes in the mechanical properties before and after leaching of the antibiotics. Pores and cracks within the BC have been reported after the elution of the antibiotics, although this may be primarily a surface phenomenon. Increasing amounts of antibiotic powder has been shown to cause gradual decreases in the compressive, tensile, and flexural strengths. However, leaching of just water does not appear to have the same effect, indicating that the degradation of mechanical properties may be dependent on the concentration of the antibiotic powder in the BC.

Curing is "triggered" by combining the dry and liquid parts of a BC kit. The resultant process has three characteristic times associated with it (Figure 6.9).

> *Dough time.* This is the time point at which, with moderate mixing, the BC will not stick to unpowdered surgical gloves. Under typical conditions (23°C–25°C, 65% relative humidity), this is 2–3 min after beginning of mixing for most BCs. Before this time point, after the components are well mixed, the BC may be loaded into a syringe or pressure gun for assisted application.

> *Setting time.* This is the time point, measured again from the beginning of mixing, when the surface temperature of the dough mass reaches one-half of its maximum value. Setting time is typically 8–10 min. The temperature increase is due to conversion of chemical to thermal energy as polymerization takes place. This produces 12–14 kcal/100 g of typical BCs. This is produced throughout the mass of the cement and then must diffuse to the outside surface. Thus, the surface temperature reached increases with the volume of the BC mass. Large balls, of 50–60 g, may reach surface temperatures of 70°C–80°C; however, *in vivo*, with the mass of the prosthetic stem to absorb heat and the heat capacity and cooling effect of circulation in the surrounding bone tissues, bone–BC interface temperatures in typical applications (cement thickness <5 mm) probably do not exceed 39°C–42°C and reach this level only for brief periods.

> *Working time.* This is the difference between setting and dough times, typically 5–8 min. Previously, this represented the full time interval available for use of a particular mix of BC. The use of mechanical introduction tools, such as syringes, and so on, extends this time by 1–1.5 min.

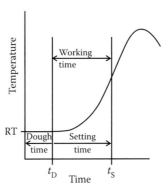

FIGURE 6.9   Phases of PMMA polymerization.

BCs are poorly adhesive to most surfaces and to themselves, especially as time after dough time increases. Thus, during the post-dough-setting period, BC should be worked and used in a single solid mass. If there is a desire to make it adhere to itself, care must be taken to assure that the interface is clean and dry, since blood, among other things, will completely prevent adhesion. Even with these precautions, BCs adhere very poorly to "old" BC, as encountered during arthroplasty revision, so that considerable attention should be given to complete removal of old BC. BCs will not adhere to metal surfaces, even when they are dry, to any great extent. If such adhesion is required, "precoat" devices should be used. These are devices in which a mantle of BC has been coupled to the metal substrate with a chemical agent, most commonly a silicon-containing compound called a silane. However, for BC to adhere even to such devices, the interface must be clean and dry. The earlier during the working period that such bonds are attempted, the greater will be their resultant strength.

The kinetics of BC curing are dictated by the chemistry and proportions of the system. These have been selected to optimize the performance of any particular BC. If smaller quantities than provided by a full kit are required, then it is better to try to get smaller packages (supplied by some manufacturers) than to try to divide the dry and liquid ingredients, which may alter the reactant ratios.

However, there are three factors that affect dough, setting, and working times:

Too rapid mixing can accelerate dough time and is not desirable, since it may produce a weaker, more porous BC.

Increased temperature reduces both dough and setting times approximately 5%/°C, whereas decreased temperature increases them at essentially the same rate.

Humidity seems to have an effect on setting time (and thus on the available working interval); high humidity accelerates setting, whereas low humidity retards it.

The combination of these factors is such that in a cold operating room on a very dry winter day, setting time may stretch out to 15–16 min and arouse concerns as to whether there is something wrong with the BC kit in use. There usually is not, but patience is required to use BC under these conditions. Water (or anything else) should never be added to BC in an attempt to modify its curing behavior. If antibiotic-impregnated BC is desired, as in revision of infected arthroplasties, commercial pre-mixes are very much preferred. If these are not available, antibiotic additions should always be in dry form, before addition of the liquid MMA, and should not exceed 10 w/o of the dry component of BC. Such an addition produces modest increases in setting and working times.

Care and technical skill are required for routine, successful use of BCs with the highest obtainable strength. Although it is hard to relate BC strength (either single-cycle or fatigue tensile strength) to clinical behavior except in cases of poor insertion technique, reason suggests the

Table 6.3   Factors in optimizing BC strength

Factors	Outcome
Uncontrollable factors	
Aging	Gradual 10% loss of strength resulting from postcuring chemical changes
Environmental temperature	10% weaker at body temperature than at room temperature
Fatigue	Fatigue strength (10^6 cycles) 20%–25% of single-cycle strength
Moisture content	Loss of 3%–10% strength owing to water absorption
Strain rate	Significant increase in strength with increasing strain rate
Partially controllable factors	
Cement thickness	Important; "intermediate" BC thicknesses minimize both fatigue stresses and shrinkage effects
Constraint	Significant; BCs far stronger in compression than tension
Inclusion of blood or tissue	Considerable effect; up to 70% loss of strength, depending on amount
Stress risers (bony bed, prosthesis)	Significant; BCs are quite notch sensitive
Fully controllable factors	
Antibiotic inclusion	5%–10% loss of strength
Centrifugation/vacuum degassing	10%–25% increase in strength, possible increase in fatigue strength
Insertion	Delay may produce up to 40% loss of strength, whereas pressurization increases strength by up to 20% by reduction of porosity
Mixing speed	Up to 21% loss of strength owing to too slow or too rapid mixing
Radiopaque fillers	5% weaker than unfilled

Note: "strength" and "fatigue strength" are in tension; behavior in compression is different and less sensitive to external conditions.

desirability of maximizing strength. The factors that contribute to BC strength optimization may be grouped into three classes: those beyond the control of the surgeon, those partially controlled by the surgeon, and those fully controlled by the surgeon. These are summarized in Table 6.3.

Despite considerable concern over the behavior of BCs *in vivo*, particularly in younger, high-demand patients, the clinical results of series with attention to cementation technique are excellent. The clinical performance of BCs in comparison with other fixation techniques will be considered in Chapter 13. However, it is safe to say that BCs will continue in wide and successful clinical use for the foreseeable future.

Poly(ethylene)

Just as the use of PMMA BCs has markedly reduced loosening and pain previously associated with total joint replacements, the introduction of high-performance polymers to replace metal–metal wear pairs with metal–polymer ones has led to markedly lower wear, and presumably has reduced the risk of both local and systemic adverse response to metal implants involving articulating interfaces.

The goal of an articulating polymer is to accomplish a material that has sufficient wear, oxidation, and fatigue resistance. Charnley originally noted the need for good friction and wear behavior in such interfaces; he called his original total hip replacement procedure "low friction arthroplasty" or LFA. The original polymer selected for this application was a poly(fluoroethylene) similar but not identical in composition and structure to modern materials. These polymers, as a group, are "slippery" and possess very low surface tensions. Thus, they appear ideal for bearing applications and are used widely in industrial and consumer product applications. However, relatively rapid wear and, more importantly, an aggressive foreign body response to the wear debris have rendered them unusable in implant applications in which wear phenomena are possible.

After the initial failure of a poly(fluoroethylene) material, Charnley then turned to PE, initially using a commercial high-molecular-weight polymer. PE was originally made by an oxygen-catalyzed addition polymerization of ethylene at high pressure and temperature, yielding an amorphous branched polymer with an average molecular weight between 300,000 and 500,000 and a relatively wide range of molecular weights. The material that was originally used in acetabular cups was a high-density polymer. This is made at relatively low pressures with metallic catalysts and, although having a similar average molecular weight and range, is highly crystalline, owing to the linearity of the polymeric molecules. However, it is mechanically inferior to the more modern UHMWPE material. This is made by extending the low-pressure process until molecular weights of 1×10^6 to 10×10^6 are reached. This produces a less dense (0.94 rather than 0.95–0.965 g/cm³) material that is extremely tough and ductile. To date, it has proven to be the best polymer for load-bearing applications in metal–polymer wear pairs, whether *in vitro* or *in vivo*. Resins for medical applications are selected by average molecular weight and weight range and by the absence of contaminating particles in a particular lot. Requirements for Medical-grade UHMWPE powders are defined in standards ASTM 648 and ISO 5834-1.

Wear properties have improved greatly since the introduction of highly cross-linked UHMWPE into acetabular bearings in the late 1990s. Cross-linking occurs in a polymer when at least two polymer chains are linked through covalent bonds. In arthroplasty applications, this will have the effect of decreasing the amount of plastic deformation on the polymer surface during articulation and will ultimately lead to less wear of the bearing. Cross-linking is implemented through chemical or radiochemical reactions and can be initiated by exposing a polymer to ionizing radiation. Irradiation cleaves the C–H and C–C bonds, forming free radicals as a by-product. Some of these free radicals can eventually recombine to form cross-links via H-linkages or long-chain branches (Y-linkages). This effect is concentrated primarily in the amorphous phases of the polymer. Recrystallization of radiation cross-linked results in a polymer with lower crystallinity compared to virgin UHMWPE, increasing the compliance of the polymer. Wear rates have been shown to decrease with radiation doses up to 100 kGy, after which the beneficial effects taper off.

Although beneficial from the perspective of wear resistance, cross-linking also reduces molecular mobility and ductility and, as a result, leaves the material with an overall reduced fatigue and fracture resistance. This is due to a reduction in chain mobility and stretch. Further, not all free radicals are sufficiently mobile to recombine into cross-links, and many end up trapped within the crystalline regions of the material. These residual free radicals may eventually react with oxygen and form unstable hydroperoxides, which will successively decay, and lead to embrittlement of the material via chain scission and recrystallization. Thermal treatment of irradiated UHMWPE may be employed to increase oxidation resistance, accomplished through either melting or annealing the material below the melt point. Heating the polymer to above its melting point can reduce crystallinity and provide enough energy for the trapped free radicals to recombine with one another. Melting also has the side effect of reducing the stiffness and fatigue strength of the material, a result of the reduction in polymer crystallinity.

Highly cross-linked and thermally treated UHMWPE is now widely accepted as the preferential form for THA. Since the introduction of first-generation, highly cross-linked implants, clinical performance is considered generally successful, though there have been a small number of reports of rim fractures on some of the thinner liners implanted at high abduction angles. On the other hand, highly cross-linked UHMWPE is currently less used in the knee owing to the inherent reduction in ductility and fracture resistance associated with the irradiation necessary to initiate the cross-links, along with questions pertaining to its clinical necessity in this application.

Currently, there are three main options for sterilization of UHMWPE, including gamma sterilization in barrier packaging, ethylene oxide gas sterilization, or gas plasma sterilization. Gamma sterilization was a controversial topic in the '90s because of findings showing that gamma sterilization in air, when followed by extended shelf storage, increased the risk for oxidation (including an increase in density and crystallinity of the material) and mechanical degradation of UHMWPE owing to the material becoming more brittle through the chemical reactions. Barrier packaging has the ability to minimize oxidative degradation during storage by limiting the access of oxygen to the polymer. The *in vivo* performance of UHMWPE sterilized with barrier packaging still remains poorly understood, though limited data suggest that oxidation may be limited for 5 to 10 years. One advantage gamma sterilization has over gas sterilization is that radiation-induced cross-linking is a by-product of gamma irradiation and can increase the tribological (wear) performance of the material. Ethylene oxide and gas plasma sterilization, on the other hand, generate no free radicals that may subsequently oxidize during shelf storage. Gas methods are currently considered the methods of choice for highly cross-linked UHMWPE materials. Gas plasma, especially, is attractive as it does not leave toxic residues or incorporate by-products that are environmentally hazardous

Despite its superior mechanical performance, UHMWPE is not a perfect material. It can absorb small amounts (<0.1 v/o) of fluids, as can be seen through the discoloration of components retrieved from infected sites. It is subject to fatigue failure and displays a tendency to creep for long-term applications, though this is reduced in its highly cross-linked form. UHMWPE is very hard to injection mold because of its high molecular weight and resulting high molten viscosity. It is for this reason that today UHMWPE is most commonly consolidated via compression molding or ram extrusion techniques. It is also difficult to machine because of its creep properties, though this is mitigated through optimization of the feed rate, cutting force, and spindle speed of the cutting tool, parameters that are often guarded as proprietary.

Silicone rubber

Silicones are differentiated from organic polymers by the configuration of their main chains. Organic molecules have covalently bonded, primarily carbon, main chains: $-C-C-C-C-$. Silicones, on the other hand, possess covalent backbones with alternating oxygen and silicon atoms: $-Si-O-Si-O-Si-$. Since each silicon atom, like carbon, can participate in two additional covalent bonds, side groups and cross-links can be attached at the silicon sites.

Silicones originate from silicon oxide (SiO_2) and are generally produced through organochlorosilanes. Depending on the number and nature of side chains and cross-links and on the average molecular weight, the resulting materials may be liquid or solid, rubbery, or brittle. Many fillers, especially SiO_2, are routinely used. They may be produced as thermoplastics or as two-part thermoset materials.

Rubbery silicones, incorrectly called silastics ("Silastic" is a trademark of Dow Corning Co., Midland, Michigan), have been widely used in implants in which large recoverable deformations at low stress are desired. Thus, they have wide applicability in cosmetic and reconstructive plastic surgery. Orthopaedic applications include use in stents to encourage reformation of tendon sheaths and in replacements for the wrist, PIP, and MCP joints. Additional, less frequent applications include "bone capping" and use as elastic bumpers, to cushion device parts at the end of the range of motion, in a number of total knee replacements.

Although improving, the poor abrasion resistance of silicone rubbers prevents their use in weight-bearing applications, either as a member of a prosthetic wear pair or against tissue. This deficiency has also produced premature failure where bony margins can abrade silicone rubber devices. However, the use of modern device designs that incorporate sheaths to separate the silicone from the surrounding bone and the development of materials with higher tear (and thus abrasion) resistance have greatly reduced this problem. The low tensile strength of silicone rubbers also prevents their use in ligament and tendon prosthetic applications, although they have been used as components in some experimental composite designs.

Silicones are modestly lipophilic, and there has been some concern that lipid absorption might degrade the properties of silicone rubber implants, as was the case with early silicone rubber heart valve poppets (balls). Although evidence for such absorption has been found, there is no convincing evidence that it has contributed to device failure.

Commercial silicones routinely use initiators containing toxic metals such as lead and tin. As a result, all silicones used in biomedical applications must be custom compounded to assure purity and nontoxicity; all of these materials are, de facto, medical grades.

PEEK

Polyarlyetheretherketone (PEEK) is a biocompatible polymer that has generated interest in orthopaedic, trauma, and, particularly, spinal applications. PEEK is associated with few toxic, inflammatory, or allergic reactions, and there is no expected cytotoxicity, mutagenicity, or immunogenicity. It also has a very high chemical resistance, being insoluble in common solvents and is resistant to attack by all substances except sulpheric acid.

The turning point with the use of PEEK for medical applications is captured within its stiffness and strength properties. PEEK is often used to capitalize on its "isoelastic" potential, creating implants with stiffness close to matching that of bone and potentially reducing adverse effects of stress shielding. While unmodified PEEK has a flexural modulus of only 4 GPa and a strength of 93 MPa, its stiffness and strength can be modified through annealing and carbon fiber–reinforced (CFR) filling, hydroxyapetite (HA) filling, and HA coating. Although there are many variations to CRF PEEK, and alterations to mechanical properties can be quite complex, the virgin material can be modified to have a flexural modulus of up to 21 GPa and a tensile strength of 225 MPa. There is some anisotropy that is introduced through the fiber reinforcement. When compared to other high-performance thermoplastic materials of polybutylene terephthalate and PS, PEEK has been found to have the highest fracture toughness and bending fatigue resistance, properties found to be insensitive to preconditioning and thermoforming. Its superior fatigue resistance is understood to be derived from its intimate bond with carbon fibers, and the matrix–fiber interfacial bond is enhanced by the creep resistance of PEEK.

PEEK is thermally stable at sterilization temperatures and will not degrade during either electron beam or gamma irradiation. PEEK will not hydrolyze and the degree of water uptake can be reduced by increasing the volume fraction of fiber-reinforced material as carbon fibers do not absorb water and do not degrade under physiological conditions. If sterility is to be achieved through gamma radiation, neither carbon fibers nor virgin PEEK degrade under gamma irradiation. In general, PEEK is resistant to all common sterilization techniques.

While its use in arthroplasty and trauma applications has been limited thus far, PEEK has found more widespread use in spinal interbody fusion cages, posterior dynamic spinal stabilization devices, arthroscopic suture anchors, and cranial defect repair. PEEK in orthopaedics is currently going through a conservative adoption period. Isoelastic hip stems made of PEEK have been cleared by the US Food and Drug Administration, and PEEK acetabular cup designs have received CE mark approval and have had limited clinical use. At this time, more long-term data are necessary to fully understand the clinical performance of these systems.

Resorbable polymers

The polymers discussed so far are intended to retain their shape and their essential properties after implantation. However, there are a number of applications in which it would be desirable to have properties change or even to have the material completely disappear with time. This principle has been long recognized in the use of absorbable sutures in deep tissue sites. One of the most challenging of these potential applications is in internal fracture fixation. It would be ideal to have a device that would slowly weaken and eventually disappear, transferring load to the healing bone and encouraging maximal Wolff's law remodeling.

There have been a number of attempts to produce such materials. The most promising absorbables today are alloys of poly(glycolic acid) (PGA) and poly(lactic acid) (PLA), particularly copolymers poylglycolide-co-polylactide and poly-L-lactide-co-DL-lactide. PLA is naturally degraded by hydrolysis *in vivo*, whereas PGA persists unchanged for long periods. Thus, alloys of these two materials may be produced that lose structural integrity over periods varying from a few weeks to 6 months. PLA–PGA alloys are very attractive as resorbable implant materials because their degradation products are indistinguishable from naturally occurring organic molecules and the evidence is that these products are handled through normal catabolic pathways.

Intentional degradation of the implant takes place through random hydrolysis of the polymer chains, enhanced by enzymes. Degradation can be affected by factors such as polymer molecular weight, molecular orientation, monomer concentration, presence of low-molecular-weight compounds, geometric isomerism, crystallinity, conformation, surface area/weight ratio, porosity, and site implantation. Generally, amorphous copolymers will disintegrate more rapidly than more crystalline compositions. As the polymeric implant begins to fragment, its molecular weight and strength properties are diminished. During this process, lactic acid and glycolic acid are metabolized into water and carbon dioxide. Eventually, macrophages will fully digest the polymeric debris. Complete resorption of commonly sized implants is highly variable depending on the polymer and may take place in between 8 months and 5 years.

The primary advantage of using resorbable material for the fixation of bone fractures is the elimination of a permanent metallic foreign implant. This is advantageous for reasons including reducing the risks of implant migration, stress shielding of the underlying bone, interference with computed tomography and magnetic resonance imaging scanning, and other aesthetic implications associated with removal of the devices. Unfortunately, the current perception is that bone plates composed of these materials do not provide enough fracture stability to be safely used in the load-bearing regions of most adult patients. Because the materials have low strength, resorbable bone plates tend to be bulky and cumbersome. The materials may also associated with a significant amount of redness and swelling, discharge, local pain, and osteolysis. These are symptoms of a transient mild microscopic foreign body reaction associated with the macrophage digestion of the polymers. Inflammation has been linked to a local acidosis secondary to an imbalance between rapid material degradation and slow material resorption. Osteolytic changes around self-reinforced polylactide screws have been demonstrated to occur in approximately a quarter of cases in some studies. Large plates have been associated with swelling recorded up to 3 years after the surgery. Resorbable materials can be self-reinforced (SR) to improve on some of the drawbacks to the material performance. But despite recent advances, absorbable plating has not seen widespread use because of the stated concerns.

Other resorbable polymeric materials, including processed collagenous allografts and xenografts, natural and synthetic suture materials, and bone void fillers, have also been used to varying degrees. Absorbable sutures and bone void fillers are currently widely available, while resorbable orthopaedic grafting materials are still on the market fringe.

Other polymers

The profusion of polymers and the growing ability to fashion them to yield specific properties have led to the experimental use of many new polymers in biomedical devices. In orthopaedic implants, this has been relatively limited. However, for completeness, several of these materials, their trade names, and their potential applications are listed in Table 6.4. Medical grades of the vast majority of these materials do not exist nor have they been approved for routine clinical use. However, some have been previously qualified for and used in food-packaging applications; these "food contact" grades are suitable for early experimental aspects of new biomaterials and implant development.

Additional problems

PROBLEM 6.4

Polymers are (select the best answer[s])

    A. Brittle, strong

    B. Ductile, weak

    C. Ductile, strong

    D. Brittle, weak

    E. None of above

Table 6.4 Other polymers

Polymer	Trade name	Application
Poly(acetal)	Delrin	Load-bearing material
Poly(amide)	Clariant, Nylon	Lipophilic; cerclage straps, bolt snubber
Poly(aramide)	Kevlar	Fiber for structural composites
Poly(carbonate)	Apec, Durolon, Makrolon, Lexan	Matrix for structural composites
Poly(cyanoacrylate)	—	Tissue adhesive
Poly(ethylene terephthalate)	Dacron	Fiber in tendon prostheses
Poly(propylene), poly(propylene oxide)	Marlex, Noryl, Huntsman Pro-fax	Matrix for soft tissue repair and structural composites, fiber in tendon prostheses
Poly(sulfone)	Udel, Thermalux	Matrix for structural composites
Poly(tetrafluoroethylene)	Proplast, Exac, Teflon	Matrix for nonrigid bony ingrowth material
Poly(etheretherketone)	PEEK-Optima, Zeniva	Load-bearing material, fixation devices
Poly(methyl methacrylate)	ACRYLITE, CYROLITE	Bone cement
Poly(styrene)	Albis, API, INEOUS, Supreme	
Poly(ethylene) (HD, UHWMPE)	Bormed, Purell	Load-bearing material, fixation devices
Poly(lactic acid)		Load-bearing material, fixation devices

ANSWER:

B.

PROBLEM 6.5

During revision of an internally fixed femoral subcapital fracture to a cemented total hip replacement, BC often extrudes through the lateral cortical defect left after nail removal (Figure 6.10). Referring to Figure 6.10 and using the data supplied, answer the following questions (disregard the curvature of the proximal femur and any stress concentration effects and remember that the bone–BC interface condition is that the strains are equal):

    A. What is the ratio of the peak tensile stresses in bone and PMMA?

    B. What percentage of the load is carried by the PMMA?

    C. What conclusion can you draw from *A.* and *B.* above?

ANSWER (B = BONE, P = PMMA):

    A. Since $\sigma = \varepsilon^* E$, then $\sigma_B = \varepsilon_B{}^* E_B$ and $\sigma_P = \varepsilon_P{}^* E_P$, then $\sigma_P/\sigma_B = E_P/E_B = 2.5/20 = 1/8$ or 12.5%.

    B. Load = stress × area, thus:

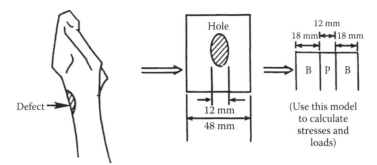

Peak load: 1100 N
Cortical thickness = 5 mm

E_B = 20 GPa E_P = 2.5 GPa

FIGURE 6.10 Lateral (proximal) cortical defect in the femur (Problem 6.5).

$Load_P = 1 \times (12 \times 5) = 60$

$Load_B = 8 \times (18 \times 2 \times 5) = 1440$

$Load_P/(Load_P + Load_B) = 60/(60 + 1440) = 0.04$

Therefore, 4% of the load is carried by PMMA.

C. It is better to leave the hole open (or bone-graft it) since the contribution of PMMA to load carriage in the defect is negligible.

PROBLEM 6.6

PMMA is an appropriate material to distribute load between a metal prosthesis and bone because (select the best answer[s])

A. Its compressive modulus is lower than that of cortical bone.

B. Its compressive modulus is higher than that of cortical bone.

C. It is a brittle material.

D. It is stronger than cortical bone.

E. None of the above.

ANSWER:

A. PMMA is both more brittle and weaker than cortical bone, which is a drawback to its use unless it can be kept fully supported and in net compression.

PROBLEM 6.7

The brittle nature of PMMA is demonstrated by its (select the best answer[s])

A. High elastic modulus

B. Lack of plastic deformation

    C. Low tensile strength

    D. Efficient load transfer to bone

    E. Exothermic reaction

ANSWER:

B.

PROBLEM 6.8

During the *in vivo* polymerization of PMMA (true or false),

1. The entire cement mass is converted from a low-molecular-weight monomeric state to a high-molecular-weight polymer.

2. Incorporation of some blood and fluid is desirable to reduce peak temperature reached.

3. Temperature elevation of surrounding tissue depends only on the total amount of cement used.

4. The bond established between PMMA and bone is simply a mechanical interlock.

5. Working time may be extended by prechilling components.

ANSWER:

F, F, F, T, T.

PROBLEM 6.9

Polyethylene, as used in joint replacements, is (true or false)

1. Low molecular weight

2. Made by condensation polymerization

3. Largely crystalline

4. A thermoset material

5. Ductile and tough

ANSWER:

F, F, T, F, T.

PROBLEM 6.10

An elastomer is a polymer (select the best answer[s])

    A. With a high T_G

    B. With a low modulus and high ductility

    C. With a large ε_y

    D. Containing silicon atoms

    E. That has a large, recoverable elasticity

ANSWER:

E.

Annotated bibliography

1. BORETOS JW: *Concise Guide to Biomedical Polymers*. Charles C Thomas, Springfield, IL, 1970.

   A short but comprehensive account of polymers used in orthotics and implants with useful information on processing and fabrication.

2. CHARNLEY J: *Acrylic Cement in Orthopaedic Surgery*. Williams & Wilkins, Baltimore, 1970.

   A highly personal account of the use of polymethyl methacrylate (PMMA) cement by one of the pioneers in total hip arthroplasty.

3. ENGLE L, KLINGELE H, EHRENSTEIN GW, SCHAPER H: *An Atlas of Polymer Damage*. Prentice-Hall, Englewood Cliffs, NJ, 1981.

   The histology of polymer failure, seen largely through the scanning electron microscope. Chapter 1 is a concise, well-illustrated review of the structure, properties, and processing of the most common classes of structural polymers.

4. HAYDEN HW, MOFFATT WG, WULFF J: *The Structure and Properties of Materials*. Vol. III. John Wiley & Sons, New York, 1964.

   Chapter 10 deals well with mechanical properties of polymers.

5. LEE H, NEVILLE K: *Handbook of Biomedical Plastics*. Pasadena Technology Press, Pasadena, CA, 1971.

   Still a standard source for compositional and performance data.

6. MATHYS R, MATHYS R, JR: The use of polymers for endoprosthetic components. In Morscher E (ed): *The Cementless Fixation of Hip Endoprostheses*. Springer-Verlag, Berlin, 1984.

   A good but brief review, with graphic figures, of polymers suitable for use in articulating implants.

7. MOFFATT WG, PEARSALL GW, WULFF J: *The Structure and Properties of Materials*. Vol. I. John Wiley & Sons, New York, 1964.

   Chapter 6 discusses structure of polymers. Excellent diagrams.

8. KURTZ S: *UHMWPE Biomaterials Handbook*, 2nd ed. Elsevier, San Diego, 2009.

   A definitive overview for UHMWPE.

CHAPTER SEVEN

Metals

Metals enjoy wide application in orthopaedics as structural, load-bearing materials in devices for fracture fixation, partial and total joint replacement devices, instruments, and external splints, braces, and traction apparatus. The principle reasons for this broad popularity are as follows:

1. Metals have high elastic moduli and reasonable yield points such that structures may be designed that will bear significant loads without large elastic deformations or any permanent deformation.

2. Metals have high enough ductility that stresses that exceed the yield point produce plastic deformation rather than sudden brittle fracture, permitting measures to be taken to modify use or to replace components before loss of integrity results.

3. Metals also possess sufficient plasticity to have fatigue endurance limits, thus suiting them for designs required to withstand great numbers of load–unload cycles, such as bone plates or proximal femoral components.

4. Metals may be fabricated into parts by a wide variety of conventional techniques and, in most cases, may have their mechanical properties adjusted before the final shape is attained.

5. When reasonable care is taken in fabrication, surface finishing, and handling, metal devices have good to excellent resistance to the variety of external and internal environments encountered in orthopaedic practice.

Basic metallurgy

The metallic elements of interest for inclusion in metallic orthopaedic biomaterials are shown in Figure 7.1, a portion of the familiar chemical periodic table. All have the ability to form interatomic metallic bonds with each other. These bonds are relatively nondirectional but strong; one may think of a metal in a simple way as an aggregation of marbles stuck together with very cold molasses. Thus, a very wide range of metallic material compositions are possible, in distinction to other

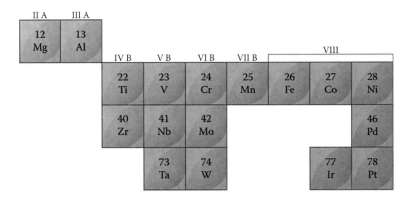

FIGURE 7.1 (See color insert.) Elements of interest in orthopaedic alloys.

types of chemical compounds, in which the nature of other bond types (ionic, covalent, etc.) dictates the inclusion of the constituent elements only in well-defined ratios. For instance, in sodium chloride, an ionically bonded compound, the combination of the two elements is only stable when they are present in a 1:1 ratio.

Metal "compounds," or more properly mixtures, are called *alloys*. The usual route to the development of an alloy of commercial value is to select a base element and then add small portions of other elements to change and enhance the properties of this base metal. The most common composition groups, that is, alloy systems, used in orthopaedics are summarized in Table 7.1.

Although metallic bonding leads to mixtures over wide possible ranges of composition, there may be preferred ratios of different elements that have some stability. These are called *intermetallic compounds*. The presence, deliberate or inadvertent, of carbon produces a range of very specific carbon–metal compounds called *carbides*. Since the metallic atoms are of different sizes, they may take up preferred minimum volume spatial arrangements when present in particular elemental

Table 7.1 Common orthopaedic alloy systems

Base element	Principal alloying elements	Generic name	Typical applications
Fe	C[a] + Cr, Ni, Mn, Mo, V	Stainless steels	Fracture hardware, braces, surgical instruments
Co	Cr, Mn, W, Mo, Ni, Nb, Ta	Super alloys or cobalt-base alloys	Joint replacement components
Ti	Al, V, Fe, Nb, Ta, Zr	Titanium-base alloys	Fracture hardware, joint replacement components
Pt	Ir, Pd	Precious alloys	Electrodes

[a] Carbon is not a metallic element; its role in determining alloy properties will be discussed later, but its controlled presence is what distinguishes steels from other iron alloys. Metallic elements are given in the approximate order of frequency of use as alloying agents.

ratios. Finally, since all of these relationships are dependent on the bonding or binding energy between atoms, they are subject to change with temperature.

Phase diagrams

All of the information about the chemical and structural relationships between metallic elements is difficult to tabulate numerically, so a graphic format was developed by metallurgists to present it in a simple manner. The resulting diagram is called a *constitution* or *phase diagram*. A *phase* is a homogeneous combination of the constituent elements that has constant structure and properties. A phase diagram is a plot of composition versus temperature for a mixture of elements, with regions of constant properties at equilibrium, defined as phases, separated by lines or surfaces, called phase boundaries.

Phase diagrams may be two- or three-dimensional or be made for two or three elements in the presence of a constant amount of one, two, or three additional elements, and so on. The simplest is the binary phase diagram, which shows the equilibrium phases possible for mixtures, that is, alloys, of two metals for compositions between 100% of one and 100% of the other.

It is unfortunate that the phase diagrams for alloys of orthopaedic interest are quite complex. Thus, for purposes of illustration of the general properties and use of phase diagrams, Figure 7.2 is an imaginary diagram, constructed for two imaginary metals, aronium and borium (A and B). This diagram obeys the thermodynamic principles of phase relationships for two metallic elements that have limited solubility in each other but possess no intermetallic compounds of fixed composition. It will be used in the subsequent discussions to illustrate the uses of phase diagrams.

This phase diagram has several important regions, labeled with Arabic or Greek letters:

$L.$ In this range of compositions and temperatures, only a homogeneous liquid is found. Note that while aronium melts at 1000°C and borium at 900°C, intermediate compositions can stay fully molten down to temperatures as low as 700°C. This type of behavior is not uncommon and is related to the presence of a eutectic composition in the system.

$E.$ The eutectic point. This composition, 65:35,* is called a *eutectic* since it melts abruptly (at 700°C) as if it were a pure metal.

$S + L.$ These two regions represent mixtures of two phases, a solid and a liquid. However, the solid phases are different in each region, being alpha (α) in the left or aronium-rich region and beta (β) in the

---

* The notation 65:35 means 65 weight percent (w/o) A, 35 w/o B including the relative structures of α and β phases.

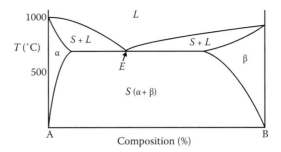

FIGURE 7.2 Aronium–borium (binary eutectic) phase diagram.

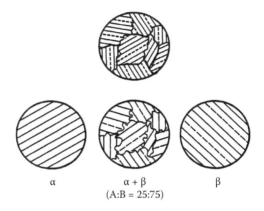

FIGURE 7.3 Phase structures.

right or borium-rich region. Thus, the left $S + L$ region might be labeled $\alpha + L$, the right one, $\beta + L$.

α, β. These are solids, with uniform, characteristic physical appearances over a range of compositions as shown. When prepared for metallographic examination, each would have a different appearance. Figure 7.3 shows schematically what each of these phases might look like. With care, materials with these compositions may be prepared as single crystals,* without grain boundaries.†

$\alpha + \beta$. This is also a solid region, with grains consisting of either α or β structure and the ratio of grain volumes depending on the distances to the α or β solid–solid phase boundaries. The size of the grains depends on thermal history and impurities, whereas the relative orientation is determined by other factors.

---

* A crystal structure of a material is defined by the arrangement of atoms or molecules.
† Grain boundaries are single-phase interfaces where crystals of different orientations meet. It is important to note that grain boundaries only divide regions of differing crystal orientation, where crystals on each side of the boundary are identical except in orientation. Grain boundaries disrupt the motion of dislocations through a material and thus tend to prevent slip. For this reason, decreasing grain size, and thus increasing the grain boundary density in a given material, will tend to increase the strength of that material.

Let us perform a thought experiment on this imaginary phase diagram to illustrate some of its uses.

PROBLEM 7.1

Suppose an 80:20 mixture were heated to 1100°C, then slowly cooled to 600°C, held there for a long time, and finally rapidly cooled to room temperature. Describe the solid structure that would result.

ANSWER:

Draw a vertical line at 80:20 (see Figure 7.4, which is a redrawn portion of the aronium–borium [A–B] phase diagram). The first material to "freeze" out, as the temperature reaches 900°C, will be particles of a phase with a composition of 97.5:2.5 (see left-pointing arrow). As the temperature decreases, the particles of a phase will grow, and through diffusion, they will gradually become more B rich, reaching 10 w/o at 700°C (right boundary of a region), while the fluid becomes more B rich, reaching 35 w/o B (right boundary of the α + L region). At 700°C, the last fluid, 35 w/o B, the eutectic composition, freezes, and the solid consists of islands of 10 w/o A α-phase in a matrix of eutectic composition (65:35). If the solid is held at 600°C for a long period, it will slowly transform through diffusion into a polycrystalline mixture of α-phase containing 92.5 w/o A (left boundary of α + β region) and β-phase containing 78 w/o B (right boundary of α + β region in Figure 7.3). The temperature for this example was picked to allow reasonably rapid diffusion for this alloy; sudden cooling to room temperature, then, will freeze it in this final structure, even though it is not the room temperature equilibrium structure.

Problem 7.1 illustrates some of the simple uses of phase diagrams. Independent knowledge of the mechanical and other properties of each of the solid phases permits estimates to be made of the properties of the resulting alloys. These properties depend on thermal history, usually

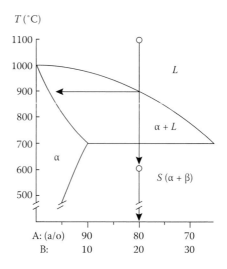

FIGURE 7.4 Detail of aronium–borium phase diagram (Problem 7.1).

called *heat treatment*. Phase diagrams exist for all of the important commercial alloys and are used as a guide in selection of materials and processing decisions.

Reflection on this example will show that the final structure would be different if the experiment in Problem 7.1 involved rapid cooling (*quenching*) from a temperature other than 600°C. The fundamental reason for discussing phase diagrams is to emphasize this point: chemical composition *alone* does not fully determine the properties of a metallic alloy.

Evolution of a metallic part

There is a long path to travel from definition of the desired chemical composition of an alloy to a final part. The major steps are as follows: alloy fabrication, casting, mechanical forming, heat treatment, and finishing (Figure 7.5).

Alloy fabrication   All alloy fabrication begins with extraction of metal ores from mineral deposits. An *ore* is a reacted compound of a metal with oxygen and other elements such as silicon, nitrogen, sulfur, and other metals. Only gold and, in very rare cases, copper occur in nature as unreacted (fully reduced) metals. Some metals exist as ions in seawater at sufficient concentrations that they may be isolated by electrochemical processes. Each component of the alloy must first be extracted from a primary source, reduced to metallic form, and cleaned of unwanted impurities. The alloy is then formed by combining the appropriate elements and melting them together under suitable conditions that prevent re-reaction with gases and other materials. The resulting liquid alloy may then be cast in suitable molds as parent or mother ingots or directly into bars or rods. By careful cooling, these primary forms attain structures defined by the relevant equilibrium phase diagram.

Thus, all alloys are first fabricated in the cast state. Some alloys are suitable to be remelted and formed into device components by molding followed by mechanical finishing. These are called casting alloys. A well-known Co–Cr–Mo (F 75*) alloy, pure titanium (F 67), and cast stainless steel (F 55) are dealt with in this way. Additional processing steps may occur before the final product is cast. The letters "VM" as part of an alloy name or designation indicate that after the initial alloy was fabricated, it was remelted in a vacuum, allowing more of the trapped gases to escape, producing a purer material. Sometimes, the removal of such material is designated by the letters "ELI," which stand for *extra low interstitials*, as commonly used in titanium alloy descriptions.

---

* The American Society for Testing and Materials (ASTM) prepares consensus standards for materials and processes. These are published annually and revised at least every 5 years. The full designation, in this case F 75-12, indicates that this specification was revised in 2012.

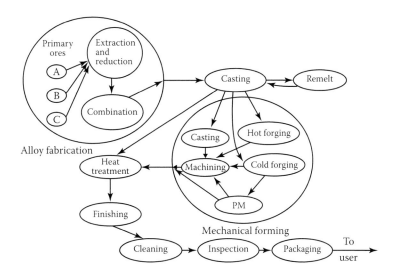

FIGURE 7.5 Processing of metal alloys.

Casting

Casting alloys may be formed into intricate shapes by a variety of processes:

Direct casting. Alloys may be cast into bars, rods, and so on, which are then machined to their final shape. This is rarely used today in fabrication of orthopaedic devices.

Die casting. Alloys may be cast in closed machined cavities (dies) in high-temperature-resistant molds. This process is usually reserved for cases in which tens or hundreds of thousands of identical parts are to be made, owing to the high cost of making the dies. Some shapes, for instance, grooves that are wider at the root than at the surface, are difficult or in some cases impossible to produce in die-cast parts, owing to the need to extract the casting easily without damaging the mold. However, die casting has the merit that it can produce extremely smooth surfaces, requiring no mechanical forming and only modest finishing. Die casting is more commonly used for polymer fabrication; it is rarely used for metallic components of orthopaedic devices.

Investment casting. In this technique, a model of the desired shape is made in wax and then invested or embedded in a suitable mold material, usually a ceramic. The wax models themselves may be made by hand or by die casting but in relatively inexpensive molds, at low temperature. The investment material is then heated in a furnace, which both strengthens it and removes the wax model by melting and vaporization. For this reason, this technique is often called *lost wax casting*. Then the metal is poured into the mold and allowed to harden, and the mold is broken away to free it. The casting surface is somewhat rough, requiring modest additional machining and finishing steps to produce a finished part. This technique permits casting of very complex shapes and is frequently used to fabricate partial and total joint replacement components.

Casting alloys are designed to be clean and to solidify without forming pores or cracks, but the resulting cast parts are relatively weak since they are relatively coarse grained and contain many defects, especially residual impurities and porosity, so they may not be highly fatigue resistant. Casting in vacuum generally improves casting cleanliness and final properties. Heat treatment, to change the phase structure, may be useful but may also result in overall grain growth, producing further reduction in strength.

Hot isostatic pressing. Hot isostatic pressing (HIPing) may be used to improve casting quality. It involves placing the castings in a suitable inert gas–filled chamber to protect the alloy and subjecting them to very high pressures at moderately elevated temperature, well below the alloy melting point, to increase diffusion rates and reduce the yield point. Since the pressure (hydrostatic) is applied uniformly through the gas surrounding the part, there are no deforming moments and shape is retained. Internal defects tend to become condensed, and the alloy is stronger after treatment. However, HIPing tends to improve only weak parts, raising the average properties of a production batch and thus reducing the incidence of service failures. It cannot radically change properties of castings.

Mechanical forming

Cast structures, even when very well designed, well made, and impurity free, are relatively weak since they contain fairly large essentially polygonal or equiaxial grains and have not been work hardened. Grain size may be controlled, to a degree, by controlled cooling through the $S + L$ region of the phase diagram, since rapid cooling produces a smaller average grain size (Figure 7.6).

However, mechanical properties of alloys may be radically improved by the use of a variety of mechanical postforming processes creating noncast materials. Many of these processes also may be used to improve the mechanical properties of devices, after a primary casting step. Some mechanical processes (other than machining) may be applied to casting alloys, but many require alloys specially designed to withstand the rigors of postcasting processing.

The principal noncasting forming processes in use are as follows:

Rolling and drawing. Ingots, bar, and rod may be converted mechanically into different shapes by rolling between smooth or shaped rollers or by pulling (*drawing*) through holes in hardened plates (to produce wire). These processes are performed at room temperature (*cold rolling*) or at elevated temperatures (*hot rolling*) to improve ductility during processing. Each produces large amounts of work hardening, depending on the amount of plastic strain and the temperature, and produces elongated, very strong grains in the direction of plastic deformation.

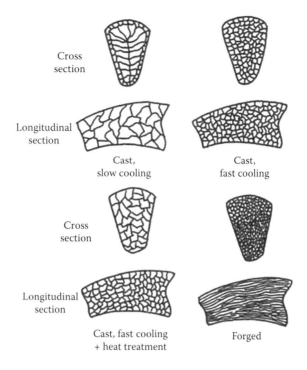

Cross
section

Longitudinal
section

Cast,
slow cooling

Cast,
fast cooling

Cross
section

Longitudinal
section

Cast, fast cooling
+ heat treatment

Forged

FIGURE 7.6 Cast alloy microstructures.

Drawing. Sheets, produced by rolling down bars or rods, may be
formed into cuplike structures by pressing between mating male
and female (open) die pairs. A great degree of plastic deformation
is required; thus, only highly ductile alloys may be formed this
way, and postdrawing heat treatment is nearly always required to
restore toughness. The process may have to be repeated, with intervening annealing steps, to produce large degrees of deformation.

Machining. Cast bars, rods, or parts may be cut and formed with
hardened tools. Machining introduces some degree of work hardening, especially at the surface, but does not change grain structure. Machining processes also include grinding with abrasive
tools and electrolytic cutting (ELOX) with a graphite cathode in
an electrolyte bath. These latter processes are useful on very hard
alloys.

*Forging.** Forging consists of gradually shaping a cast ingot, bar, or
rod into a final shape by successive compression between mating
negative dies. A series of three or more die pairs may be used, with
each set nearer to the final desired shape than the previous one.
The metal is usually worked hot (*hot forging*); *cold forging* is also

---

* There is a general confusion between the terms "forging" and "working" (past tense:
"wrought"). The former should be used to describe the forming of components; the latter, to describe preprocessing of alloy before final forming.

possible but more difficult. In either case, annealing (controlled heating and cooling that does not enter the $S + L$ region) between forging episodes (*reductions*) is used to control the degree of work hardening and the grain size. During forging, grain size may be reduced and desirable elongated grain structures are formed (Figure 7.6). Final machining then produces the desired closely controlled dimensions and surface finish.

Working. (See footnote to *Forging,* above.) Forging is a very expensive process since several dies are required for each part and die life is fairly short. An alternative, which is somewhat less expensive, is to forge a rod or bar that is later machined to the final shape; such material is often referred to as having been wrought, to distinguish it from cast material or forged parts of the same composition.

Powder metallurgy. This is an alternative route to formation of fine-grained strong materials. A fine, homogeneous powder, with particle sizes typically between 50 and 100 μm, is produced by grinding an ingot or preferably by injecting a melted primary alloy into a stream of inert gas, such as nitrogen or argon. The resulting powder is placed in closed dies and then heated to cause bonding of the particles through solid-state diffusion, termed *sintering.* The final part may require additional heat treatment and HIPing. It is strong, fine grained, and fatigue resistant, but lacks the longitudinal bending resistant fiber texture of a forged part. Not all alloys may be handled this way, but the result may be an extremely fine-grained structure in large complex parts that cannot be economically formed in any other way. The abbreviation *PM* is often used to describe such parts.

Welding. It is generally considered undesirable to "mix" metals in a corrosive environment, such as the human body, so as to avoid galvanic corrosion (see Chapter 12). However, there are occasions, especially in surgical instrument fabrication, when it is necessary to join two or more parts with similar composition but different degrees of cold working or heat treatment. This is done by welding, which is generically local melting, resulting in fusion by liquid phase diffusion and solidification. A protective inert gas (argon, etc.) "blanket" may be used to protect the molten metal from oxidation. If an additional metallic filler material of a different composition is added, the process is called *brazing.* Because welding and brazing change the phase structure in the vicinity of the joint between parts, these processes must be very carefully selected for biomedical applications. Perhaps the best one is *electron beam welding* in which a very narrow, energetic beam of electrons produces local melting in a vacuum. This, combined with the rapid cooling possible in a vacuum, produces the narrowest possible weld zone with the least disturbance of the phase structures of the base alloys and without introduction of impurities.

Heat treatment   The ability to regulate mechanical properties without changes in overall composition is the key to the high desirability of metals in fabrication of artifacts such as surgical devices. Thus, parts may be formed easily while the alloy is relatively deformable, and then the yield point and ductility may be adjusted thermally to produce the final required mechanical behavior.

In thermal processing, metallurgists are guided by what are called *time–temperature–transformation* or *TTT* diagrams, which describe the interrelationship between time, temperature, and transformation of phase structure for each alloy. In general, the time and temperature required for a structural change vary inversely, but the exact relationship may be complex.

The principal applications of heat treatment are as follows:

Annealing. Working alloys at low temperatures above their yield points produce work hardening and thus loss of toughness and ductility. If large changes in cross section are required by the forming process, this may result in cracking of the part, since the ultimate strain may be exceeded locally. This may be prevented by heating to between one-third and one-half of the melting temperature followed by controlled cooling. This cycle relieves the cold work, restoring unworked properties, but results in modest grain growth. Sometimes, it is used deliberately for this purpose to eliminate so-called "duplex" structures: ones that contain both large and small grains rather than a normal distribution around a single average grain size. Duplex structures are relatively weak; annealing tends to normalize them by removing the small grains since large grains grow at the expense of small ones. A related process called *tempering* is a partial annealing used to slightly toughen very brittle strong alloys used for cutting edges. Tempering generally requires extremely rapid cooling (*quenching*).

Aging. Aging is storage for long periods at slightly elevated temperatures (below annealing temperatures) to permit the formation of intermetallic, carbide, or oxide precipitates. These very small, very strong crystals internally stress the alloy, raising both yield and ultimate strengths without affecting moduli. The resulting alloy is said to be *aged* or *precipitation hardened*.

Phase transformation. The great power of modern metallurgy comes from the discovery that some alloys, particularly many steels, can have phases of identical compositions but with different local arrangements of atoms, resulting in different densities and mechanical properties. The change from one structure to another, in the solid state, is called a *phase transformation*. We distinguish between two general types of phase transformation: those requiring diffusion, as in the formation of interposed lamellae of α + β from a eutectic composition, and those that do not require diffusion but occur owing to a very local rearrangement of atoms. Phase transformations may be orchestrated in many alloys by very careful and complex cycles of heating, storage, and cooling.

Composition, *fabrication*, and *heat treatment* all affect mechanical and, to a degree, chemical properties of alloys and should be fully described in materials selection processes.

Finishing

Many steps are required to produce the ideal structures desired for satisfactory performance in biomedical applications. In addition to bulk processing, there is usually a requirement to adjust or finish the surface of a part. The processes used may result in mechanical or chemical modification or both.

The following are the principal surface-finishing techniques used in the manufacture of orthopaedic devices, in alphabetical order. More than one may be used on any one component, and the order may be varied. Finishing is still not an exact science, and commercial process details tend to be guarded.

Anodization. Formation of a strong oxide surface film on aluminum-base and titanium-base alloys by placing the parts in a suitable conductive (electrolyte) bath and rendering them anodic (in this case, positively charged) with an external power supply. This essentially converts the surface of the part from a metal to a ceramic and improves corrosion and wear resistance very significantly.

Carburization. Deliberate reaction of carbon with steel surfaces produces local carbide precipitation and very great hardness, although corrosion resistance may be reduced. This produces a very hard, tough surface layer over a ductile base, a perfect combination for a cutting edge. This process was one of the secrets in making the famous Damascus steel and is still widely used in the manufacture of scalpel blades, osteotomes, saws, and so on.

Electroplating. Metals may be deposited in a surface film from a suitable solution by rendering the part cathodic (in this case, negatively charged). This is frequently done commercially to improve corrosion resistance, as in the electroplating of chromium onto automobile bumpers, which are made of non-stainless steel alloys. This is rarely used in orthopaedic devices for a number of reasons (see Chapter 10), but electroplated gold coatings are seen on the handles of some surgical instruments.

Grinding. Physically removing the surface layers by abrasion with aluminum oxide or silicon carbide on papers or in bonded grinding tools. This may be used as a primary forming process for hard-to-machine alloys such as the cobalt-base ones or merely to remove surface impurities, as after investment casting or welding.

Nitriding. Steels and titanium-base alloys may have a portion of their surface iron or titanium atoms, respectively, converted to nitrides by reaction with gaseous ammonia or molten potassium cyanate, both at elevated temperatures. This greatly hardens the surface and, in the case of titanium-base alloys, imparts a pleasant golden color.

Passivation. All orthopaedic alloys may be passivated by acid treatment, which converts surface elements, particularly chromium and titanium, to oxides or hydroxides. Although many alloys will passivate spontaneously in air or water, deliberate acid treatment, as described in ASTM F 86, produces more adherent passivation layers with better structure and corrosion resistance. All metallic implants in use today are routinely passivated during manufacture. Passivation also performs a crucial cleaning function in terms of reducing the organic and inorganic residues on the implant surface.

Polishing. A smoothing process, using very hard, finely divided polishing materials, such as aluminum oxide, silicon carbide, or industrial diamond, sometimes suspended in an oil or grease and carried on supporting media such as paper or cloth. The aim is to remove unwanted surface materials, such as casting investment debris, dirt, and so on, and to smooth out surface defects including marks left by machining. The quality of the final surface is dependent on the hardness and the size of the successively used polishing agents. Mirror finishes are possible, as on the femoral head of a total hip replacement (THR).

Sand blasting and shot peening. Bombarding the surface with a stream of foreign particles. These may be done to clean and remove small amounts of the surface, in which case coarsely divided grinding agents may be used. However, larger particles, such as ceramic beads or steel balls (shot), may be used in a deliberate move to work harden the surface. This latter process is called *shot peening* and can be used with great success to produce hardening in a confined region, as on the tip of a screwdriver or the striking face of a mallet, without any chemical modification.

Surface alloying. It may be desirable to actually change the metallic composition of the surface to produce different properties from those in the bulk alloy. This may be done by electroplating or vacuum deposition followed by heat treatment, by electrodiffusion from a molten (fused) salt bath (*metalliding*), or by direct implantation of ionized species from gas phase (*ion implantation*). Surface alloying techniques are relatively new to orthopaedic applications and are in various stages of development and qualification testing.

Many common commercial surface-finishing processes, such as galvanizing, painting, and polymer coating, are not suitable for orthopaedic applications because of both material and host response requirements.

Stainless steel

Compositions

Historically, steels were the first modern metallic alloys to be used in orthopaedics. Dissatisfaction with the "rusting" of early implants led to the use of so-called stainless steels. These are iron-base alloys with a relatively low carbon content and high chromium content. The low carbon content controls the formation of carbides, which are needed for strength but are more easily corroded *in vivo* than the alloy matrix, whereas the chromium permits the formation of a stable chromium oxide–containing surface layer during passivation. Molybdenum also controls corrosion in stainless steels but is much less effective than chromium. It is generally used only in small quantities since it is expensive and it greatly hardens the alloy, making it difficult to work. Other elements are added to control mechanical properties and, in casting alloys, to control structure and prevent cracking during solidification.

Stainless steels consist of four basic types, depending on the appearance of characteristic phases at room temperature:

Austenitic. Steels containing a solid phase, γ-Fe, called austenite, which is a solid solution of Fe with 2% or less C. This phase is stabilized by the presence of Ni.

Ferritic. Steels with a low Ni content in which the austenitic phase formed at high temperatures dissociates to Fe + C at low temperatures.

Martensitic. Steels in which rapid heating and cooling may produce an internal nondiffusional phase transformation of the austenite phase to a new phase, martensite, without precipitation.

Precipitation hardenable. Steels with a high enough C content that a carbide precipitate, Fe_3C, may be formed by heat treatment.

The martensitic stainless steels, such as American Iron and Steel Institute (AISI) type 420, are hard and tough and thus are favored for fabrication of surgical instruments such as osteotomes and scalpel blades. However, the superior corrosion resistance of austenitic alloys, such as AISI 316L, has led to their present dominance in implant applications.

The compositions of the principal implant alloys in use today are given in Table 7.2. (In this and subsequent composition tables, the ASTM standard or commercial compositions are given. Other standards, noted for comparison [e.g., ISO (International Standards Organization), AISI], may vary slightly.)

F 55 and F 138 describe the popular alloy referred to by its AISI designation as 316L. This is a casting alloy with high ductility, which can undergo extensive postcasting mechanical processing and which is the most common stainless alloy in use in orthopaedic applications as a wrought material. It is descended from earlier alloys EN85J, 18-8sMo, and AISI 316 by a gradual process of improvement to reduce the corrosion rate. The "L" designation (equivalent to F 55, Grade 2) refers to a C content below 0.03, which is modern practice. F 138 has a slightly tighter control of impurities and standards for the number of visible impurity inclusions. A variation of 316L, known as 316LVM (low carbon vacuum remelted) has been developed to provide more reliable corrosion resistance.

F 745 is a modern high-strength casting alloy, whereas F 2229, F 1586, and F 1314 are high-strength forging alloys, all with nitrogen added to further stabilize the austenite phase and improve strength. All four alloys may be wrought and hot and cold forged. In the annealed state or after relatively low work hardening, stainless steels, although

Table 7.2 Stainless steel alloy compositions

Alloy					
ASTM	F 55[a], F 138[a]/139	F 2229	F 1586	F 1314	F 745
ISO	5832-1				
Other	AISI 316L				
Elements (%)					
C	0.03	0.08	0.08	0.03	<0.06
Cu	0.5	0.25	0.25	0.5	
Cr	<19	<23	<22	<23.5	17–19
Fe	>58	>58	>58	>58	>58
Mn	2	<24	<4.25	<6	<2
Mo	<3	<1.5	<3	<3	2–3
N	0.1	>0.9	<0.5	<0.4	
Nb			<0.8	<0.3	
Ni	<15	0.1	<11	<13.5	11–14
P	<0.025	0.03	0.025	0.025	<0.045
S	0.01	0.01	0.01	0.01	<0.03
Si	0.75	0.75	0.75	0.75	<1
V				0.1–0.3	

[a] Grade 2.

on the whole more difficult to form than most non-stainless steels, may be fabricated by virtually all machining and finishing processes. This combined with the relatively low price of their elemental components (compared with cobalt-base, titanium-base, and various precious alloys) contributes to their wide popularity in orthopaedic applications.

Mechanical properties

The properties of all alloys are sensitive to differences in processing (Table 7.3). The elastic moduli (tensile, compressive, etc.) are set by the chemical composition and are relatively insensitive to changes of composition within an alloy system. However, yield, ultimate, and fatigue properties are strongly affected by small changes in chemical composition and even more so by the phase structure created during fabrication. In addition, fabrication may involve some degree of work hardening, which may or may not be relieved by later annealing and which may have residual effects on the grain structure. Hardness is extremely variable depending on, in addition to these factors, mechanical and chemical finishing steps. All stainless steel components used in orthopaedic applications are chemically passivated.

In comparison with other alloys of orthopaedic interest, austenitic stainless steels have moderate yield and ultimate strengths combined with high ductility. This high ductility and, in particular, the significant retention of ductility after large amounts of cold work, combined with relatively low cost, render them excellent for use in fracture fixation devices. The newer forging alloys show exceptional mechanical

Table 7.3   Stainless steel alloy mechanical properties

Alloy					
ASTM	F 55, F 138	F 2229	F 1586	F 1314	F 745
ISO	5832-1				
Other	AISI 316L, UNS S31673	UNS S29108	UNS S31675	UNS S20910	
Mechanical properties					
	Fe-17Cr-14Ni-2.5Mo	23Mn-21Cr-1Mo	21Cr-10Ni-3Mn-2.5Mo	22Cr-12.5Ni-5Mn-2.5Mo	
Tensile modulus (Y, GPa)	192–201	#	#	#	#
0.2% Yield strength ($\sigma_{0.2\%}$, min, MPa)	170 a 250 hf 310 cw 1200 cf[a]	586 a 1227 cw	430 a	380 a 862 cw	205 c
Ultimate strength (σ_u, min, MPa)	480 a 550 hf 655 cw 1300 cf[a]	931 a 1496 cw	740 a	690 a 1035 cw	480 c
Strain to failure (ε_u, min, %)	40 a 55 hf 28 cw 12 cf[a]	52 a 19 cw	35 a	35 a 12 cw	30 c
Hardness	85 RB a 30 RC cw				

Note: a, Annealed; c, as cast; cw, 30% cold worked; cf, cold forged; hf, hot forged; RB, Rockwell B; RC, Rockwell C; #, not reported, close to F 55.

[a] F 138.

properties and are resulting in a resurgence of interest in the use of stainless steel in joint replacement components. Although cast stainless steel was used in early joint replacement prosthesis components, this has been largely abandoned since early casting alloys displayed inadequate yield and fatigue strengths, resulting in unacceptable incidences of medullary stem bending and component fatigue fracture.

Cobalt-base alloys

Compositions   F 75 is the traditional cast alloy and is probably the one in most common use today. It was originally called Vitallium (Howmedica, Inc., Rutherford, New Jersey), and unfortunately this name is frequently used incorrectly to refer to the whole class of cobalt-base alloys. There is a modified version, F 799, which is used both as a hot forging alloy and as a base material for powder metallurgic processes (Table 7.4).

Table 7.4 Cobalt-base alloy compositions

Alloy					
ASTM	F 75	F 90	F 563	F 562	F 1537, F 799
ISO	5832-4	5832-6			
UNS	R30075	R30605		R30035	R31537–R31539
Elements (w/o)					
C	<0.35	0.05–0.15	<0.005	<0.025	<0.35
Co	Balance (>34)	Balance (>34)	Balance (>34)	Balance (29–39)	Balance (>34)
Cr	27–30[a]	19–21	18–22	19–21	26–30
Fe	<0.75[a]	<3	4–6	<1	<0.75
Mn	<1	<2	<1	<0.15	<1
Mo	5–7		3–4	9–10.5	5–7
Ni	<1	9–11	15–25	33–37	<1
P				<0.015	
S			<0.01	<0.01	
Si	<1	<1	<0.5	<0.15	<1
Ti			0.5–3.5	<1	
W		14–16	3–4		

[a] F 799: Cr 26–30, Fe < 1.

F 90 is a wrought alloy with 15% tungsten, reduction in chromium, and changes in other elements making it more suitable for hot rolling. F 563 is occasionally used in Europe as a forging alloy, whereas F 562 is coming into fairly common use, despite some concern about its high nickel content. F 562 possesses many of the desirable strength properties of the cobalt-base system while retaining a higher-than-typical ductility.

The phase structure of these alloys is very complex. In general, they are austenitic, can undergo partial conversion to produce a strengthening martensitic phase, and can also be precipitation hardened by suitable heat treatment. (The austenitic and martensitic phases of cobalt chrome alloys have the same crystalline structure, unlike stainless steels where these phases have different structures.)

Mechanical properties

The mechanical properties of cobalt-base alloys are given in Table 7.5. In comparison with stainless steels, cobalt-base alloys have slightly higher moduli and much higher strengths but lower ductilities. Although these properties may be regulated to a great degree by heat treatment, the alloys are relatively more difficult to machine since they have high intrinsic hardnesses. On the other hand, high hardness is a characteristic that is looked upon as being favorable for a bearing surface. Furthermore, their constituent elements, particularly cobalt and tungsten, are quite expensive, so that base alloy costs are significantly higher than for stainless steels.

Table 7.5   Cobalt-base alloy mechanical properties

Alloy ASTM	F 75	F 799	F 90	F 563	F 562
Mechanical properties					
Tensile modulus (Y, GPa)	195	195	210	220–234	232
0.2% Yield strength ($\sigma_{0.2\%}$, min, MPa)	450 ac 890 f	900 f	310 a	276 a	240 a 1585 cw*
Ultimate strength (σ_u, min, MPa)	655 ac 1400 f	1400 f	860 a	600 a 827 cw	795 a 1790 cw*
Strain to failure (ε_u, min,%)	8 ac 28 f		30 a	50 a 18 cw	50 a 8 cw
Hardness	25 RC ac 38 RC f				

Note: a, annealed; ac, as cast; cw, 30% cold worked; cw*, 48% cold worked; f, forged; RB, Rockwell B; RC, Rockwell C.

Titanium-base alloys

Compositions

Titanium-base alloys have entered commercial use much more recently than stainless steels and cobalt-base alloys, so there are far fewer choices. There are two major alloys in use today whose compositions are given in Table 7.6. Pure titanium is relatively soft compared to stainless steel and cobalt chromium alloys, although its strength and ductility can be seen as advantageous and may be varied over a broad range by control of its oxygen content. Interstitial elements such as oxygen and nitrogen are readily absorbed at elevated temperatures and can increase strength and reduce ductility. To date, both F 67, Grade 4, the commercial grade with the highest oxygen content, and F 136, more commonly known as Ti6A14V, have seen considerable use.

Titanium compositions are classified as near-alpha (α) alloys (<10% β), beta alloys (>25% beta), and alpha–beta ($\alpha + \beta$) alloys (10% to 25% β). Pure Ti exists as an allotropic metal with a hexagonal close-packed α-phase at room temperature which transforms to a cubic β-phase (body centered cubic) above 882°C. Because α-titanium cannot be significantly strengthened using heat treatments, β stabilizers are alloyed into pure titanium to improve material properties. Ti6A14V, an $\alpha + \beta$ alloy, is the most common commercial form of Ti, accounting for approximately 45% of total titanium production, including extensive use in aerospace applications. The addition of Al tends to stabilize the α-phase, whereas V stabilizes the β-phase. The presence of these two major phases and

Table 7.6   Titanium-base alloy compositions

Alloy			
ASTM	F 67	F 136	
ISO		5832-3	
Other	Pure Ti	Ti6Al4V	Ti-5Al-2.5Fe
Elements (w/o)			
Al	—	5.5–6.5	4.5–5.5
C	<0.1	<0.08	<0.08
Fe	<0.5	<0.25	2–3
H	<0.015	<0.015	<0.0125
N	<0.05	<0.05	<0.05
O	<0.4	<0.2	<0.2
Ti	>99	Balance	Balance
V	—	3.5–4.5	—

the ability to manipulate their microstructure by chemical additions and heat treatment permit the generation of a very wide range of microstructures and mechanical properties. Because of concerns with the toxicity of vanadium and aluminum, alternative alloys of Ti6Al7Nb (ASTM F 1295) and Ti-5Al-2.5Fe have been developed with a similar metallurgical structure.

In a continued search for a Ti alloy with high corrosion resistance, good toxicity, low modulus (to minimize stress shielding), high strength, and good notched fatigue strength, alternative β-Ti alloys are being developed. β-Ti does not alloy with Al or Va, thus reducing concerns with cytotoxicity. The principal alloying elements in β-Ti include tantalum, iron, niobium, zirconium, and molybdenum. The most notable of the β alloys include Ti-13Nb-13Zr, Ti-12Mo-6Zr-2Fe (ASTM F 1813), and Ti-15 Mo. All except Ti-6Al-7Nb have a low elastic modulus designed to combat stress shielding.

Titanium in a porous form has been developed to reduce the stiffness mismatch between the alloy and its supporting bone and to facilitate ingrowth of new bone tissue. Porous titanium has been prepared via slurry foaming, plasma spray coating, sintering of titanium fibers or powder, and the space holder method. Each fabrication technique has unique advantages and disadvantages. Material properties for Ti in its porous form are presented in Chapter 13.

Mechanical properties

Titanium is lighter than stainless steel and cobalt chromium alloys, with a density of 4.5 g/cm^3. Titanium and its alloys have moduli that are roughly half those of stainless steel and cobalt-base alloys, combined with relatively high strengths (a higher strength-to-density ratio than any other metal) and low ductilities. In fact, F 136 is a relatively brittle material (Table 7.7). Another of the attractions of alternative Ti alloys is the potential for greater ductility, producing easier formability, thus making Ti suitable for a greater range of applications. Because of the formation

Table 7.7   Titanium-base alloy mechanical properties

Alloy				
ASTM	F 67	F 136		F 1813
ISO		5832-3		
Other	Pure Ti	Ti6Al4V	Ti-5Al-2.5Fe	Ti-12Mo-6Zr-2Fe
Mechanical properties				
Tensile modulus (Y, GPa)	100–104	101–114	112	74–85
0.2% Yield strength ($\sigma_{0.2\%}$, min, MPa)	170–485	795–875	895	1000–1060
Ultimate strength (σ_u, min, MPa)	240–550	860–965	1020	1060–1100
Strain to failure (ϵ_u, min, %)	15–24	6–15	15	18–22

of a thin oxide layer (TiO_2), all Ti alloys exhibit very good biocompatibility. Further, Ti is amenable to direct apposition of bone minerals on its interface, which leads to good osseointegration.

Shape memory and superelastic alloys

Shape memory alloys are metals that exhibit two properties: pseudoelasticity and shape memory. Shape memory refers to the ability of a material to remember its original cold-forged shape, whereas superelasticity is a state where a material may be deformed well beyond its typical breaking point without fracturing. Both shape memory and superelasticity are features stemming from the same mechanism, though we will refer to these alloys as "shape memory" alloys for simplicity.

The unique properties were first observed in 1938 by Arne Olander, though serious research advances were not realized until the 1960s. The shape memory alloy family includes NiTi (Nitinol), CuZnAl, CuAlNi, and MgSi. Nitinol (National Bureau of Standards, Washington, DC), an alloy with roughly equal atomic percentages of Ni and Ti, is currently considered the most promising of the shape memory alloys for orthopaedic applications.

Shape memory in Nitinol is made possible through a solid-state phase change from martensite to austenite. Phase changes are most commonly recognized in the transition from solid to liquid, as in ice melting. A solid-state phase change is similarly a reorganization of the arrangement and position of molecules within the crystal structure of the material—it is unique in that the molecular arrangement remains closely packed and therefore the substance remains a solid. At high temperatures, Nitinol exists as the cubic structure called austenite. When cooled below a transformation temperature, which can be tuned, it becomes monoclinic martensite.* Martensite is relatively soft and easy to deform and tends

---

* A monoclinic structure is described as a rectangular prism, with a parallelogram as its base. Describing the crystal system with three vectors, two of the vectors intersect obliquely and are perpendicular to the third.

to exist at lower temperatures. Its properties are derived from its low-symmetry twinned close-packed monoclinic (hexagonal) crystalline structure. Austenite has a more compact and regular pattern, typically owing to its rigid body–centered cubic arrangement. We will see that transition between martensite and austenite phases is dependent only on temperature and stress. There is no diffusion, and therefore time is not a factor (i.e., the transformation is instantaneous).*

Starting at point A_f in Figure 7.7 and decreasing the temperature through the critical transformation temperature range (TTR) past M_s, the material begins to transform from austenite to martensite until it is 100% twinned martensite at M_f. Martensite deforms by moving twin boundaries, whereas most metals deform by slip or dislocation. The stress required to "detwin" is very low as twin boundaries are highly mobile and of very low energy. Upon deformation, the structure will remain in its deformed state until heat is applied, which provides enough energy for the molecular structure to find its rigid body–centered austenitic crystalline structure. The transformation to austenite will take place through the curve starting at A_s and continuing through the reverse transformation temperature range (RTTR) to A_f where the material will be in a fully austenitic structure.† The shape of curve in Figure 7.7 depends on material properties such as the composition of the alloying elements and the degree of work hardening. Figure 7.8 is a diagrammatic representation of the shifts occurring in the atomic structure through TTR and RTTR.

The transformation from austenite to martensite may also take place as a result of an application of stress. The application of a stress favors the martensitic phase because it has an ability to easily adapt its shape. Upon the application of stress, the material is continuously deformed (strained) up to a limit. Once the deforming force stops, the materials will "spring back" to its pre-deformation austenitic shape without any permanent strain. This phenomenon is termed *pseudoelasticity* or *superelasticity* and is displayed when a material in the austenitic phase is deformed while the temperature is held above that which martensite is stable (i.e., martensite is only stable at low temperatures). As much as 8% strain may be fully recoverable in a superelastic material. In Figure 7.7, superelasticity may take place up to temperature M_d.

Mechanical properties

Select mechanical properties for "55 Nitinol" (56% Nickel, 44% Ti), a common medical-grade Nitinol alloy, are given in Table 7.8. All mechanical properties of Nitinol are subject to a discontinuous change at the point of transformation between martensitic and austenitic phases. The chemical, physical, mechanical, and metallurgical requirements

---

* A shape memory material needs to be shape set annealed before it will exhibit shape memory properties. Shape setting is accomplished by firmly constraining the material into a desired "memory" shape using a fixture or mandrel and annealing. After heating in an oven to between 500 and 550°C, the material is quenched to avoid aging effects.

† It is clear from Figure 7.7 that the path is unique in both heating and cooling; that is, there exists transition temperature hysteresis. For most Nitinol alloys used in medical applications, this hysteresis is around 20°C to 30°C.

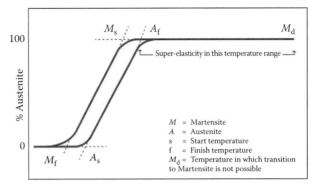

FIGURE 7.7 (See color insert.) Phase transformation and hysteresis in a shape memory alloy.

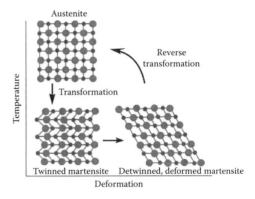

FIGURE 7.8 (See color insert.) Atomic structure in a shape memory alloy through transformation and reverse transformation.

for Nitinol are guided by ASTM F2063-05. In its austenitic phase, the mechanical behavior of Nitinol is similar to a β-titanium alloy with low work hardening and ductility. In its martensitic phase, deformation occurs via the movement of twin boundaries, accommodating large strains with low stress. At the end of its superelastic range, martensitic NiTi will deform in a conventional manner. Fatigue life prediction for Nitinol alloys is extremely difficult owing to the nonlinear stress–strain response and the stress-induced phase transformations.

Nickel release owing to corrosion may induce allergic response, cellular hypersensitivity, cytotoxicity, and genotoxicity. Nitinol forms a passive titanium oxide layer that resists corrosion, and further surface modifications can reduce the nickel release rate to below normal daily Ni intake. Clinical cytotoxicity has been shown to be comparable to other implantable alloys. Some current orthopaedic uses of Nitinol include

Table 7.8 Platinum and platinum-base alloys, nitinol, tantalum, and magnesium: composition and mechanical properties

Property	Pt (99.85%)	Pt101r	55-Nitinol (austenite)	55-Nitinol (martensite)	Tantalum	Magnesium
Tensile modulus (Y, GPa)	147	#	120	50	186	41
Ultimate strength (σ_u, min, MPa)	152 a	275 a / 485 cw	690–1380	–	285 a / 650 cw	86.8 ac
Strain to failure (ϵ_u, min, %)	35 a	35 a	13–40	<60	30 a / 5 cw	13 ac

Note: a, Annealed; cw, cold worked; ac, as cast; #, not reported, similar to Pt.

spinal correction rods, fracture fixators, and compression staples, while other widely used applications include cardiovascular stents.

Tantalum

Tantalum is a refractory metal that has found some use as a medical material in vascular ligation clips, arterial stents, wire mesh, and sutures. It is the material's physical resemblance to cancellous bone in terms of porosity and stiffness that has shown the greatest potential for orthopaedic use. The material is an excellent surface for integration with bone and soft tissue. Zimmer currently markets a tantalum "Trabecular Metal" as a surface material to promote bone ingrowth for total joint arthroplasty components and as a scaffold for biologic ingrowth (Figure 7.9). Trabecular metal is a metallic strut configuration that is similar to trabecular bone, which ideally makes it conductive to direct bone apposition. Tantalum's high strength-to-weight ratio, low stiffness in a porous state, and high coefficient of friction facilitate physiologic load transfer and minimize stress shielding. It is noted that tantalum is not the only alloy used for porous coatings, as titanium and titanium alloys, magnesium and magnesium alloys, and cobalt–chromium alloys have all found use as porous metal matrices.

Tantalum has a body-centered cubic α-phase and a meta-stable tetragonal β-phase that rarely exists in the bulk form. In its α-phase, tantalum is characterized as being hard, dense, and very ductile. It has a passive oxide surface (Ta_2O_5) that has a high resistance to chemical attack in the physiological environment, leading to a very high resistance to corrosion. It is also considered good in the soft tissue environment as it is nonferromagnetic and thus will not displace, rotate, or heat up during MRI diagnostic scanning. Tantalum coatings are typically fabricated through pyrolysis of a thermosetting polymer foam. Pure tantalum deposited on the surface of a vitreous carbon skeleton using chemical vapor deposition. The resulting composition of the structure is 99% tantalum, 1% vitreous carbon by weight. Average pore sizes of 400 µm to 600 µm are typical.

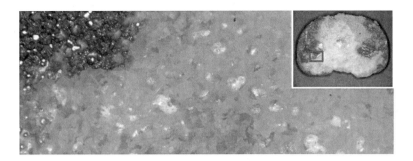

FIGURE 7.9   (See color insert.) Microscopic view of bone ingrowth on a tantalum tibial knee component.

Mechanical properties

Tantalum, along with other refractory metals, including tungsten and molybdenum, are characterized by their very high melting points. They are highly corrosion resistant under *in vivo* conditions and have excellent mechanical properties. Comparatively, it has been reported that tantalum has greater volume porosity, a lower bulk stiffness, and a higher coefficient of friction with bone when compared to similar porous foam materials. The characterization of tantalum is guided by ASTM F560-08, which covers the chemical, mechanical, and metallurgical requirements for unalloyed tantalum plate, sheet, strip, rod, and wire for the manufacture of surgical implants. Table 7.8 gives the basic mechanical properties for tantalum. Chapter 13 discusses the properties of porous tantalum, including typical porosity, modulus of elasticity, compressive strength, and coefficient of friction of tantalum in comparison to other porous materials.

Magnesium

Magnesium has the unique capability to biodegrade *in vivo* through the mechanism of surface pitting corrosion. The intended application for Mg is as a temporary supportive structure, in the form of biodegradable metal bone fixtures or bone scaffolds. The earliest recording of magnesium as an implant material was in 1907, when a French surgeon named Lambotte used the material to fixate a lower leg fracture. Currently, Mg is being used in cardiovascular stents and fracture fixation devices. Viable fabrication methods include plaster casting with polyurethane foam and powder metallurgy with space holding particles.

Unlike corrosion in other common biomaterials, corrosion products of Mg have minimal caustic effects and are non-toxic. Magnesium is essential to the human metabolism. It is found naturally in bone tissue and required for healthy skeletal development and maintenance. The body is capable of tolerating large amounts of Mg without toxicity, and excess ions are excreted through urine with no known damage to the liver or kidneys. It has even been proposed that Mg may have an effect of stimulating new bone growth by enhancing osteoblastic activity around the implant.

Its corrosion resistance and mechanical properties can be improved through alloying and surface treatments. Mg alloying elements include Zn, Mn, Al, Ca, Li, Zr, Y, Cu, GD, Ni, Nd, and rare earth. Corrosion can be increased when elements Fe, Ni, and Cu are present, all of which are common impurities found within refined Mg. Alloying with Zn, an essential trace mineral, can increase its yield strength and potentially reduce the risk of hydrogen gas evolution. Copper can increase the strength of an Mg alloy but it is unclear about the cytotoxicity of excessive amounts of copper. Manganese can improve corrosion resistance by reducing corrosion potential caused by impurities such as Fe (Mn separates Fe and Mg). Like Mg, Mn is an essential mineral, though excessive amounts may lead to neurological disorders.

There still remain a number of challenges to the widespread use of Mg for orthopaedic applications. Controlling the corrosion rate in electrolytic, aqueous environments when chloride is present can be difficult. Excessive corrosion can cause any implant to lose mechanical integrity early. In some cases, the implant may not retain sufficient strength through the healing process. Compounding the problem of strength, alloys currently in use tend to be relatively brittle. Alloying is one avenue to affect the corrosion rate, though there are limits in element selection owing to potential systemic affects. New processing techniques also continue to be developed to improve upon the materials' ductility.

Perhaps more problematic is the production of hydrogen gas as a byproduct of the reaction with aqueous solution, attributed to the high oxidative corrosion rates of Mg. This may increase the pH locally and lead to the formation of potentially harmful hydrogen pockets, which can overwhelm the host response and increase the potential for gas gangrene when corrosion is too fast. The clinical effect of hydrogen evolution on the local tissue response is still uncertain.

Mechanical properties

Magnesium is an exceptionally lightweight material with approximately one-third the density of titanium. As a bioabsorbable material, it has a distinct advantage in that it is on average over twice as strong as most polymers. Its primary advantage is in its reduced stiffness which may minimize risks from stress shielding in load-bearing implants, as it has a modulus that is about half that of titanium. Table 7.8 gives the basic mechanical properties for magnesium. Material properties for porous Mg are discussed in Chapter 13.

Platinum-base alloys

Platinum-base alloys are not used for device fabrication because of their high cost, but they are used as electrodes in electrical stimulation apparatus, for example, in faradic stimulation of bone growth. They are popular for this application since they are highly corrosion resistant with good mechanical properties. Platinum may be used by itself or alloyed with 1–10 w/o of rhodium or iridium. The composition and mechanical properties of pure platinum and of a common alloy are given in Table 7.8.

TRIP steels

There is a continuing interest in alternative alloys for orthopaedic applications. The principal driving forces are the designers' wishes for improved properties, especially in fatigue; the manufacturers' concerns over limiting costs, both of raw materials and of manufacturing processes; and the researchers' concerns over the biologic activity of components of present alloys. TRIP (transformation-induced plasticity) steels are a class of steels that may be cold worked after heat treatment to produce significantly higher strengths for a given degree of work hardening while retaining greater ductilities than can be achieved in austenitic stainless steels. Unfortunately, they have somewhat higher corrosion rates than stainless steels; additional alloy improvements will be necessary before clinical use.

Fatigue strength

The typical orthopaedic application may be characterized as involving low-stress, high-cycle fatigue loading. Thus, the fatigue behavior of implant alloys has taken on great importance. The endurance limit is frequently defined as the *residual strength* (alternate term for fatigue strength) after 10^7 load–unload cycles. Since a typical lower extremity device experiences 1 to 2 million cycles per year, this reflects 5–10 years of service and has come to be a routine comparative measure of fatigue behavior. Table 7.9 is a tabulation of the fatigue strength limits for some of the alloys previously discussed.

These values should be interpreted with some caution as they are somewhat test dependent and are *all* measured in air. The fatigue resistance superiority of titanium and its alloys becomes clearer in corrosive environments: under these conditions, as *in vivo*, the ratio of σ_f/σ_u tends to fall for stainless steels and cobalt-base alloys but is essentially unaffected for titanium-base alloys.

Trade names

Table 7.10 gives a compilation of past and current trade names for orthopaedic alloys, their manufacturer's names, and the ASTM standards that they meet. Although two alloys that meet the same standard may have very similar compositions, a fairly wide range of properties is possible since different starting material purities, manufacturing techniques, and finishing techniques, especially different degrees of cold work, different annealing cycles, and different surface treatment methods, all contribute to a broad range of possible mechanical properties in any one system. However, there are no clear "winners"; each manufacturer has had to develop his material types to suit their designs and vice versa, so that performance is satisfactory and failure rates are acceptably low.

Table 7.9 Fatigue strength of orthopaedic alloys

Material	Ultimate strength (MPa)	Fatigue strength (10^7 cycles, $R = -1$) (MPa)	σ_f/σ_u
Stainless alloys			
F 55 a	480	240	0.5
F 55 cw	655	310	0.47
Ortron 90 a	834	459	0.55
Ortron 90 cw	1035	640	0.62
Co-base alloys			
F 75 c	793	310	0.39
F 75 pm	1300	765	0.61
F 75 f	1400	793	0.56
F 90 f	860	485	0.56
F 90 pm, f	1240	825	0.6
F 562 cw	1200	500	0.42
F 799 f	1400	900	0.64
Ti and Ti-base alloys			
F 67 af	550	240	0.44
F 136 f, a	985	520	0.53

Note: a, Annealed; af, as fabricated; cw, cold worked; pm, powder metal-lurgical; f, forged; data from various sources, all in air.

Modification of surface geometry

Current interest in the replacement of poly(methyl methacrylate) bone cements with implant fixation by direct biologic means has led to the development of numerous techniques to modify the surfaces of ortho-paedic implants. There are four principal types of surface structural modification in use in implant fabrication today (some are in routine use; others are still in the pre-market approval stage).

Cast structures. Devices that are cast may easily have a grooved, pebbled, or beaded surface formed during initial fabrication. The advantage of such surfaces is that they have the same composition and properties of the base material; the disadvantage is that they must have very simple geometry with no real possibility for internal porosity (Figure 7.10).

Sintered structures. Cast and forged devices may have a surface coating attached by sintering. This involves placing beads or particles in close approximation to the surface and then heating both components to produce diffusion bonds, both within the coating and between the coating and the surface. This is the most popular

Table 7.10   Trade names of orthopaedic alloys

Trade name[a]	Base	ASTM Type	Manufacturer	Comment
Alivium	Co	F 75	Biomet	
Biophase	Co	F 562	Richards	
CoCroMo	Co	F 75	Biomet	
Endocast SL	Co	F 75	Krupp	No Ni
Francobal	Co	F 75	Benoist-Girard	
Isotan	Ti	F 136	Aesculap-Werke	
Metasul	Co		Zimmer	
Multiphase MP35N	Co	F 562	Latrobe Steel	
Orthochrome	Co	F 75	DePuy	
Orthonox	Fe		Howmedica, UK	Low O_2
Ortron 90	Fe		Chas. F. Thackray	
Protosul 2	Co	F 75	Sulzer	Cast
Protosul 10	Co	F 562	Sulzer	Forged
Protosul 64WF	Ti	F 136	Sulzer	
Syntacoben	Co	F 563	?	Wrought
Tilastan	Ti	F 136	Waldemar Link	
Tivaloy 12	Ti	F 136	Biomet	ELI grade
Tivanium	Ti	F 136	Zimmer	
Trabecular metal	Ta		Zimmer	
Tritanium	Ti		Stryker	
Vinertia	Co	F 75	Deloro	
Vitallium-C	Co	F 75	Howmedica	Cast
Vitallium-FHS	Co	F 75	Howmedica	Forged
Vitallium-W	Co	F 90	Howmedica	Wrought
Zimaloy	Co	F 75	Zimmer	
Zimaloy Micro-grain	Co	F 75	Zimmer	PM type
TiOsteum	Ti	F 136	ATI Allvac	Low Modulus

[a]   Registered trademarks; not to be used as common names.

technique in use today and permits fabrication of structures with wide ranges of bead or particle size and internal porosity.

Direct coatings. It is possible to apply a surface coating directly, without significant substrate heating, by a variation of a welding process. In this technique, called *plasma spraying* or plasma coating, a stream of particles is "sprayed" on the surface in a protective high-temperature gas stream. The particles partially melt and are very rapidly chilled when they contact the surface, but not before welding to it. This process is very difficult to control and may be used successfully only with certain selected alloys. However, it can produce a coating with a very high specific surface area that may closely resemble cancellous bone in structure and produces minimal heat-related property changes in the base material.

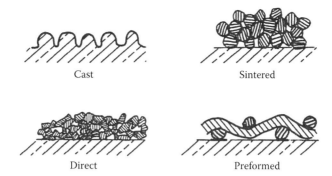

Cast   Sintered

Direct   Preformed

FIGURE 7.10   Surface structures.

> *Preformed structures.* The last approach has been to form pads of
> material, either in a random mesh or felt or in an orderly woven
> structure, and then to bond the resulting "preform" to the surface
> by diffusion. This approach has the advantage over a pure sintering
> process in that the resulting coatings may be made much stronger,
> and shorter periods at high temperature are required, thus better
> preserving the properties of the base material. A design disadvan-
> tage is the difficulty in coating complexly shaped surfaces.

These surface structural modification processes have profound consequences on the behavior of the finished device for two reasons.

1. The interface between the surface structure and the base material
   produces regions of stress concentration, greatly degrading fatigue
   resistance. This effect may be reduced by careful design and control of processing but cannot be eliminated.

2. Thermal requirements of the processes for surface structure formation may severely degrade the properties of the base material.
   This is especially pronounced in the use of sintering for which temperatures must be maintained at a high level to permit sufficient
   diffusion between substrate and coating for adequate bonding.

It appears experimentally that all surface structural modification
reduces fatigue resistance. This reduction has been reported to be up to
75% in some materials systems. Significant design and process development efforts are under way to reduce this effect to an absolute minimum,
but it will continue to be with us for the foreseeable future.

Comparison of orthopaedic alloys

It is clear that composition, properties, and processing of these alloys
vary widely. It is difficult to make generic comparisons because of the
previously stated close relationship between mechanical design and
selection of materials. However, as a general guide, Table 7.11 presents

Table 7.11   Comparison of properties of orthopaedic alloys

Property	Stainless steel	Co-base	Ti-base	Pt-base
Modulus	2	1	4	3
Yield strength	2	1	2	3
Ultimate strength	1	1	2	3
Endurance limit	3	2	1	4
Ductility	1	3	4	2
Machinability	1	4	2	3
Corrosion resistance	4	3	2	1
Cost	4	3	2	1

Note: 1 = highest, 4 = lowest. When the same number appears more than once in the same row, ranges overlap.

relative alloy system ratings with respect to some principal design considerations.

Additional problems

PROBLEM 7.2

In comparison to polymers, metal alloys (true or false)

1. Are stiffer
2. Are less dense
3. Are more ductile
4. Have higher melting points
5. Have a greater variety of fabrication techniques

ANSWER:

T, F, F, T, T.

PROBLEM 7.3

Rank cortical bone (CRB), titanium alloy (Ti), bone cement (BC), and cast stainless steel (SS) in *increasing* order of

A. Elastic modulus
B. Ductility
C. Strength

ANSWER:

A. BC, CRB, Ti, SS
B. CRB, BC, Ti, SS
C. BC, CRB, SS, Ti

PROBLEM 7.4

Compared with stainless steels and cobalt-base alloys, pure titanium is (select the best answer[s])

A. Relatively flexible

B. Weaker

C. Heavier

D. Easier to machine into complex shapes

E. Nonelastic

ANSWER:

A (poor term, but refers to modulus). Titanium has a higher σ_u than cast stainless steel (not *B*), is less dense than either stainless steel or cobalt-base alloys (not *C*), is relatively difficult to machine (not *D*), and is obviously elastic (not *E*).

PROBLEM 7.5

The most important theoretical advantage of titanium alloy over stainless steel internal fracture fixation plates is (select the best answer[s])

A. Titanium alloys are lighter than stainless steel.

B. Fracture healing rates are somewhat improved by the use of titanium alloy plates.

C. Titanium alloy plates are considerably less costly.

D. There is less bone loss under titanium alloy plates during healing and remodeling.

E. Greater screw torque and therefore better fixation stability can be achieved with titanium alloy parts.

ANSWER:

It has been reported that less rigid plates, within limits, do produce less resorption and remodeling in an animal model (Moyen BJ-L, Lahey PJ Jr, Weinberg EH, Harris WH: Effects on intact femora of dogs of application and removal of metal plates. A metabolic and structural study comparing stiffer and more flexible plates. *Bone Joint Surg* 60A:940–947, 1978); thus, *D* is the best answer. Titanium is lighter than stainless steel, but this apparently does not affect fracture healing (not *A*). A large comparative clinical study between stainless steel and titanium alloy plates (Holzach P, Matter P: The comparison of steel and titanium dynamic compression plates used for internal fixation of 256 fractures of the tibia. *Injury* 10:120–123, 1978) showed no advantage in healing time for titanium (not *B*). Titanium alloy components are typically two to three times the cost of stainless steel ones (not *C*). Maximum achievable screw torque depends on bone strength rather than on the metal used, given an adequate screw design (not *E*).

PROBLEM 7.6

The relative disadvantage of annealed cast stainless steel as an implant material is that it (select the best answer[s])

A. Has a low elastic modulus

B. Deforms plastically at low stress

C. Has poor ductile properties

D. Has too high an elastic modulus

E. Has an ultimate strength below standards

ANSWER:

Fully annealed cast stainless steel has the lowest yield stress of any implant alloy. This produced varus deformation in the stems of early THR devices, leading to increased bending moments and stem fatigue failure; thus, *B* is the best answer. All implant alloys have moduli well above that of bone; this must be accounted for in design (not *A* or *D*). Fully annealed stainless steel may have greater than 50% ductility (not *C*). An individual part may have strength "below standards," owing to poor manufacture; however, there are no categorical standards for minimum strength of implant materials (not *E*).

PROBLEM 7.7

A 14-year-old girl is treated for a distal femoral osteosarcoma by en bloc excision of the distal third of the femur followed by prosthetic reconstruction of the knee 1 year later. The best metal for the prosthesis would be

A. Cast stainless steel

B. Wrought stainless steel

C. Cast cobalt-base alloy

D. Pure titanium

E. HIP cobalt-base alloy

ANSWER:

One cannot say categorically which metal alloy would be best for this application, in absence of design details. Alloys *C* and *E* would probably be satisfactory, *B* would be marginal, and *A* and *D* would not be recommended.

PROBLEM 7.8

Phase diagrams (true or false)

1. Predict ductility

2. Allow calculations of time and temperature required for alloy heat treatment

3. Permit determination of possible phase structures

4. Permit calculation of melting points

5. Predict corrosion rates

ANSWER:

F, F, T, T, F.

PROBLEM 7.9

A vertical line on a phase diagram connects points with _____ weight composition (fill in the blank).

ANSWER:

Identical.

PROBLEM 7.10

Match the following terms (when possible):

1. Aging	A. Casting technique
2. Martensite	B. Ti–Al phase
3. Passivation	C. Fe–C phase
4. Annealing	D. Heat treatment
5. Duplex	E. Grain structure

ANSWER:

1, *D*; 2, *C*; 4, *D*; 5, *E* (there are no matches for 3, *A* and *B*).

Annotated bibliography

1. BANSIDDHI A, SARGEANT TD, STUPP SI, DUNAND DC: Porous NiTi for bone implants: A review. *Acta Biomater* 4:773–782, 2008.
   A thorough review of the fabrication, biocompatibility, *in vitro* studies, and implant applications of porous NiTi.

2. DOBBS HS, ROBERTSON JLM: Alloys for orthopaedic use. *Eng Med* 11(4):175–182, 1982.
   A good, easy-to-understand study of the effects of processing on properties of cobalt-base and titanium-base implant alloys.

3. DUERIG T: Shape memory alloys. In Narayan R (ed): *ASM Handbook, Volume 23, Materials for Medical Devices*. ASM International, 2012.
   History, metallurgy, and properties of nitinol.

4. ENGEL L, KLINGELE H: *An Atlas of Metal Damage*. Prentice-Hall, Englewood Cliffs, NJ, 1981.
   Chapter 1 deals very briefly with structure of metals. Chapters 2–4 are given over to scanning electron microscopic views of manufacturing and service-produced defects.

5. HAYDEN HW, MOFFATT WG, WULFF J: *The Structure and Properties of Materials*. Vol. III. John Wiley & Sons, New York, 1964.

  Chapter 8 is a brief but clear discussion of strengthening mechanisms.

6. LAMPMAN S: Titanium and its alloys for biomedical implants. In Narayan R (ed): *ASM Handbook, Volume 23, Materials for Medical Devices*. ASM International, 2012.

  A good synopsis of the properties of many Ti alloys available for medical device use.

7. LEVINE BR, SPORER S, POGGIE RA, DELLA VALLE CJ, JACOBS JJ: Experimental and clinical performance of porous tantalum in orthopaedic surgery. *Biomaterials* 27:4671–4681, 2006.

  A review of the basic science, mechanical, and biologic properties of porous tantalum.

8. LUCKEY HA, KUBLI F, JR (eds): *Titanium Alloys in Surgical Implants*. STP 796. American Society for Materials and Testing, Philadelphia, 1982.

  Refereed papers drawn from a 1981 conference; includes a good cross section of discussions of both titanium-base and cobalt-base alloy fabrication and properties.

9. MOFFATT WG, PEARSALL GW, WUIFF J: *The Structure and Properties of Materials*. Vol. I. John Wiley & Sons, New York, 1964.

  Chapters 6–8 deal with phase structures in metals and the design and use of phase diagrams. Easy to follow.

10. NARAYAN R: Medical applications of stainless steels. In Narayan R (ed): *ASM Handbook, Volume 23, Materials for Medical Devices*. ASM International, 2012.

  Physical and mechanical properties of numerous SS alloys, along with a good discussion of the effect of surface treatments on properties.

11. NASSER S: TANTALUM. In Narayan R (ed): *ASM Handbook, Volume 23, Materials for Medical Devices*. ASM International, 2012.

  Properties and applications for tantalum in medical devices.

12. NIINOMI M, NAKAI M AND HIEDA J: Development of new metallic alloys for biomedical applications. *Acta Biomaterialia* 8(2012):3888–3903.

  An overview of recent advanced research in metallic implant materials. Of particular interest for orthopaedic applications are the low-modulus B alloys, improvements in shape memory alloys, and the emergence of resorbable magnesium- and iron-based alloys with mechanical properties that are superior to many resorbable polymers.

13. OLDANI C, DOMINGUEZ A: Titanium as a biomaterial for implants. In Fokter S (ed): *Recent Advances in Arthroplasty*. ISBN: 978-953-307-990-5, InTech, 2012.

  A good review of various titanium alloys for potential use in orthopaedic implants.

14. PILLIAR R, RAMSAY SD: Cobalt-base alloys. In Narayan R (ed): *ASM Handbook, Volume 23, Materials for Medical Devices*. ASM International, 2012.

  Commonly used cobalt alloys, their properties, applications, and processing.

15. PILLIAR RM, WEATHERLY GC: Developments in implant alloys. *CRC Crit Rev Biocompat* 1(4):371–403, 1986.

  A contemporary review, with an extensive bibliography, emphasizing the role of details of metallurgical structure in producing properties.

16. SEAL CK, VINCE K, HODGSON MA: Biodegradable surgical implants based on magnesium alloys—A review of current research. In *Processing, Microstructure and Performance of Materials, IOP Conf. Series: Materials Science and Engineering* 4, 2009.

  A discussion of the potential and challenges of applying Mg-based materials for biomedical applications.

17. SEMLITSCH M: Metallic implant materials for hip joint endoprostheses designed for cemented and cementless fixation. In Morscher E (ed): *The Cementless Fixation of Hip Endoprostheses.* Springer-Verlag, Berlin, 1984.

A review of the properties of metallic implant alloys by an investigator who has been involved in optimizing many of them. Very clear comparative bar charts of mechanical properties.

18. SHARMA D, McGORAN A: Bioedegradable magnesium alloys: A review of material development and applications. *J Biomim Biomater Tissue Eng* 12:25–39, 2012.

A review of potential alloying elements for Mg-based medical applications.

19. STAIGER MP, PIETAK, AM, HUADMAI J, DIAS, G: Magnesium and its alloys as orthopaedic biomaterials: A review. *Biomaterials* 27:1728–1734, 2006.

A review of the biological and mechanical properties of magnesium, along with discussion of its potential applications.

20. TARNITA D, TARNITA DN, BIZDOACA N, MINDRILA I, VASILESCU M: Properties and medical applications of shape memory alloys. *Romanian J Morphology Embryology* 50:15–21, 2009.

A basic discussion of shape memory behavior, along with a review of current clinical applications in orthopaedics and trauma.

21. THOMPSON SA: An overview of nickel–titanium alloys used in dentistry. *Int Endodontic J* 33:297–310, 2000.

An excellent conceptual description of the structure of nickel titanium, its phase transformations, and superelasticity and shape memory properties.

CHAPTER EIGHT

Ceramics and composites

Ceramics, as a class, tend to be defined by exclusion. The classes of materials called metals on the one hand and polymers on the other hand are easy to determine, both by the predominant interatomic bonding mechanism and by class properties (mechanical, electrical, etc.). Ceramics are primarily those essentially homogeneous materials left out of the previous two classes.

The word *ceramic* comes from the Greek *keramos* meaning "burnt stuff" or, more generally, pottery. The classical definitions state that ceramics are composed of inorganic, nonmetallic materials. A traditional list of ceramic materials would include abrasives, bricks, cement, enamels, nonmetallic ferromagnetic materials, gem stones both natural and artificial, glasses, plaster, and porcelain as well as pottery. A modern list would add glassy and vitreous carbons, graphites, and nonmetallic single-crystal filaments. More formally, ceramics can be classified within the following five types: glass, plasma-sprayed polycrystalline ceramic, vitrified ceramic, solid-state sintered ceramic, and polycrystalline glass ceramic.

There are a few features common to all of these materials. Most ceramics contain one or more metallic oxide or other compounds and are generally dominated by ionic bonds. They may be crystalline—either single crystals or polycrystalline—and may contain a glassy phase, reminiscent of polymers, but made up of inorganic chains, most commonly silicon dioxide (SiO_2). Such inorganic polymerizable materials are often called *glass formers*. As a class, ceramics are stiff, hard, brittle, and water insoluble. However, there are so many exceptions to each of these attributes that they are not unique identifiers.

The interest in ceramics as candidate biomaterials stems from several origins, as will be seen later in this chapter. However, efforts to use some of their desirable properties, such as stiffness and strength, while minimizing their primary drawbacks, lack of plasticity and ductility, have led naturally to design of composite materials.

Properties of ceramic materials

General considerations

Ceramics are complex materials, in terms of both composition and structure, consisting of metallic oxides and other compounds and often combining multiple phases with different properties. The individual phases may be amorphous (glassy), polycrystalline, or single crystal, producing materials with mixed structures.

Processing is equally complex. Traditionally, ceramic materials are made in a four-step process:

1. *Compounding*, mixing and homogenizing primary materials into a water-based suspension, termed a *slurry*, or into a solid plastic water-containing mass, termed a *clay*.

2. *Forming* into parts by various physical means, including molding and casting.

3. *Drying*, usually in air but frequently with controlled humidity, into the so-called "green" or "leather" condition, for ease of handling. Because of the difficulty of machining the final product, most forming processes are performed at either the clay or leather stage.

4. *Firing* by heating in a furnace to drive off the remaining water, melt glassy phases, and foster grain growth. Firing usually produces shrinkage, so careful design is required for "engineering" parts that must have accurate final dimensions.

After firing, a limited variety of polishing and surface modification processes are possible. A second material, called a *glaze*, may be applied in a slurry and the part is refired at a lower temperature to produce a glassy surface finish.

There are too many variations of these steps to list here. Carbon materials are made by controlled oxidation of resin preforms. Single crystals may be "grown" by drawing a seed crystal out of a bath of molten material. Some materials, such as silicon carbide, are grown directly from a vapor phase in a high-temperature furnace or a vacuum furnace.

Ceramic materials share a propensity for containing impurities, since the starting materials are usually reacted elements derived from natural mineral or plant sources and rarely achieve theoretical density, owing to inclusion of internal porosity. Thus, there has been a difficulty in developing materials that are sufficiently pure and strong for surgical implant applications. During *chemical processing*, the required compounds are formed from pure elements or compounds, processed into a gel, and then converted to a solid by thermal treatment. In addition to having much higher purities, chemically processed ceramics may be made at almost theoretical density, thus overcoming the problems of porosity in materials fabricated by older, conventional techniques.

Ceramic materials intended for surgical implant applications are further classified in two ways: by their microstructure and by their material response to implantation.

As previously stated, structurally, these materials are termed glassy (or vitreous), polycrystalline, or single crystal. In general, high-density polycrystalline materials, with small, controlled-size crystallites, are the strongest and toughest, but defect-free single crystals may be stronger, if they lack notch sensitivity.

The following terms are used to describe material response (to implantation):

Nonresorbable (or "bioinert"): Essentially unaffected by chemical effects of implantation.

Reactive (or "bioactive"): React with the local host environment to produce altered surface properties, which may elicit a desired host response.

Resorbable (or "bioresorbable"): Dissolve with time in vivo. For reasons discussed in more detail later (see Chapter 12), the compound "bio-" form terms are unsatisfactory and should be avoided in common usage; none of these material responses are apparently cell mediated.

Inert ceramics

Ceramics currently used in orthopaedic applications include alumina (Al_2O_3), zirconia (ZrO_2), and hydroxyapatite $Ca_{10}(PO_4)_6(OH)_2$. Hydroxyapatite is a reactive ceramic and will be discussed in the next section. Alumina and zirconia, on the other hand, are both bioinert and are continuing to find use as articulating components in hip arthroplasty for select patient profiles. Both of these ceramics have enormous potential to reduce wear rates relative to metallic and polymeric articulating surfaces, though they also carry risks of sudden fracture that are the focus of continual improvement in the materials and design. Intolerable squeaking is also a risk with ceramic implants, which has been attributed to edge loading, potentially from malpositioning of the implant and other causes, such as rim design.

Alumina. High-density alumina (Al_2O_3) is a fine-grained polycrystalline ceramic that has found use for load-bearing prosthesis for large joint arthroplasty over the last 30 years. The material, standardized in 1984 (ISO 6474), is produced by sintering alumina powder at temperatures between 1600°C and 1800°C. A small amount (<0.5%) of magnesia (MgO) is added to limit grain growth during sintering. The advantages to alumina include its good biocompatibility, high hardness, and low coefficient of friction, leading to exceptionally low wear rates in arthroplasty devices. The low coefficient of friction for alumina and other ceramics is attributed to its hydrophilic surface, high wettability, and fluid-film lubrication capability. Linear wear rates of current-generation alumina-on-alumina total hip arthroplasty (THA) components are 4000 times lower than traditional metal-on-polyethylene components.

The use of alumina ceramics in orthopaedics is extensive, particularly in total hip replacements. This has been traced back to 1970 when the first all-ceramic total hip replacement prostheses were introduced in France. In the early 1980s, the US Food and Drug Administration approved the first ceramic hip (Mittelmeier); however, by the mid-1980s, it was no longer accepted clinically in the United States. This was attributed primarily to the high mechanical/fixation failure rates. Then, in the late 1980s, ceramic as an articulating surface came back into the United States in the form of a ceramic head combined with ultrahigh-molecular-weight polyethylene insert, as well as with metal-backed ceramic cups.

Alumina has a high compression strength but is considered to be somewhat limited in terms of its bending strength. Early generations of alumina components were subject to unacceptable fracture rates. Over time, the manufacturing techniques have improved the quality of alumina by increasing the density, reducing the size and "distribution" of the grains, decreasing the number of stress risers, and resultantly reducing the propagation of fractures. Manufacturing processes of alumina implants have also improved, including the use of laser markings instead of the earlier engraving method, which may have been a source of stress risers. Refinement of three-dimensional stress models also led to a better understanding of the trunnion taper designs and the various stress states in ceramic ball designs. In the mid-1990s, the hot-isostatic hipping process was introduced to ceramic implant technology, which increased its density, produced smaller grain size, and subsequently improved its mechanical properties. Currently, the fracture risk for the existing generation of alumina heads is less than 0.004%. Despite improvements in the material, fracture concerns continue to limit the use of alumina components in THA, with use depending on patient factors including age, activity level, and joint biomechanics.

Zirconium oxide. Zirconium oxide (ZrO_2) is an alternative for alumina ceramic in the search for a ceramic with improved strength, stiffness, and fracture toughness. ZrO_2 tetragonal zirconia polycrystals (TZPs) were introduced to the market in the late 1970s as a high-density, fine-grain-size, and high-purity ceramic. The toughness of zirconia is due to a unique phase change characteristic of the material. Naturally, zirconia is unstable with three different crystalline phases: monoclinic, tetragonal, and cubic. After manufacturing, and at high temperatures, zirconium oxide exists in its tetragonal phase featuring cubic lattices that will transform into the monoclinic phase upon cooling with an associated volume expansion. These phase changes will break down the material and can produce cracks. It is for this reason that the addition of oxides, such as yttria (Y_2O_3), calcium oxide (CaO), or magnesium oxide (MgO), is used to give zirconia a metastable state by maintaining the tetragonal phase through cooling to room temperature. Once stabilized, the lattice volume expansion associated with a change to the monoclinic structure is used to prevent crack propagation. As a crack tip hits a tetragonal grain, the metastable lattice is immediately transformed into a stable monoclinic phase, accompanied by the aforementioned volume expansion that will compress against the crack tip and dissipate its energy.

There is interest in a number of forms of zirconia, including stabilized zirconia, partially stabilized zirconia, yttria-stabilized TZP (Y-TZP), and zirconia-toughened alumina. Of these, fine-grain Y-TZP currently offers the best mechanical properties, including a strength and toughness that are twice that of alumina. Y-TZP was standardized in 1997 (ISO 13356). Zirconia can further be incorporated into alumina matrix (up to 25% ZrO_2), to act as a toughening agent, sometimes termed zirconia-toughened alumina. In a similar manner as Y-TZP, controlled phase transformation of zirconia particles stops subcritical crack propagation.

The major shortcomings with zirconia use for articulating bearing surfaces are due to degradation and aging through low-temperature phase transformation in wet environments, grain pullout, roughening, and poor wear properties. These materials are currently only recommended for use with ultrahigh-molecular-weight polyethylene (UHMWPE) liners, as ceramic–ceramic combinations with zirconia have shown very high wear rates. When paired with UHMWPE, wear rates, although one-half or less than that for metal–UHMWPE pairings, are still higher than articulations with alumina components. Mixed oxide ceramics are being developed with the aim of combining the mechanical properties of Y-TZP and the tribological properties of alumina. Currently, mixes of 25% to 80% zirconia have exhibited in vitro wear comparable to alumina.

An oxidized zirconium-layered countersurface on metallic bearing surfaces has also been developed for clinical use. This has resulted in enhanced abrasion resistance of metallic counterfaces. The processing method entails nitrogen ion implantation, thermally driven diffusion hardening, vapor deposition of an oxide surface, and transformation of the substrate metal surface into a ceramic layer. Use of an oxidized zirconium counterface has been shown to effectively reduce total knee arthroplasty wear in vitro. Analyses of explants have also shown less UHMWPE wear damage with a hardened scratch-resistant counterface compared to cobalt chrome.

Mechanical properties

As discussed in Chapter 3, ceramic materials as a class are extremely stiff and strong in compression but weak in tension, owing to their extreme brittleness. For this reason, the primary mechanical parameters used to describe them are the elastic modulus and the ultimate strength. The tensile elastic modulus (Young's) is usually given in engineering tables, although it is usually calculated from a four-point bending test and should more properly be called a *flexural* modulus. The compressive modulus may be assumed to be equal to the tensile modulus. The strength is usually reported as the *flexural* strength, again for ease of determination. This is usually close to the tensile strength and may be as little as 5%–10% of the compressive strength owing to the inherent brittleness of ceramics and the resultant sensitivity to structural defects.

Nonresorbable, or bioinert, materials are the only class of ceramics currently used in strictly structural or load-bearing applications in orthopaedics. Care must be taken during design to minimize the effects of their inherent notch sensitivity and to encourage upon them net compressive loading. Representative properties of some nonresorbable ceramics used in medical applications are given in Table 8.1. It must be stressed that these are *typical* values since both stiffness and strength depend strongly on small differences in composition, processing parameters, and final porosity.

As discussed previously, ceramics tend to behave in a brittle manner, and sudden fracture is a continual risk. Brittle materials are very

Table 8.1 Mechanical properties of some inert ceramic materials

Material	Density (g/cm^3)	Average Grain Size/ Crystallite Size	Tensile Modulus (GPa)	Flexural Strength (MPa)	Compressive Strength (MPa)	Fracture Toughness (K_{Ic}) (MPa·m$^{0.5}$)
Isotropic LTI carbon	1.5–2.2	3–4 nm	17–28	275–550	400	
Vitreous (glassy) carbon			24	170		
Silicon alloyed LTI carbon	2.0–2.2	3–4 nm	18–41	550–620		0.9–1.1
Aluminum oxide (>99.8%)	3.98	3.6 μm	380	595	4250	5–6
Zirconia	6.1	0.2 to 0.4 μm	210	1000	2000	7
Carbon–silicon carbide composite (50:50)	3.1		410	550	1000	4.6
Carbon–carbon fiber composite (30:70)			140	800	800	

sensitive to the flaw size and distribution in the material. In comparison, ductile materials can deform around microscopic stress concentrations, minimizing the contribution of flaws to fracture propagation. Brittleness as a property is characterized by the fracture toughness (K_{Ic}) of the material. A fracture in the material will occur if a stress intensity factor in a region of the material is larger than K_{Ic}. This stress intensity factor is calculated using the following equation:

$$K_I = Y\sigma a^{0.5}$$

where a is the size of initiating crack, σ is the region stress, and Y is a factor dependent on the crack shape and geometry of the part.

When K_I exceeds K_{Ic}, sudden crack propagation will occur. As a direct result, strength and fracture toughness of any sintered ceramic are dependent on grain size, porosity, and purity.

Further complicating matters, fracture loads for ceramics in vivo tend to be much less than those measured in static burst tests. It is thought that this is due to subcritical crack growth during the life of the implanted ceramic, which can begin as imperfections in the material or at the component surface. Glasses and ceramics are susceptible to stress-corrosion cracking, which can occur as water molecules cleave the metal–oxygen–metal bonds. In cases where stress-corrosion cracking is an issue, subcritical cracks will grow slowly above a threshold stress, K_{th}. (For alumina, this value has been reported to be 2.5 MPa·m$^{0.5}$.) As subcritical cracks grow, K_I will increase and lead to sudden fracture in the case that $K_I > K_{Ic}$.

Wear properties are particularly important for ceramics in THA applications, and generally it can be stated that they are directly dependent on the grain size of the material. Some grain sizes are also reported in Table 8.1.

Two composites are included in Table 8.1: carbon–silicon carbide (50:50) and carbon–carbon fiber (30:70). These are examples of ceramic–ceramic composites. They are discussed here since, unlike most composites, which are formed with the final part configuration in mind, these are frequently made as bulk materials and machined to shape.

Carbons and graphites, unlike most ceramics, may be fairly easily machined to close tolerances. Thus, both of these carbon matrix materials may be machined much like isotropic carbon, but possess superior mechanical properties as shown. They also have fatigue endurance limits that exceed 70% of their flexural strength and, in common with high-purity aluminum oxide, show extremely low wear rates against UHMWPE. Other carbon forms listed in Table 8.1 are more commonly used in the cardiovascular arena, but may have potential applicability in certain aspects of orthopaedics. Carbon materials are extremely tough compared to alumina, have a much higher strain to failure, and a very good wear resistance. The opportunities for incorporating carbon-based material into orthopaedics could certainly expand with changing technologies.

PROBLEM 8.1

Aluminum oxide is an unsuitable material for fabrication of fracture fixation hardware because

A. Its elastic modulus is too high

B. It displays no plastic deformation

C. It is difficult to machine

D. It will dissolve in vivo

E. It is a glassy material

ANSWER:

B and *C*. The modulus does not represent an intrinsic problem but does limit design choices. Aluminum oxide (Al_2O_3, also called *alumina*) may possibly release ions at a very low rate, especially if impure, but it is nonresorbable. It is a polycrystalline material.

Reactive ceramics The presence of a ceramic phase in bone (calcium hydroxyapatite; CaHAP or HA) accomodates attachment with collagen and external soft tissues. Given this character, it has been suggested that ceramic implants may be designed to bond with tissue. There have been a number of approaches to this idea.

Titanium. Although thought to be a metal, titanium should be considered a ceramic insofar as local host response is concerned, since it has a fairly uniform surface layer of TiO_2. Under certain controlled conditions, bonds will form in vivo between bone and high-purity titanium with appropriate surface preparation (passivation).

Tantalum. This is another metal with a surface layer of Ta_2O_5. Tantalum has been used as a surface coating, applied by a variety of techniques, and as high surface area porous material resembling cancellous bone. Its high strength, hardness, and cost rule out its use as a bulk implant material.

Hydroxyapatite. HA is a calcium phosphate ceramic having a close association with collagen in normal bone. Some workers report bond formation with bone; this depends apparently on HA grain size and purity and on the experimental model. In some cases, bone growth on or near implanted HA is more rapid than in association with control implants of similar composition or of metal. Thus, HA is commonly known as being "osteoinductive." This is probably incorrect; a better term might be "osteoconductive" since HA has not been shown to have any specific stimulating effect on osteoblasts as does bone morphogenetic protein or similar biologic molecules. Osteoconductive materials can encourage bone formation in an osseous environment, while osteoinductive materials can elicit bone formation in an extraosseous environment.

HA is currently used most extensively as a plasma spray coating on joint prosthesis. Its use here provides a solution for fixation without having to deal with complications from PMMA debris. It also provides a bone-conserving alternative to cement fixation. The consensus among studies is that bone ingrowth or ongrowth is enhanced with HA, though it is still uncertain whether HA improves fixation when compared to bone cement. HA may have some advantages over cement fixation in younger patients whereas cement fixation may provide improved fixation in more elderly, severely osteoporotic patients. The main drawbacks to HA are its brittle behavior and poor tensile strength, which have limited its applicability as a bone graft substitute.

There is a further caution necessary concerning the literature on HA and its biologic performance. Strictly speaking, HA is calcium hydroxyapatite, with the chemical formula $Ca_5(PO_4)_6(OH)_2$ and a Ca/P ratio equal to 1.67. "HA-type" materials used in research activities vary widely in composition, with Ca/P ratios as low as 1.5, and are rarely well characterized. These latter materials are usually mixtures of CaHAP and octacalcium phosphate, $Ca_8H_2(PO_4)6.5H_2O$, a more soluble ceramic. Thus, it is extremely hard to compare and rationalize the results of studies by different investigators.

Surface-active glass. A number of glasses and ceramic bodies with glassy phases have been developed that encourage direct bonding by bone and, in some cases, soft tissues after implantation. In some cases, the bond strength may exceed that of the adjacent bone. The necessary precursor to bonding is a surface reaction that releases Ca^{2+}, P^{4+}, and Na^+ ions and produces a water-rich gel on the implant surface. This gel is chemically inhomogeneous, usually presenting a silicon-rich surface layer over a calcium- and phosphorus-enriched underlayer.

The best known of these materials is Bioglass 45S5 (University of Florida, Gainesville, Florida), developed by L.L. Hench and coworkers. It contains SiO_2, P_2O_5, CaO, and Na_2O in a 45:6:24.5:24.5 weight percent (w/o) ratio. This is a glass, with no crystalline phase, but it may be combined with other less reactive materials to produce a glass phase–containing ceramic. Bioglass has not yet been used as a load-bearing material owing to its poor mechanical properties.

There are several known polycrystalline surface-active materials, the best known being Ceravital (E. Leitz, Wetzlar, FRG). This material has a similar composition to 45S5, but with more P_2O_5, less Na_2O, and the addition of K_2O and MgO. Recent innovations have seen the development of sol-gel processed glasses in the SiO_2–CaO–P_2O_5 system. These bioactive gel-glasses are hydrolyzed at ambient temperatures and have improved reactivity and degradability through an initial high specific surface area. They are currently being investigated as coatings on alumina implants. Osteoconductive properties of sol-gel processed glasses are similar to melt-derived glasses. Within this group of materials, apatite wollastenite glass ceramic ($CaOSiO_2$) is an alternative to Bioglass with increased mechanical strength.

Resorbable ceramics

There has been a continual fascination with the concept of providing a ceramic material for filling bony defects or augmenting bone healing that would be gradually resorbed and replaced by tissue and that would release only normal physiologic ions. Sterile plaster of Paris, sometimes called surgical plaster (($CaSO_4)_2$ *H_2O), has been used in this application since the 19th century, continuing up to today. It is usually preformed into fully hydrated ("set") pellets. However, it resorbs slowly and is relatively weak. Thus, there has been a continual search for an alternative material.

Most materials in development today are in the calcium–phosphorus system, with Ca/P ratios varying from 1 (brushite) to 1.5 (tricalcium phosphate), although others incorporate alumina and other nonresorbable or partially resorbable phases. The most exciting aspect of calcium phosphate–based materials is their excellent biocompatibility and compositional similarities to natural bone. Doping these ceramics with various metal ions has significantly influenced their properties. Resorbable bioactive silica–calcium phosphate nanocomposite (SCPC75) has been investigated as a novel controlled release carrier of antibiotics for the treatment of osteomyelitis. It is believed to be viable for eradicating infection and stimulating bone cell differentiation and new bone formation.

Composite materials

A *composite* (material) is a material in which two or more different phases are deliberately combined to obtain a material whose properties are a mixture or composite of those of the individual materials. Thus, carbon fibers may be placed in an epoxy matrix in an effort to obtain a material with strength and stiffness (from the fibers) combined with toughness and ductility (from the matrix). This is a common practice with ceramics owing to their brittle nature.

Although any materials may be combined into a composite, the most successful generic combination has been the ceramic reinforced polymer matrix composite (PMC). PMCs are usually referred to in the engineering literature as fiber-reinforced polymer composites or FRPs. This is undesirable as the reinforcing phase may be in other forms (granules, microspheres, whiskers, etc.) than fibers. These are widely used in industrial applications, appearing in consumer products such as tennis racquets, automobile body parts, and sailboat hulls. PMCs have been widely adopted in military applications, despite their high cost, because the combination of their high strength and toughness with their being lightweight can radically improve the performance of vehicles and airplanes historically fabricated almost entirely from metals.

Hydroxyapatite-reinforced high-density polyethylene is one example of a composite material that has been used clinically. A major concern with composite materials is the quality of mechanical properties found at the interfacial bond between the hydroxyapatite-reinforcing particles and the polyethylene. In nonmedical applications, various sizing or adhesive agents are used to improve the mechanical behavior of this interface. However, most of such agents provoke unsatisfactory local host responses; thus, the direct use of composites previously developed for other applications may not necessarily be suitable for biomedical tissue-contacting applications.

Properties of PMCs

General considerations

Composites gain their mechanical properties from a combination of the properties of the individual components (filler[s], matrix) and from interactions between these components. Although there are traditional combinations, such as glass fibers in epoxy, there are essentially an infinite number of possible composite materials. This complexity is further increased by the ability of the designer and engineer to vary composite properties in different parts of a component by altering the filler-to-matrix ratio and, in some cases, the internal orientation of the filler.

For this reason, and for two others, there are no "off the shelf" composites waiting for application to orthopaedic problems, as there have been in the case of metal alloys and polymer compositions. These additional reasons are as follows:

1. Most industrial composites are not designed for continuous service immersed in water.
2. Industrial composites contain large amounts of chemical agents (for priming, bonding, mold lubrication, sealing, etc.) such that might produce adverse host responses.

However, a number of matrix–filler combinations have been tried to a limited extent in implant applications (Table 8.2). As previously noted,

Table 8.2 Present composite applications in orthopaedics

Matrix	Filler	Application
Carbon	Carbon fiber	TJR[a] component
Epoxy	Graphite fiber	Fracture fixation plate, TJR component
UHMWPE	Carbon fiber (CH)[b]	TJR component
UHMWPE	HA	TJR component
Polylactic–polyglycolic acid	Carbon fiber	Partially resorbable fixation plate
Polymethyl methacrylate	Carbon fiber (CH)	Bone cement
Polytetrafluoroethylene	Carbon fiber (CH)	Porous TJR coating
Polyhydroxyethyl methacrylate	Polyethylene terephthalate	Tendon prosthesis
Silicone rubber	Polyaramid	Tendon prosthesis

[a] TJR, total joint replacement.
[b] Chopped (short staple) fiber.

there are challenges with reacting or bonding these phases/combinations together. Such bonding may be promoted by altering the surface texture of the filler and, in some cases, by introducing one of a very limited range of *coupling* agents—molecules that can react with both filler and matrix, such as silanes.

Thus, the composite designer must select materials from "scratch," as it were. Tables 8.3 and 8.4 present candidate matrices and fillers that

Table 8.3 Candidate matrices

Resin	Unfilled		30% S-glass fill	
	E (GPa)	σ_u (MPa)	E (GPa)	σ_u (MPa)
Epoxy	3.1	90		
Polyacetal	2.6	97	5.0[b]	103[b]
Polyamide	2.7	96	10.3	227
Polycarbonate	2.3	65	7.6	130
UHMWPE	0.9	39	5.5	62
Polyethylene terephthalate	2.4	59	9.2	160
Polymethyl methacrylate	2.8	90		
Polypropylene	1.2	41	4.5[a]	72[a]
Polypropylene oxide	2.5		8.3	
Polystyrene	3.1	49	6.6[b]	69[b]
Polysulfone	2.7	106	7.2	140
Polyvinyl chloride	0.3			
Polyetheretherketone	3.9	160	11	265

Note: Values are generic in flexion; actual individual resins may vary significantly in properties.

[a] 40% glass.
[b] 20% glass.

Table 8.4 Candidate fillers

Material	E (GPa)	σ (MPa)	E_f/E_m^a
Fibers			
Graphite (high E)	577	1725	192
Tungsten	400	4000	133
Alumina	380	1725	126
Zirconia	345	2050	125
Graphite (high σ)	250	2350	83
316L stainless steel	193	1000	64
Polyaramid (high E)	131	3800	45
Ti6Al4V	115	930	38
Titanium	115	280	38
S-glass[b]	86	4500	29
Aluminum	73	90	24
E-glass[c]	72	3500	24
Polyaramid (low E)	62	3800	21
Whiskers			
Carbon	980	21,000	327
Silicon carbide	840	11,000	280
Boron carbide	483	13,800	161
Alumina	429	20,700	142
Titania (alpha rutile)	380	4000	127
Silicon nitride	379	13,800	126
Aluminum nitride	320	5000	107

Note: Values are generic (in tension); actual individual materials may vary significantly in properties.

[a] $E_m = 3$ GPa.

[b] Composition: SiO_2, Al_2O_3, CaO; balance, 52–56:12–16:16–25:balance.

[c] Composition: SiO_2, Al_2O_3, MgO; balance, 65:25:10:trace.

are being considered for design of PMCs for orthopaedic applications. Table 8.3 includes typical values of flexural stiffness and strength with a 30% glass fiber fill for comparison. Note in Table 8.4 that whiskers have significantly higher values of tensile strength and stiffness than fibers. This is due to the relatively defect-free nature of whiskers; however, they are, in general, extremely brittle.

PMC fabrication

PMCs may be distinguished with respect to processing by whether their fillers are particulate (grain, whisker, short fiber, etc.) or continuous. PMCs with particulate fillers are fabricated in much the same way that polymeric components are (Figure 8.1; see also Figure 6.6), depending on whether the matrix is a thermoset or a thermoplastic. Three additional problems arise from the addition of the filler:

1. The fluid matrix must be able to "wet" the filler, that is, to form a stable phase interface. Matrix–filler combinations that do not meet this requirement will produce only extremely weak PMCs.

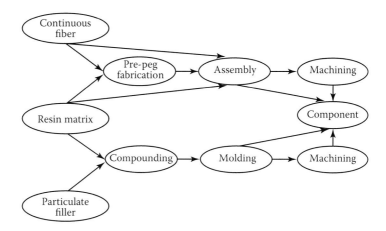

FIGURE 8.1   Processing of composites.

2. The filler must have a density near enough to that of the matrix that "settling" of the filler during processing does not occur. There is no firm rule for this; matrices with high viscosities and good wetting abilities may be successfully used in the face of large density differences.

3. The matrix–filler composition must be able to be processed. Addition of the filler to the matrix rapidly increases the viscosity of the mixture. Thus, some processes, such as injection molding, may become very difficult or impossible when large amounts of filler are used.

Continuous fiber fillers are used primarily with thermoset matrices, such as epoxies. It is the usual practice to form sheets with fibers in a single orientation, called *pre-pregs*, and then to combine the sheets as is called for in the design. The final body then may be machined, as in the production of screw holes in a fracture plate (Figure 8.2). Care must be taken with such steps, as they break fibers and may produce areas of relative weakness in the finished devices. One mode of failure of such devices is separation along pre-preg interfaces, called *delamination*, resulting from inadequate cohesion of the overall part.

Mechanical properties

There are many possible structures that a composite material may take, depending on the shape of the reinforcing phase (particles, fibers, etc.) and its spatial arrangement within the matrix. The simplest of these is a random arrangement of short fibers in a uniform matrix. The properties of such PMCs are difficult to predict exactly, but some indication may be obtained from examination of matrices with 10–30 volume percent (v/o) chopped S-glass filler. Table 8.3 provides a sampling of such data.

Although composite materials and structures must be tested for accurate determination of mechanical properties, mathematical analyses have been performed on a variety of defined structures with extremely complex and relatively accurate solutions derived for elastic moduli and failure strengths. The simplest solution, but one that illustrates most of

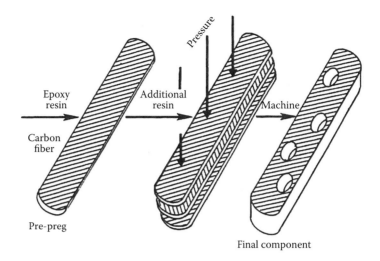

FIGURE 8.2   Fabrication of composite bone plate.

the important principles, is that for a composite consisting of parallel continuous fibers in a ductile matrix (Figure 8.3).

Such a composite has two different sets of mechanical properties, depending on whether the external loads are applied *parallel* to the fibers or *perpendicular* to them (in *serial*). In the following analysis, the following terms will be used:

V_f = the volume fraction of fiber in the composite

E_m, E_f, E_c = the tensile elastic moduli of the matrix, fiber, and composite (at some value of V_f), respectively

$\sigma_{u(f)}$, $\sigma_{u(m)}$ = the ultimate tensile strengths of the fiber and the matrix, respectively

σ_{max} = maximum strength of the composite (at some value of V_f)

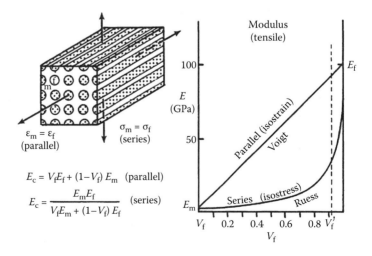

FIGURE 8.3   Tensile moduli of two-phase continuous fiber PMC.

Elastic modulus, "parallel" loading   The continuous fiber model with loading *parallel* to the fiber direction is called the *Voigt* model. So long as the fibers are intact, it is assumed that the *strain* will be *equal* in both phases; thus, this is also called an *isostrain* model.

In this case, the modulus of the composite is given by:

$$E_c = V_f * E_f + (1 - V_f)E_m$$

The dependence of E_c on V_f is shown in Figure 8.3 for a hypothetical case for which E_f = 100 GPa and E_m = 4 GPa. It can be seen that E_c increases linearly with increasing V_f. Such a relationship is often called a "law of mixtures" since the components of the "mixture" (in this case, the composite is a "mixture" of fiber and matrix) contribute to the overall property (in this case, elastic modulus) in proportion to their concentration. This is the case here, since V_f and $1 - V_f$ are the volume proportions of fiber and matrix, respectively, in the composite.

There is a limit on the ability of the fiber to stiffen the matrix. At some value of $V_f (= V_f')$, the fibers would come into contact and no more fibers could be added to the matrix. For a continuous parallel fiber composite, $V_f' = 0.907$. Practically, composites begin to lose their integrity as V_f approaches two-thirds of this value. Other shapes of reinforcing phases (discontinuous fibers, whiskers, spheres) possess lower values of V_f', down to as low as 0.5.

Elastic modulus, "perpendicular" loading   The continuous fiber model with loading *perpendicular* to the fiber direction is called the *Reuss* model. So long as the fibers are intact, it is assumed that the *stress* will be *equal* in both phases; thus, this is also called an *isostress* model. Since load passes alternately through matrix and fiber, this arrangement is a *series* configuration. There is an additional assumption that must be made in a series configuration: the interface between fiber and matrix is assumed to have the same failure strength as the weaker of the two phases (usually the matrix).

In this case, the modulus of the composite is given by:

$$E_c = \frac{E_f \cdot E_m}{V_f \cdot E_m + (1 - V_f)E_f}$$

The dependence of E_c on V_f is shown in Figure 8.3 for the same hypothetical case for which E_f = 100 GPa and E_m = 4 GPa. It can be seen that E_c increases almost linearly with increasing V_f (but less rapidly than for the Voigt model) for low values of V_f, but then increases very rapidly as V_f exceeds 0.5. This is difficult to see graphically at low values of V_f; thus, Table 8.5 provides calculated values of both the parallel (Voigt) and series (Reuss) moduli for the case shown in Figure 8.3. In addition, the ratio E_c/E_m expresses the proportional stiffening of the matrix by the fiber.

These two models, Voigt and Reuss, form an "envelope" for the tensile moduli of all composites. The values for other spatial configurations,

Table 8.5 Tensile moduli of model composite material

	Parallel (Voigt)		Series (Reuss)	
Volume fraction (V_f)	E_c (GPa)	E_c/E_m	E_c (GPa)	E_c/E_m
0.1	13.6	3.4	4.4	1.1
0.2	23.2	5.8	5.0	1.2
0.3	32.8	8.2	5.6	1.4
0.5	52.0	13.0	7.7	1.9
0.8	80.8	20.2	17.2	4.3
0.907($= V_f'$)	91.1	17.8	30.9	7.7

Note: $E_m = 4$ GPa; $E_f = 100$ GPa; $E_f/E_m = 25$.

with the same phase moduli as given here, will lie between the two curves shown in Figure 8.3.

Materials that possess mechanical properties dependent on the direction of loading are called *anisotropic* materials. A previous example is cortical bone (see Chapter 5). This is a natural composite, with a ductile matrix (collagen) and a brittle reinforcing phase (calcium HA). In fact, most tissues are composites; this is a primary source of their anisotropic mechanical behavior.

PROBLEM 8.2

What is the range of percent stiffening (compared with unreinforced matrix material) that can be displayed by composites fabricated from the fiber and matrix used to form the composite shown in Figure 8.3, for $V_f = 0.2$?

ANSWER:

20% to 480%. This may be obtained directly from Table 8.5 or calculated from the two equations given for the composite moduli of the Voigt and Reuss models.

Problem 8.2 illustrates both the great reinforcing ability of fibers or other fillers in low-modulus matrices and the range of options available to materials designers, even with a fixed value of V_f (constant chemical composition). In addition, both the values and the range of values increase rapidly as E_f/E_m increases. Actual engineering fibers and polymer matrices suitable for biomedical applications may produce combinations with this ratio as high as 350 (see Table 8.4). For this reason and others associated with failure and processing considerations, most composites have a V_f below 0.4, with a range of 0.1–0.2 being a common design target.

Strength It is extremely difficult to calculate the ductile and failure behavior of composites. In particular, the theoretical solutions are very much dependent on assumptions about the properties of the phase inter-face between filler and matrix, sometimes called the *mesophase*. Since the structure and mechanical properties of the mesophase are largely unknown for the vast majority of potential matrix–filler combinations, yield, maximum, ultimate, and fatigue strengths are usually determined experimentally, in the proposed operating environment.

One case that may be analyzed fairly easily illustrates the point that composite materials design, like all design processes, requires a "trade-off" in properties. This is calculation of the maximum tensile stress in the Voigt (parallel) model with a continuous fiber filler.

The result is strongly dependent on the ratio of fiber to matrix strength, $\sigma_{u(f)}/\sigma_{u(m)}$. For this example (see Figure 8.4), this ratio is chosen to be 4. The resulting strength has two ranges, defined by three relationships, depending on the value of V_f:

For $V_f \leq 1/(1 + \sigma_{u(f)}/\sigma_{u(m)})$:

$$\sigma_{max} = (1 - V_f)\sigma_{u(m)}$$

For $V_f > 1/(1 + \sigma_{u(f)}/\sigma_{u(m)})$:

$$\sigma_{max} = V_f\sigma_{u(f)}$$

For $0 < V_f < 1$:

$$\sigma_{u(c)} = (1 - V_f)\sigma_{u(m)}$$

These solutions produce the paradox that small amounts of a rein-forcing phase actually *weaken* a Voigt composite. This arises because the fibers are extremely brittle and fail at a low strain ($\varepsilon_{u(f)}$) at which the stress in the polymer is below $\sigma_{u(m)}$ (see Figure 8.4, lower left). Thus, until the fibers, by themselves, can sustain a greater load than a pure matrix ($V_f = 0$) component of the same external dimensions, they pro-duce a weakening rather than a strengthening effect. Although this effect is somewhat moderated by use of a ductile fiber (Figure 8.4, right

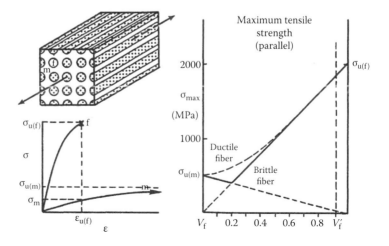

FIGURE 8.4   Maximum tensile strength of two-phase Voigt composite.

side, upper curve), it is often said that the strength of a composite is the strength of its *stronger* phase.

Stress–strain curve for a composite material   The result of the effects of the matrix and the fiber on composite strength may be seen in the stress–strain curve of a composite, as shown in Figure 8.5. The same matrix and fiber properties assumed in Figures 8.3 and 8.4 were used to construct this curve. For a composite with $V_f = 0.5$, at low strain, the curve is well behaved. However, when the strain exceeds $\varepsilon_{u(f)}$, fibers begin to fracture sequentially and the sustainable stress decreases. Finally, an ultimate stress is reached. This cannot exceed $(1 - V_f)\sigma_{u(m)}$ and may be much less if the matrix is notch sensitive. For the same reason, $\varepsilon_{u(c)}$ is usually less than $\varepsilon_{u(m)}$.

The point P marked on the stress–strain curve is one at which the stress has declined to approximately 80% of maximum with a strain approximately 50% greater than $\varepsilon_{u(f)}$. If the "modulus" is calculated continuously ($= \sigma/\varepsilon$) while the stress–strain curve is generated, it will be approximately 30% less here than in the initial elastic region. Since σ_{max} has been exceeded and significant numbers of fibers have broken, the decrease in instantaneous modulus (in this case, 30%) is often used as an indication of failure of composites, rather than $\sigma_{u(c)}$. This is particularly useful in fatigue studies during which the peak value of σ/ε is usually plotted continuously as a function of the number of load–unload cycles, and a predetermined modulus decrease, usually between 10% and 30%, is selected as a failure criterion.

It is clear that there are large numbers of trade-offs to be made in composite design. Is maximum stiffness required? Is maximum strength required? What is the minimum toughness? And so forth. Combined with anisotropy effects, it is obvious that composites must be designed for each application and cannot be kept "on the shelf" in the manner of more conventional metallic and polymeric materials.

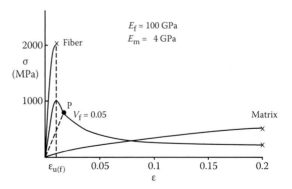

FIGURE 8.5   Stress–strain curve for two-phase Voigt composite $(V_f = 0.5)$.

Casting materials

Composition

"Plaster bandage" and its modern replacements represent interesting examples of nonimplantable composites. They are peculiar in design also, since neither of their components is very strong. However, they are combined to form a strong, tough composite.

The reinforcing or "fabric" component (cotton gauze in older products; fiberglass, polyester mesh, or a fiberglass–polyester interweave in more modern products) is weak and flexible in compression but fairly strong in tension. By comparison, the matrix ("plaster" [calcium sulfate], a thermoset polymer, or a polymer–plaster mixture) is weak and flexible in tension but quite strong in compression. Thus, the composite combines these properties to produce a material that is fairly strong and tough. It is highly "defective" in terms of the interfaces or voids, and although the tensile strength of the fibers produces reasonable single-cycle strength, these materials are fairly poor in resisting fatigue. However, the more modern materials have high strength-to-weight ratios, permitting multiple layers to be built up to overcome this fatigue weakness.

The matrices "set" or harden by two different processes.

1. Plaster is usually partially anhydrous calcium sulfate, ground to a fine powder. It sets owing to the recombination of water with the $CaSO_4$ powder and the growth of an interlocking matrix of crystals. The typical reaction is

$$(CaSO_4)_2 \cdot H_2O + 3H_2O \rightarrow 2[CaSO_4 \cdot 2H_2O] + \text{heat}$$

Too little water may prevent stoichiometric rehydration or adequate crystal growth; too much water or early motion may produce many small, weak crystals.

2. Resins are a variety of materials including low-molecular-weight polyesters and polyurethanes. They harden by either addition or condensation polymerization, initiated by water, heat, or ultraviolet illumination or some combination, forming interlocking polymer networks. The setting of resins (and plasters) is modestly accelerated by elevated temperature. However, both types of material release heat during setting so that temperature elevations may produce unacceptable temperatures at the patient's skin, especially if applied over insufficient padding material.

Table 8.6 lists some of the many casting materials currently available. They may be grouped into three main categories by matrix type: plaster, plaster–resin, and resin. These groupings are shown in Table 8.7 with some of the principal advantages and disadvantages of each system.

Despite the generic differences recited in Table 8.7, familiarity in use may be the chief factor in selecting a casting material. This is the case, even though there are significant differences in handling among apparently similar synthetic (resin matrix) materials. After fabrication, materials within each of the three generic categories are difficult to distinguish except by appearance (color, etc.). However, isolated properties such as

Table 8.6 Casting materials

Trade name	Fabric[a]	Matrix[a]	Cure	Manufacturer
Plaster matrix types				
Carapace	Cotton	Plaster	Water	Carapace
Cellona	Cotton	Plaster	Water	Sellomas
Firstcast	Cotton	Plaster	Water	AOA Professional Medical Products
Gypsona	Cotton	Plaster	Water	Smith and Nephew
Specialist	Cotton	Plaster	Water	Johnson & Johnson
Orthoflex	Cotton–rubber	Plaster	Water	Johnson & Johnson
Plaster–resin matrix types				
Cellamin	Cotton	Plaster–resin	Water	Sellomas
Crystona	Cotton	Resin–filler	Water	Smith and Nephew
Resin matrix types				
Caraglass	FG	PU	Water	Carapace
Cuttercast	PES–cotton	PU	Water	Cutter Biomedical
Deltacast	Cotton	PU	Water	Bayer
Deltalite				Johnson & Johnson
Black label	PES	PU	Water	
Red label	FG	PU	Water	
Green label	FG	PU (S)	Water	
Blue label	FG–rubber	PU (S)	Water	
K-Cast	FG	PU	Water	Kirschner
Hexcelite	PES	PCL	Thermo-plastic	Hexcel
Maxcast Plus	FG	PU	Water	Cutter Biomedical
Roycecast	FG	PU	Water	Royce Medical
Scotchcast	FG	PU	Water	3M
Scotchcast II	FG	PU	Water	3M
Scotchcast Plus	FG	PU (S)	Water	3M
Tufstuf II	FG	PU	Water	DePuy
Zim-Flex F	FG	PU	Water	Zimmer

[a] FG, Fiberglass; PCL, polycapralactone; PES, polyester; PU, polyurethane; S, smooth, high conformability.

water resistance or weight may suggest the use of particular materials in any single orthopaedic application.

Evaluation

Casting materials are difficult to evaluate since they possess their service properties only *after* being formed into a splint, cast, or brace. Thus, their mechanical properties depend both on design and manufacturing features *and* on technical aspects of application. After many attempts at producing evaluation procedures, in the American Society for Testing and Materials and elsewhere, present activities are focusing on two methods:

1. A "handleability" or "conformability" evaluation that involves forming a standard shape about a mandrel or constructing a standard structure, such as short forearm cast, and awarding points for

Table 8.7   Advantages and disadvantages of casting materials

Matrix type	Advantages	Disadvantages
Plaster	Low cost	Slow setting
	Familiarity	24 h to maximum strength
	Easy revision	Heavy/bulky
	Weight restricts patient activity	Significant heat generation during setting
	Good conformability	Radiopaque
		Not waterproof
		Low fatigue resistance
		Impervious
Plaster–resin	Intermediate cost	Slow setting
	Handles like plaster	Heavy/bulky
	Weight restricts patient activity	Radiopaque
	Water resistant	Impervious
Resin	Lightweight	Higher cost
	Rapid setting	Poor conformability
	Waterproof	Possible hazard to cast technician
	Permeable	Resin adheres to skin and clothes
	Radiolucent	Some flammable when impregnated with flammable liquids
		Tissue irritation (adjacent skin)

Note: These are generic advantages and disadvantages; they may not all be possessed by any particular product.

relative abilities of the layers to adhere, to be able to form a tuck, to turn at an angle, and so on. The points are then combined into an overall score or index number.

2. A single-cycle diametral "crush strength" test of a cylinder formed, usually of 5 to 10 layers around a 2- to 3.5-inch-diameter mandrel (removed after setting, before mechanical testing).

Neither of these two techniques has become recognized standard practices; thus, reliable comparative data on casting materials are not available. In addition, a reliable consensus test of fatigue properties is needed for realistic functional comparison of these various materials.

Casting materials with plaster matrices typically display crush strengths of 175–250 N (3.5 inch mandrel, 6 layers, 1 week after fabrication), whereas those with plaster–resin or resin fillers may be expected to be two to three times stronger. Plaster and, presumably, plaster–resin matrix casting materials have strengths that are strongly dependent on their water content and time after setting. They are usually "optimized" for equilibrium water contents of 20% of initial dry weight; higher or lower water contents or excess water content during setting will produce a weaker material.

The elastic moduli of most casting materials are not well known. However, modulus is not an important parameter since cast stiffness is increased by the surgeon or cast technician adding extra layers of material and the final cast is "decoupled" from the patient's limb by a highly compliant layer of padding.

Additional problems

PROBLEM 8.3

Compared with metals, nonresorbable ceramics are (select the best answer[s])

    A. More ductile

    B. Tougher

    C. Stiffer

    D. More brittle

    E. Less chemically reactive

ANSWER:

C, *D*, and *E*.

PROBLEM 8.4

Bioactive ceramics are (select the best answer[s])

    A. Resorbable

    B. Ductile

    C. Osteoinductive

    D. Osteoconductive

    E. Able to form bonds to tissue

ANSWER:

E. This is one of the properties of some bioactive materials. They are not ductile; their other properties depend on composition and structure.

PROBLEM 8.5

Polymer matrix composites (true or false)

    1. Are always anisotropic

    2. Are less stiff than pure alumina ceramics

    3. Are fatigue resistant

    4. May be made from any polymer–fiber combination

    5. May be made with a wide range of stiffnesses

ANSWER:

F, T, F, F, T.

PROBLEM 8.6

Carbon fiber has all of the following desirable characteristics as a PMC-reinforcing phase *except*

    A. High tensile strength

    B. High bending strength

    C. Nonresorbability

    D. Little immunogenic activity

    E. Cost

ANSWER:

B. Carbon fibers are strong in tension and relatively low in cost compared with other, higher-performance materials, especially whiskers. They are quite chemically inert and thus invoke very modest host responses.

PROBLEM 8.7

A continuous fiber two-phase Reuss PMC has the same _____ in each phase (complete the sentence).

ANSWER:

Stress.

PROBLEM 8.8

An epoxy-carbon fiber fracture fixation plate such as that shown in Figure 8.2 is tested in an animal long bone osteotomy model in comparison with a stainless steel plate with the same bending stiffness. A greater degree of callus hypertrophy is noted in fractures treated with the PMC plates than in those treated with the stainless steel plates. Why?

ANSWER:

A possible explanation is that creep under the screw heads may have caused premature "decoupling" of the PMC plate from the bone. This may be a generic design problem with such devices; perhaps it could be solved by replacing the outer pre-pregs with thin metal sheets.

PROBLEM 8.9

Compared with casts made from "plaster" bandage, those made from synthetic casting materials are (select the best answer[s])

A. Lighter

B. More radiopaque

C. More air permeable

D. More expensive

E. Better fitting

ANSWER:

A and *C*. Synthetic casting materials are relatively radiolucent. Although they are more expensive, on a roll-for-roll basis, less material is needed than for plaster casts to produce equal-strength structures, so cost may be comparable. Plaster bandage is still more "conformable" than synthetic materials; thus, well-fitting plaster casts are easier to fabricate.

PROBLEM 8.10

A cast room technician is instructed to "strengthen" a long leg cast. The cast was made from a synthetic cast material with an average of six layers; the technician adds two additional layers. The resulting case is

A. 33% stiffer

B. 75% stiffer

C. 135% stiffer

D. 215% stiffer

E. No stiffer

ANSWER:

A. What is desired is an increase in stiffness. A cast acts as a thin-walled cylinder; the most important deformation mode is bending (see Table 2.4). Note: The result depends on bonding of the new material to the old material. Actual "strength" increase may be determined experimentally.

PROBLEM 8.11

Compared to metallic and polyethylene components, the drive to use ceramics for load-bearing arthroplasty components is due to the following material characteristics (true or false):

1. High hardness

2. High strength

3. Low wettability

4. Low coefficient of friction

ANSWER:

T, F, F, T.

PROBLEM 8.12

Compared to alumina, zirconia is considered an improvement in terms of the following properties (true or false):

1. Stiffness
2. Wear
3. Toughness
4. Bending strength

ANSWER:

T, F, T, T.

Annotated bibliography

1. DE GROOT K (ed): *Bioceramics of Calcium Phosphate*. CRC Press, Boca Raton, FL, 1983.
   Useful collection of chapters about the most common chemical system of resorbable ceramics for orthopaedic applications.
2. HAMADOUCHE M, SEDEL L: Ceramics in orthopaedics. *J Bone Joint Surg* 82-B: 1095–1099, 2000.
   A review of the material properties and characteristics of ceramics used and proposed for use in arthroplasty components.
3. HAYDEN HW, MOFFATT WG, WULFF J: *The Structure and Properties of Materials*. Vol. III. John Wiley & Sons, New York, 1964.
   Chapter 9 deals very briefly with the mechanical properties of ceramics and composites, proving how difficult it is to generalize about these materials.
4. HUET R, SAKONA A, KURTZ SM: Strength and reliability of alumina ceramic femoral heads: Review of design, testing, and retrieval analysis. *J Mech Behav Biomed Mater* 4: 476–483, 2011.
   An in-depth review of the testing, mechanics, and fractography of fractured ceramic alumina heads.
5. HUTTNER W, HUTTINGER KJ: The use of carbon as an implant material. In Morscher E (ed): *The Cementless Fixation of Hip Endoprostheses*. Springer-Verlag, Berlin, 1984.
   Despite the misleading title, a good short review of the application of isotropic carbon, carbon–silicon carbide alloys, and carbon fiber–reinforced polymer composites to total hip replacement design.
6. JONES RM: *Mechanics of Composite Materials*. CRC Press, Boca Raton, 1998.
   Discussion of the mechanical design of composite materials. Many problems to be solved, some of which are fairly easy; a teacher's manual with worked solutions is available for the previous (McGraw-Hill) version.
7. KINGERY WD: *Introduction to Ceramics*. John Wiley & Sons, New York, 1961.
   Still the standard work. Chapter 17 deals well with elasticity and fracture.
8. OSAKA A: Ceramic materials. In Narayan R (ed): *ASM Handbook, Volume 23, Materials for Medical Devices*. ASM International, 2012.
   Physical characteristics of ceramic materials used in orthopaedics.

9. ROWLEY DI, PRATT D, POWELL ES, NORRIS SH, DUCKWORTH T: The comparative properties of plaster of Paris and plaster of Paris substitutes. *Arch Orthop Trauma Surg* 103:402–407, 1985.

Useful comparative data on a number of commercial casting materials.

10. SCHWARTZ MM: *Composite Materials Handbook*. McGraw-Hill, New York, 1984.

Discussion of composite material design, fabrication, and applications. Many useful tables.

11. WEHBE MA: Plaster uses and misuses. *Clin Orthop* 167:242–249, 1982.

An interesting, practically oriented discussion of the properties of "plaster bandage."

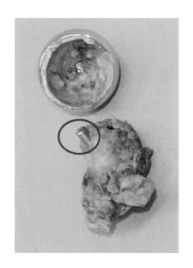

FIGURE 3.7 Fatigue failure in a hip resurfacing stem.

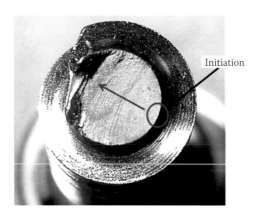

FIGURE 3.10 Low-stress, high-cycle-number fatigue failure in metal component.

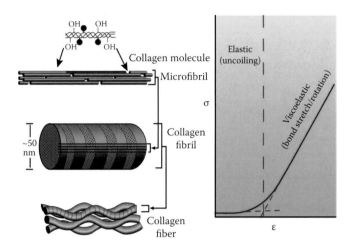

FIGURE 5.1 Structure and mechanics of collagen.

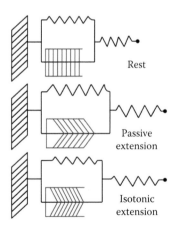

FIGURE 5.4 Model representation of muscle.

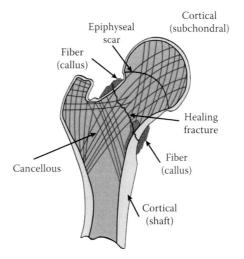

FIGURE 5.10 Microstructural elements of bone.

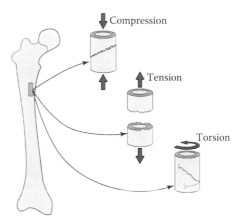

FIGURE 5.13 Fracture of cortical bone.

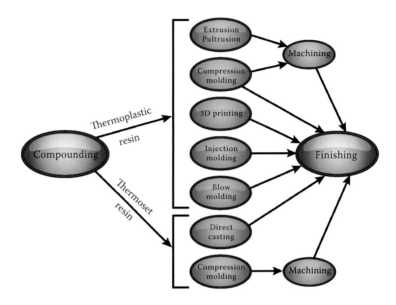

FIGURE 6.6 Processing of polymers.

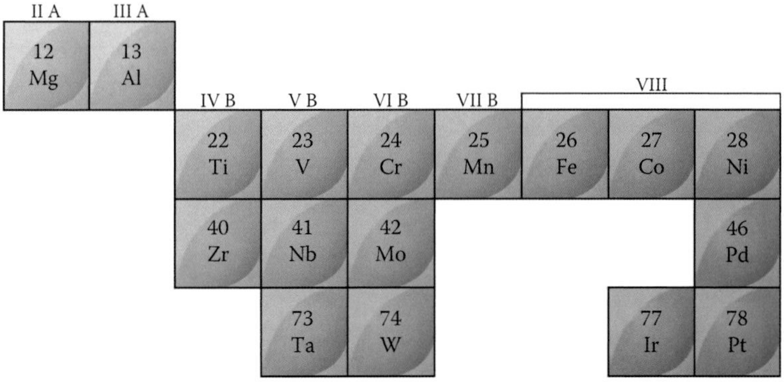

II A	III A							
12 Mg	13 Al							

		IV B	V B	VI B	VII B		VIII	
		22 Ti	23 V	24 Cr	25 Mn	26 Fe	27 Co	28 Ni
		40 Zr	41 Nb	42 Mo				46 Pd
			73 Ta	74 W			77 Ir	78 Pt

FIGURE 7.1 Elements of interest in orthopaedic alloys.

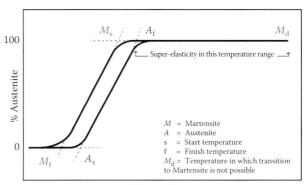

FIGURE 7.7 Phase transformation and hysteresis in a shape memory alloy.

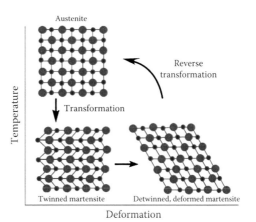

FIGURE 7.8 Atomic structure in a shape memory alloy through transformation and reverse transformation.

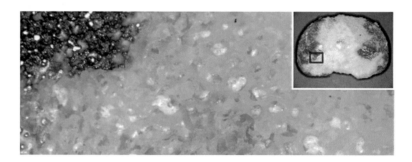

FIGURE 7.9 Microscopic view of bone ingrowth on a tantalum tibial knee component.

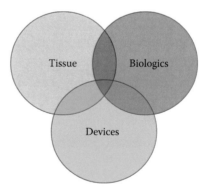

FIGURE 9.1 The intersection of tissue, biologics, and medical devices in the field of tissue engineering.

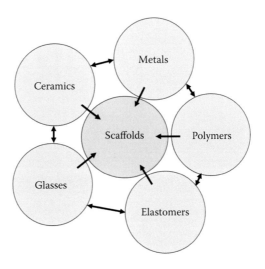

FIGURE 10.1 Combination of materials to form multiphase scaffolds.

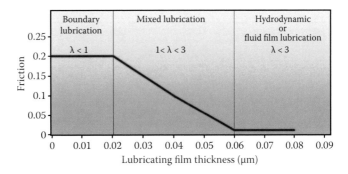

FIGURE 11.4 Mechanisms of lubrication as dependent on film thickness and friction.

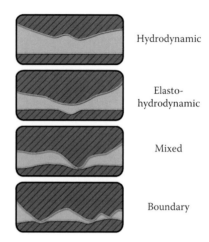

FIGURE 11.5   Principal mechanisms of lubrication.

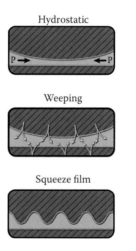

FIGURE 11.6   Alternative mechanisms of lubrication.

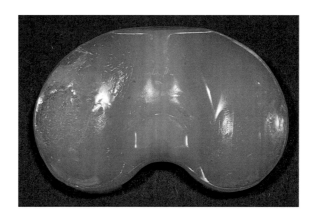

FIGURE 11.14   Wear of tibial plateau (UHMWPE).

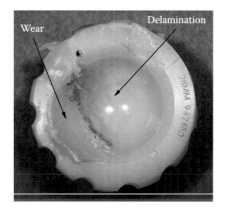

FIGURE 11.15 Wear and delamination of an acetabular cup (UHMWPE).

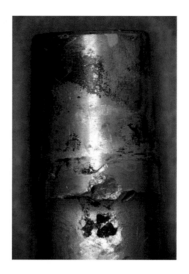

FIGURE 12.1 Corroded hip stem taper.

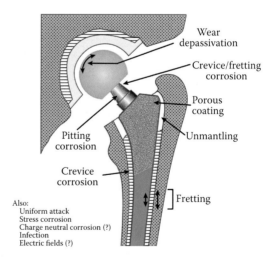

FIGURE 12.16 Types of corrosive attack on proximal femoral THR component.

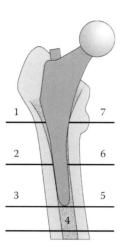

FIGURE 14.6 Gruen zones for sectionalizing bone resorption in the proximal femur.

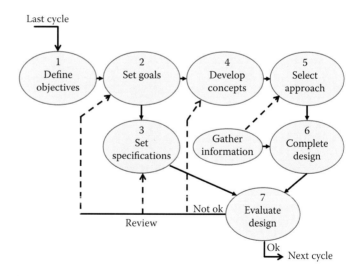

FIGURE 15.1 The design cycle.

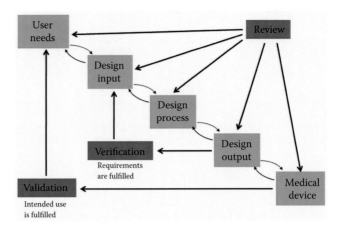

FIGURE 15.2 The waterfall model for the design process.

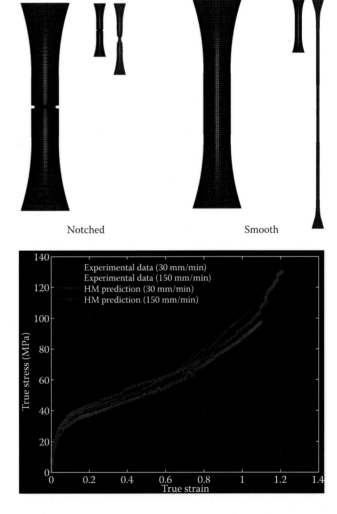

Notched   Smooth

FIGURE 15.3 Finite element models (top) to simulate tensile testing of smooth and notched rod biomaterial samples, with corresponding finite element results and physical experiments demonstrating good concordance.

Tissue engineering

Synthetic materials such as metals, ceramics, and polymers are widely used in the medical devices. However, it is a desire of designers to design and develop intermediate treatments that are more "natural," which has ushered "tissue engineering" into the biomedical field. Tissue engineering,* as a discipline, is "an interdisciplinary field that applies the principles of engineering and life sciences toward the development of biological substitutes that restore, maintain, or improve tissue or organ function." The objective of the field is the use of a combination of cells, engineering and materials methods, and biochemical and physiochemical factors to improve or replace biological functions. Most tissue-engineering applications involve the repair or replacement of portions of or whole tissues, such as bone, cartilage, blood vessels, bladder, skin, and so on. These tissue-engineered devices are required to meet certain mechanical and structural property specifications for proper functioning. Other terms have been used synonymously with tissue engineering, such as regenerative medicine or engineering, or genetic engineering. However, there are some subtle but distinct differences between these terms. For example, regenerative medicine places more emphasis on the use of stem cells to produce tissues. Also differentiated, genetic engineering involves altering the genetic makeup of an organism by removing DNA material or by introducing DNA prepared outside the organism either directly into the host or into a cell that is then fused or hybridized with the host.

Significance of tissue engineering

The concept of tissue engineering involves creating more complex organisms from simpler pieces of living specimens. Historically, some may say that tissue engineering was rooted in the Biblical account of Eve being created from Adam's rib, which in modern times may be a form of hybrid cloning. The growth of tissue engineering can be seen

---

* Langer R, Vacanti JP (May 1993). Tissue engineering. *Science* **260**: 920–926.

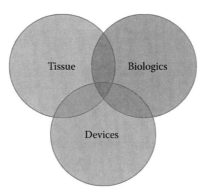

FIGURE 9.1   (See color insert.) The intersection of tissue, biologics, and medical devices in the field of tissue engineering.

as the merging of clinical medicine (such as prosthetics, reconstructive surgery, transplantation medicine, and microsurgery) and biology (cell biology, biochemistry, molecular biology, and genetics). As such, tissue engineering can be defined as the application of the principles and methods of engineering and life sciences toward the fundamental understanding of structure–function relationships in normal and pathologic mammalian tissue and the development of biological substitutes to restore, maintain, or improve function (Figure 9.1). Tissue engineering has evolved from cell biology and *in vitro* cell culture in plastic and reconstructive surgery to microvascular tissue transplantation in whole organ transplantation surgery.

Tissue-engineered medical products are evolving treatment options for musculoskeletal conditions and diseases. The products include cells, tissues, and inorganic and organic substances used alone or in combination with other factors that are manufactured, manipulated, or altered in a laboratory. They may be used for the repair, restoration, or regeneration of living tissue. They also may include substances that are not found naturally in tissues or whose normal physiologic concentration has been altered.

Synthesis methods

Tissue-engineered products are often built from three-dimensional (3D) structures known as scaffolds. Cells are implanted or seeded onto these scaffolds, which help with cell attachment, delivery and retention of cells and biochemical factors, and diffusion of cell nutrients and cell-expressed products.

Cells are cultured by controlling the oxygen, pH, humidity, temperature, nutrients, and osmotic pressure. Nutrient and metabolic transport via diffusion is a necessary condition for maintaining culture conditions. The functionality of a tissue culture may also require a capillary network or the introduction of growth factors, hormones, chemical stimuli, and physical stimuli. Some cells respond positively to mechanical stimuli that mimic their natural environment. For example, endothelial cells respond to shear stress from fluid flow, which is present in blood vessels. Because pressure pulses are encountered in heart valves and blood vessels, this form of stimuli is essential to the maintenance of phenotypic behavior of cardiovascular tissue cells.

There are many considerations for a scaffold onto which the cultured cells are seeded. In addition to the obvious need of biocompatibility, some of the key features of feasible scaffolds include high porosity and adequate pore size, biodegradability, and injectability. The porosity and pore size help facilitate cell seeding and diffusion of cells and nutrients. Biodegradability is a key feature so that it can be absorbed and does not require surgical removal. It is preferred that degradation occurs at a similar rate to tissue formation so that the cells can form their own natural matrix around themselves while the scaffold provides structural integrity and stability. For example, in a regenerating bone environment, the scaffold aims to mimic the extracellular matrix. Once the cell matrix is sufficiently mature and developed, it can then sustain the mechanical load, while the scaffold breaks down. In some applications, it may also be important that the scaffold can be injected into the body.

Various materials have been investigated as tissue scaffolds. Carbon nanotubes have been considered because they are biocompatible and resistant to biodegradation. However, the toxicity of nonbiodegradable nanomaterials may not have been fully characterized. Polylactic acid (PLA), which is a polyester, has been commonly used for synthetic scaffolds. An advantage is that it degrades in the body to form lactic acid, which is a naturally occurring chemical that is easily removed from the body. Polyglycolic acid (PGA) and polycaprolactone (PCL) have also been considered. These have similar degradation characteristics as PLA, but at different rates (faster for PGA and slower for PCL). Poly(ethylene glycol) (PEG), which is a hydrophilic biocompatible polymer, has also been considered as a scaffold to promote osteoblastic differentiation for bone or cartilage tissue.

Natural materials can also be used to construct scaffolds. Components of the extracellular matrix, such as collagen, fibrin, and glycosaminoglycans, have been investigated for their support of cell growth and cell compatibility. Decellularized tissue matrices have also been used.

For these various scaffolds, different synthesis methods have been employed and are described below:

Textile Fabrication: For example, building on the successful use of non-woven polymeric meshes, textile fabrication methods have been tested for tissue-engineering applications. However, the ability to obtain sufficiently porous scaffolds is unclear.

Molecular Self-Assembly: Molecular self-assembly has been shown to produce biomaterials with properties similar in scale and chemistry to that of natural extracellular matrix.

Casting and Leaching: Combined casting and leaching techniques is an alternative approach that involves dissolving the polymer into an organic solvent. The solution is then casted into a mold that is filled with porogen particles. After this has been casted, the solvent is allowed to evaporate, and then the composite structure in the mold is immersed in a liquid for dissolving the porogen to obtain the porous structure. Although this method provides scaffolds with regularly organized pores, these structures have limited thickness. In addition, confirmation of the evaporation of the organic solvent can sometimes be uncertain; these could cause potential damage to the seeded cells.

Gas Foaming: An alternative method, which is similar to casting and leaching, is gas foaming whereby gas is used as a porogen. This technique begins with disc-shaped compression-molded polymers that are exposed to high-pressure carbon dioxide. As the exposed pressure is lowered to atmospheric levels, pores are formed in these discs. These are formed by the carbon dioxide molecules dissipating from the polymer, which leaves behind a porous structure. Concerns with potentially excessive exposure to heat, which could disrupt or destroy any temperature-sensitive material that is seeded into the polymer matrix, and potential lack of connectivity of the scaffold could inhibit widespread adoption.

3D Printing: The advancement of 3D printing technologies has opened the doors to its use in tissue engineering. Scaffolds can be formed from "printing" or deposition of layers of polymer powders. The use of computer-aided design methods is particularly appealing because of its ability to fully control the design of the scaffold's structural characteristics. These processes are sufficiently gentle that it is possible to fabricate "tissue" with one or more viable cell types incorporated.

Lyophilization: Lyophilization or freeze-drying is a common approach for synthesizing scaffolds. For example, collagen sponges are fabricated using this method. Collagen is first dissolved in an acid that is cast into a mold. This is then frozen using liquid nitrogen and then lyophilized by removing the dispersed water and solvent from the frozen emulsion.

Electrospinning: Polymeric fibers can be constructed using electrostatic methods. This is known as electrospinning, whereby a solution is fed through a spinneret with a high-voltage tip. The buildup of electrostatic repulsion within the charged solution causes the ejection of a thin fibrous stream, which is drawn into a collector plate or rod with an opposite or grounded charge. This is collected in the form of a highly porous matrix. This method has the benefits of being simple and easy to vary or adjust to change the architecture of the matrix.

Cell types

Living cells are the building blocks for tissue-engineered products. These include fibroblasts for skin replacements or repairs and chondrocytes for cartilage repair. Thus, there many different types of cells that can be used. Cells can be classified based on their source:

- Allogenic cells: cells from the donor of the same species; for example, dermal fibroblasts from human foreskin have been shown to be viable for engineering of skin.

- Autologous cells: cells from the same individual in which the cells will be reimplanted. Since the cells are from the same individual, they pose the least risk of rejection and pathogen transmission. However, the challenge is that autologous cells are not always available. For example, individuals that are very ill, or who have a genetic disease, may not be able to provide useful cells. The need to surgically remove these cells may also expose these individuals to surgical site infections or postoperative pain.

- Xenogenic cells: cells from the donor of another species; for example, animal cells such as bovine, equine, and porcine tissues have been used extensively for cardiovascular implants.

Other categories of cells include stem cells, syngenic cells, primary cells, and secondary cells. Stem cells are undifferentiated cells that can be divided in culture into different specialized cells. These may be used for repairing diseased or damaged tissue or used to grow new organs. Syngenic cells, which are also known as isogenic cells, are those derived from genetically identical donors, such as twins or clones. Primary and secondary cells refer to the source, where primary ones are from an organism compared with secondary ones, which are from a cell bank.

Skin grafts

One of the milestones of tissue engineering is the development and widespread use of skin grafts. Part of the drive and desire to develop skin grafts for plastic and reconstructive surgery was to help treat injuries from military wars. Extensive investigation of tissue healing through cellular effects, as well as through the cultivation of cells outside the body, has helped fuel growth in this area. As such, cell biology and especially *in vitro* cell culture became the mainstay of what can be considered tissue engineering.

In the 1950s, animal studies showed that the products of a culture of epidermal cells could be applied to a graft bed to reconstitute an epidermis. However, a challenge at that time was the inefficient means of cell cultivation, which provided insufficient cells to sustain transplantation. Then, in the 1960s and 1970s, growth factors were found to promote greater proliferation of epidermal cells when the factors were added to the culture medium. In the late 1970s, cultured cells were shown that they could be grown in sheets in a petri dish and transferred intact, rather than as disaggregated cells, to a graft wound bed. During that same period, the use of fibroblasts to condense a hydrated collagen lattice to a tissue-like structure was shown to be potentially suitable for wound healing. This development led to the first functional living skin equivalent in 1981, consisting of fibroblasts suspended in a network of collagen and glycosaminoglycan. On the basis of knowledge of the components of the underlying matrix structure of skin, dermal regeneration template, when implanted and seeded with autologous basal cells, showed regrowth of functional skin. All of these advancements proceeded to the development of commercial products.

Several tissue-engineered skin products have completed clinical trials, met US Food and Drug Administration (FDA) approval, and were released to the market. In 1997, the FDA approved a skin replacement tissue made by Advanced Tissue Sciences, which consists of dermal keratinocytes grown on a biodegradable polymer. This replacement tissue serves as a temporary wound cover for burns as new tissue forms. Live human skin cells have also been used commercially to form a dual-layer skin equivalent to treat diabetic leg and foot ulcers. Other commercial products include grafts grown from hair follicle stem cells to treat chronic skin ulcers; cryopreserved human fibroblast–derived dermal substitute composed of fibroblasts, extracellular matrix, and a bioabsorbable scaffold; and autologous skin graft that can permanently close a burn wound. In addition, human dermal collagen seeded with allogenic fibroblasts has been used for patients with third-degree burns and limited donor-site tissue and then further indicated for abdominal wall reconstruction and breast reconstruction postmastectomy. Porcine dermis has also been used for a range of breast reconstruction and revision surgery cases.

Wound coverings   Skin grafts have viability not only for wound reconstruction but also in burn wound management. For the latter application, a full-thickness burn during battlefield injuries results in complete destruction of the epidermis and dermis, which leaves no residual epidermal cells to repopulate. The current focus of burn wound care is to improve long-term function and appearance of the healed or replaced skin cover. This has generated a significant interest in the use of skin grafts and skin substitutes to improve wound healing, control pain, create more rapid closure, and improve functional and cosmetic outcomes.

Advancements in skin graft tissue engineering have included the adoption of 3D printing techniques with the intention of treating soldiers wounded in the battlefield. Cells are placed in the printers and then used to rebuild damaged or burned skin. Preclinical evaluations are ongoing. Scarless wound healing is another area of focus in the field. This is an attempt to understand the molecular basis of scar formation, which is the major complicating factor of musculotendinous injury to the extremities. This is intended to help spur the development of adjunctive molecular therapies to surgery. For example, PEG-ylated matrix metalloproteinase-1 is being investigated to mitigate scar tissue formation.

Vascular grafts

One of the landmark developments about a century ago was the demonstration of successful techniques for the anastomosis of blood vessels and the extension of these techniques from the transplantation of vessels to the transplantation of entire solid organs. In the 1950s, tubes of synthetic fabric were shown to have viability as arterial prostheses. As the knowledge of thrombogenesis and the interaction between synthetic materials, blood flow, and vascular tissue became better understood, resorbable vascular grafts were developed and introduced into clinical practice. The improved healing process of Dacron vascular grafts via pre-seeding with endothelial cells in the late 1970s bestowed even more popularity to graft use.

Contemporary research has experimented with using porcine intestine as a graft base for endothelial cell seeding, which is intended to grow and develop into vessel-like structures. Other sources for graft bases have also been explored, including fibrillar collagen and bovine collagen gels. However, there have been challenges adapting the mechanical properties and strength of graft material in relation to native blood vessels. Clotting and scar tissue formation are challenges in cellular replacements and limit the transition of *in vitro* products for evaluations in clinical trials. Another challenge is the ability to create a functional nerve supply and capillary network *in vitro* to support live vascular tissues.

Organs

There is continued promise in the engineering of entire organs, such as the kidney, pancreas, and liver. The primary challenge with engineering whole organs is that cells, and resultantly the organ, tend to lose their function when taken outside of their usual microenvironment. Success so far has been mixed. The following sections detail some of the highlights.

Pancreas

The first pancreas transplant, in conjunction with a simultaneous kidney transplant, was performed in 1966. Additional development resulted in isolated pancreas cells being first transplanted in 1970, although the problem of immune rejection was not resolved. The ability of beta cells cultured on synthetic semipermeable hollow fibers to restore glucose homeostasis in animals was demonstrated in the 1970s.

Kidney

The first kidney dialysis machine was used in patients for the first time in the late 1940s, and subsequently the first successful transplant of a donated kidney occurred in the mid-1950s. Further advances in immunosuppression for transplantation and refinement of dialysis technology made both techniques practical for widespread and routine use, transforming the management of end-stage renal disease. During the late 1960s and early 1970s, the combination of kidney cells with hollow synthetic fibers was first used as a medium for nutrients and waste.

Subsequent research on growing liver cells on the outside of hollow fibers led to the demonstration of hollow-fiber bioreactors. In the mid-1980s, further development of the bioartificial kidney concept was accomplished through the use of hollow-fiber bioreactors employing renal epithelial cells. Whole kidney replacement organs are still being researched. In the meantime, temporary replacement devices, such as extracorporeal kidney assist devices, have shown some success.

Liver

The first successful liver transplant was also carried out around the same time as the first pancreas transplant. Continued research was focused on providing extracorporeal support to patients suffering from liver failure. Research on cell-based therapies and bioartificial systems followed a similar path as that of pancreatic cells. Rat hepatoma cell line was first shown to be able to be cultured on the surface of semipermeable hollow fibers within a plastic housing in the mid-1970s. In 1977, transplanted hepatocytes were used to treat drug-induced liver failure in rats. Bioartificial liver bioreactor designs have been developed in the laboratory to replace liver function. The basic design of such devices is composed of circulating patient plasma extracoporeally through a bioreactor that houses liver cells, which are sandwiched between artificial plates or capillaries. Desirable properties for such devices include having a spherical shape, having a large surface area, having large pores or high porosity, and being hydrophilic and biocompatible, which serve to improve their efficiency and efficacy. However, the complex synthetic and metabolic functions of the liver are a challenge to replicate. In addition, human hepatocytes are limited in supply, which makes their harvest and culture for liver assist devices challenging. Furthermore, hepatocytes are extremely difficult to stabilize and maintain in culture and thus tend to lose their specificity relatively quickly.

Bone and cartilage

Synthetic materials such as metal alloys and polymers have traditionally been used to replace damaged bone and joints. With the increasing incidence of osteoporosis and extensive healthcare resources being used to treat osteoporotic fractures and fractures resulting from trauma, there has been great interest in bone substitutes. It is estimated that more than half a million bone graft substitutes are used annually in the United States. Current therapies include autografts and allografts, but the increasing demand for alternatives have been fueled with the growth of the tissue engineering.

Bone

Bone tissue engineering typically involves the use of harvested cells, recombinant signaling molecules, and 3D matrices. One common approach involves producing highly porous biodegradable matrices/scaffolds in the shape of the desired bone and then seeding the matrices/scaffolds with cells and signaling molecules (e.g., protein growth factors). The cells are cultured and the matrix/scaffold is then implanted into the defect to induce and direct the growth of new bone. The goal is for the cells to attach to the scaffold, multiply, differentiate (i.e., transform from a nonspecific or primitive state into cells exhibiting the bone-specific functions), and organize into normal, healthy bone as the scaffold degrades.

Interest in using components from bone to provide a more "natural" alternative led to the development of bone morphogenetic proteins (BMPs), which were initially discovered by Marshall Urist in 1965. These are growth factors that are capable of inducing the formation of new bone. As an alternative to autologous bone graft, which is associated with significant donor site morbidity, recombinant versions of BMPs, rhBMP-2 and rhBMP-7, have been shown clinically to be beneficial in treating a variety of bone-related conditions including delayed union and non-union. Although BMP has demonstrated extensive popularity, growing substantially in use after its clinical introduction, recent years have brought controversy with its use. For example, there are concerns with swelling after its use in anterior cervical fusion. The development and use of BMPs are further discussed in Chapter 10.

Other areas of development pertain to treating injuries from combat situations. Although the current gold standard for replacing bone is autograft material, the intent is to provide off-the-shelf materials containing biological factors (e.g., hemostatic agents, analgesics, antibiotics, drugs, hormones, and cells) and biodegradable scaffolds to stabilize, protect, minimize tissue damage, and promote tissue repair. This avoids the need to harvest autograft bone from a wounded individual or to remove excessive bone when the supply may be limited because of extensive bone injuries. Off-the-shelf calcium aluminate materials have been investigated on the basis of hydratable formulations that are engineered with antimicrobial and bone regeneration–enhancing activities. These grafts are intended for use as an easily castable/moldable bone implant material for a variety of reconstructive orthopaedic (e.g., implants for critical-sized fractures, hip and knee replacements).

Cartilage

Cells from cultured periosteum have the ability to form new bone, as well as cartilage. However, articular cartilage has limited capacity to regenerate itself compared to bone. Even minor lesions or injuries to cartilage may lead to progressive damage, and in case of articular cartilage, these can lead to subsequent joint degeneration. Autologous chondrocyte implantation for cartilage repair was first performed in 1987. Damaged knee cartilage has been replaced by harvesting autologous chondrocytes, growing them in a biodegradable matrix, and then transplanting them in place of the damaged tissue. However, some concerns with the formation of fibrocartilage and progression of degenerative changes in the joint have been raised. Cartilage repair and restoration is a relatively new advancement and is becoming an increasingly important part of orthopaedic care. Knowledge and understanding of the available surgical techniques are critical to the appropriate use of these interventions. Further discussion of cartilage materials is included in Chapter 10.

Osteochondral allografting emerged in the 1970s as an option for treating large post-traumatic injuries, osteonecrosis, and tumors adjacent to articular joints. Osteochondral allografting involves transplanting mature hyaline cartilage containing living chondrocytes that can support the hyaline cartilage matrix indefinitely. The osseous portion of the graft serves as an osteoconductive scaffold for graft incorporation and for restoring absent bone.

Other approaches to the use of tissue engineering for bone and soft tissue healing involve concentrated platelets in plasma-rich platelet injections. Plasma-rich platelet has been used in rotator cuff surgeries, meniscal repairs, and allograft anterior cruciate ligament reconstructions to accelerate healing. However, the positive actions of plasma-rich platelet are still unclear. The findings in the literature are mixed. Some researchers have reported no benefits for bone healing in animal models, while others have found effective augmentation of porous biomaterials after plasma-rich platelet use. Some commercially available plasma-rich platelet preparation systems include gravitational platelet separation by Cell Factor Technologies/Biomet Biologics, Magellan by Medtronic, and Symphony II by DePuy. The potential role of plasma-rich platelets in healing musculoskeletal injuries is an exciting frontier that may even lead to newer improved therapies, but studies are still being conducted to establish effectiveness, indications, and protocols.

Stem cells

Over the last decade, there has been considerable interest in the use of mesenchymal stem cells and tissue-engineering principles in orthopaedics and musculoskeletal sciences. Stem cells are an attractive option because of their potential for a high rate of proliferation, with the ability to undergo chondrogenic, osteogenic, and adipogenic differentiation. Cells with mesenchymal stem cell characteristics can be isolated from different adult tissues, such as bone marrow, periosteum, skin, adipose tissue, skeletal muscle, synovial tissue, the infrapatellar fat pad, and cartilage. Stem cells have demonstrated excellent gene transfer with the capability to be transduced for the tissue engineering of bone. Gene transfer could enable growth factors and bone morphogentic proteins to enhance bone repair. Stem cells are implanted onto scaffolds, which help support tissue formation by allowing cell migration, proliferation, and differentiation. These scaffolds are required to deliver and retain cells, allow for cell attachment, and have adequate biodegradability, biocompatibility, and nonimmunogenicity.

Cell-based clinical therapies using mesenchymal stem cells have used several approaches. Tissue-engineering approaches have been used where stem cells are seeded into 3D scaffolds in order to generate functional tissues for replacement of defective tissues. Another approach has used stem cell transplantation to replace defective host cells. The properties of stems acting as cytokine/growth factor producers have also been investigated to stimulate repair or inhibit degenerative processes.

Regenerative medicine/engineering

While tissue engineering is more clearly defined, regenerative medicine is more difficult to differentiate from tissue engineering and to define. It is widely characterized as a field where stem cells drive embryonic formation, or where inductive organizers induce a blastema to regenerate a tissue, ultimately aimed at reforming damaged tissues and organs in humans. Regenerative medicine concerns itself primarily with stem cell plasticity and cloning, when nuclear transfer, transdifferentiation, and cell fusion are measures to modulate the stem cell differentiation pathway. Experiments in the cloning of animals, such as frogs, lambs, and sheep, have shown how genetic material from an adult cell can be used to re-express every gene to build an entirely new animal. However, the possibility of cloning humans raises extreme ethical concerns. Commercial development has been inhibited by inefficiencies in the cloning process owing to problems with reprogramming a cell's DNA in the search for new eggs. During cloning, an adult nucleus is implanted into an egg, which must erase the adult genome's epigenetic marks in order to re-express them. The addition of chemicals or proteins to adult cell nuclei to bypass the need for eggs may help accelerate development in this field.

Regenerative medicine, sometimes known as reparative medicine, is also defined as the regeneration and remodeling of tissue *in vivo* for the purpose of repairing, replacing, maintaining, or enhancing organ function, and the engineering and growing of functional tissue substitutes *in vitro* for implantation *in vivo* as a biological substitute for damaged or diseased tissues and organs.

Genetic engineering

Genetic engineering has also been used to describe some aspects of tissue engineering. Genetic engineering is a process in which recombinant DNA technology is used to produce certain desirable traits into organisms. For example, a genetically engineered animal is one that contains a recombinant DNA construct producing a new trait. Conventional breeding methods have been used to produce more desirable traits in animals, but genetic engineering is a much more targeted and powerful method of introducing desirable traits. The first known experiments in genetic engineering brought engineered human insulin in the late 1970s. Since then, there has been work to create animal models of human diseases, as well as gene therapy where defective human genes are replaced with functional copies.

In simple terms, the first step in the genetic engineering process is to isolate the selected gene that is intended for insertion into an organism. There are two options for isolation. The first uses restriction enzymes to cut the DNA into fragments and gel electrophoresis to separate them out according to length. An alternative employs polymerase chain reaction to amplify up a gene segment, which can then be isolated through gel electrophoresis. If the DNA sequence of the gene is known, then it can also be artificially synthesized. The gene to be inserted must be combined with other genetic elements for it to work properly.

Genes may also be modified for better expression or effectiveness. The most common form of genetic engineering involves inserting new genetic material within the host genome at a random or specific location. When inserted at a specific location, the effect is to generate mutations at desired genomic loci capable of knocking out endogenous genes.

Although genetic engineering opens the door to many opportunities, the efficacy of these methods is still unclear. In addition, there are ethical concerns that the technology may be used for more than just treatment of diseases, namely, for enhancement or modification of non-medically related characteristics, such as appearances or behavior.

Regulatory pathway and regulations

Because tissue-engineered constructs involve the use of biological elements such as cells or tissue, the regulatory process for these products is more complex than for a "standard" synthetic product, such as a hip prosthesis. In a typical medical device, the indication, application, construction, and behavior are relatively more predictable. Tissue-engineered products may be regulated by the FDA under several different pathways because they often contain components from different product categories of tissue, device, and biologics. For example, tissue-engineered products that fall under the medical devices category are often classified as a Class III device and reach the market via the premarket approval process in the United States. Conversely, pharmaceuticals typically require an investigational new drug application/biologic license application in the United States.

The FDA's regulation of tissue-engineered products has been continuously evolving. Detailed discussion of the regulatory history is included in Chapter 10. In brief, the jurisdiction of combination products is based on the determination of the *primary mode of action* (PMOA), through which the product achieves its therapeutic effect. In products where the mode of action is derived through multiple methods, the single PMOA that provides the most important therapeutic action or provides the greatest contribution to the overall therapeutic effect is scientifically identified. The following sections discuss segments of potential regulatory requirements of a tissue-engineered product.

Regulation

After the initial toxicity, pharmacology, and pharmacokinetic studies, the IND application may include chronic toxicity, carcinogenicity, special toxicity, and drug metabolism studies. Special toxicity evaluations include assessment of mutagenicity and reproductive and development toxicity. After *in vitro* assessment, clinical trials are conducted in a series of steps or phases (Figure 9.2). These are conducted in phases because each is designed to answer separate research questions. During Phase I, researchers test the product in a small group of people for the first time to evaluate its safety, determine a safe dosage range, and identify any side effects. This initial phase can take several months to complete and usually includes a small number of healthy volunteers (20 to 100). Once the product has demonstrated its initial safety in a small group of patients, the product is then given to a larger group of patients to test safety AND effectiveness in Phase II trials. This second phase may last from several months to 2 years and involves up to several hundred patients. Most Phase II studies are randomized trials where one group of patients receives the experimental product, while a second "control" group receives a standard treatment or placebo. During Phase III, the treatment is given to large groups of people to confirm its effectiveness, monitor side effects, compare it to commonly used treatments, and collect further information that may guide the use of the product. This large-scale phase, which can include several hundred to several thousand patients, can last several years. If all Phase III requirements are met, the product can be considered for market approval by the FDA. A fourth phase of clinical trial is also performed later to gather information on the product's effect in various populations and any side effects associated with long-term use. This is also known as "post-market" surveillance trials. In the case that there are unintended or unforeseen events that are observed during the post-market phase, the device may be taken off the market or subjected to some restrictions to its use.

Basic characteristics of the tissue-engineered components are also required, as is expected with any other classes of products. For example, for cell-device combination products, characterization of the cells and scaffold is necessary. The source of the cells (auto-, allo-, or xenograft), along with their sterility, purity, viability, cell number, stability, and potency/biologic activity, is specified. This also includes the identity of the cells, that is, morphologic evaluation, unique biochemical markers, phenol-type specific cell surface antigens, and gene and protein expression analysis. The characterization of the scaffold includes evaluation of

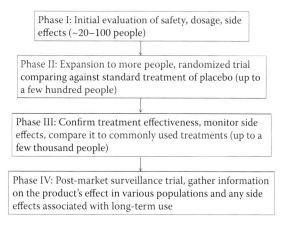

FIGURE 9.2   Clinical trial phases.

the chemistry such as the material source and the impact of the material on cells, the testing materials and the leachables/extracts for biocompatibility, decomposition products, and assembling materials, and, lastly, the sterilization conditions and the impact on the product and residue's impact on cells. Other categories of scaffold characterization include the design and physical attributes, such as mass, volume, density, pH, porosity, particle size, resorption kinetics (mechanism and pathway of decomposition, kinetics of cell in-growth), and mechanical properties (e.g., structural strength, modulus, fatigue/abrasion resistance, fixation strength). Considerations for the characterization of cell-scaffold constructs include the appropriate *in vitro* and *in vivo* testing and characterization method owing to the complexity in 3D structure, heterogeneity in composition, small lot sizes (single lots due to biological nature of some products), and remodeling of product post-implantation. Since the product is not designed to be stable in the intended decomposition sense, the final product specification from *in vitro* testing may not necessarily be representative of the full spectrum of the product performance. Additional complexity may result from the specificity of the product type and intended use, as well as some products involving multiple modes of action.

Tissue-engineered device regulation

Tissue-engineered products, as with other medical devices, are regulated by the Code of Federal Regulations (CFR), Title 21 (Food and Drugs), Parts 1270 (Human tissue intended for transplantation) and 1271 (Human cells, tissues, and cellular and tissue-based products). The regulations in 21 CFR Part 1270 apply to banked human tissue and to establishments or persons engaged in the recovery, processing, storage, or distribution of banked human tissue. These provide regulations for donor testing and screening, as well as their corresponding written procedures and records. As for 21 CFR Part 1271, the regulations are to establish donor eligibility, current good tissue practice, and other procedures to prevent the introduction, transmission, and spread of communicable diseases by human cells, tissues, and cellular and tissue-based products. Regulated products, as defined by the CFR, include items containing or consisting of human cells or tissues that are intended for implantation, transplantation, infusion, or transfer into a human recipient. Examples include bone, ligament, skin, dura mater, heart valve, cornea, hematopoietic stem/progenitor cells derived from peripheral and cord blood, manipulated autologous chondrocytes, epithelial cells on a synthetic matrix, and semen or other reproductive tissue. However, this regulation does not cover vascularized human organs for transplantation; secreted or extracted human products, such as milk, collagen, and cell factors; animal-derived cells, tissues, and organs; and blood vessels recovered with an organ. Whole blood or blood components or blood derivative products are regulated by CFR Parts 207 (Registration of producers of drugs and listing of drugs in commercial distribution) and 607 (Establishment registration and product listing for manufacturers of human blood and blood products).

Standards

Tissue engineering is still relatively nascent in terms of its development. The testing and evaluation of tissue-engineered products are extremely varied owing to the numerous classes of products, indications, and approaches to design and production. The standards process for tissue-engineered medical products first began in 1997, when categories of importance were developed. Since then, several standards have been developed by the American Society for Testing and Materials (ASTM). For example, the ASTM has provided guidance on writing materials specification for raw or starting biomaterials, which are intended for use in tissue-engineering scaffolds for growth, support, or delivery of cells or biomolecules (ASTM F2027: Standard guide for characterization and testing of raw or starting biomaterials for tissue-engineered medical products). This standard takes advantage of existing test methods and standards for contemporary biomaterials and covers the specifications and characterizations of these biomaterials. However, because the focus of this standard is on the raw or starting materials, this standard does not provide safety and biocompatibility requirements for evaluations that are typically performed on the final form of the product. Guidance for the characterization and testing of biomaterials after they have been formed into 3D scaffolds is provided by ASTM F2150 (Standard guide for characterization and testing of biomaterial scaffolds used in tissue-engineered medical products). This will be discussed in Chapter 10, along with other relevant standards ASTM F2212 (Standard guide for characterization of Type I collagen as starting material for surgical implants and substrates for tissue engineered medical products [TEMPS]) and ASTM F2347 (Standard guide for characterization and testing of hyaluronan as starting materials intended for use in biomedical and tissue engineered medical product applications).

The physicochemical attributes of the raw or starting biomaterial used in tissue-engineered scaffolds carry significant potential to affect product performance through affecting cell behavior or the release of bioactive molecules or drugs. Thus, ASTM F2027 seeks to recommend specifications or characterizations of raw or starting biomaterials to ensure reproducibility prior to their fabrication into implantable tissue-engineered scaffolds or controlled release matrices. The specified chemical requirements for the biomaterials depend on the class of material (ceramics, metals, polymers, composites) (Table 9.1). Natural materials made of proteins, nucleic acids, or polysaccharides are classified as polymers, while anorganic bone and other naturally occurring inorganic substances are classified as ceramics. All classes of materials require information about the chemical formula or composition. In addition, for ceramics, chemical specifications include, but are not limited to, phase content, purity, major/minor elemental constituents, processing aids, and the allowable amount of foreign material contaminants. For metals, typically specified chemical requirements include phase content, purity, major/minor elemental constituents, corrosion susceptibility, and

Table 9.1 Chemical, physical, and mechanical requirements per ASTM F2027

Requirements	Ceramics[a]	Metals	Polymers[b]	Composites
Chemical	• Chemical formula or composition • Phase content • Purity • Major/minor elemental constituents • Processing aids • Allowable amount of foreign material contaminants	• Chemical formula or composition • Phase content • Purity • Major/minor elemental constituents • Corrosion susceptibility • Surface modification	• Chemical formula or composition • Unreacted monomer content • Synthesis method • Source (if harvested) • Viscosity • Use of additives/ fillers/ contaminants • Use of curing agents/catalysts/ initiators/ accelerators • Co-polymer ratio • Extractables • Degradation products (including mechanism and kinetics) • Residual moisture or solvent content • Contact angle/ surface tension	• Requirements per components (ceramics, metals, polymers) • Phase content • Characterization of the bonding process between phases • Chemical content at the interface
Physical and mechanical	• Particle and crystal size distributions • Density • Specific surface area • Crystallinity • Particle porosity	• Material microstructure (grain size and orientation) • Condition (hot-worked, annealed, or cold-worked) • Melting point • Hardness • Elastic modulus • Yield/ultimate tensile/ compressive strengths	• Primary/ secondary structures • Powder size distribution • Water absorption or swelling percent • Glass transition temperature/ melting point • Crystallinity • Density • Elastic modulus • Ultimate tensile/ compressive strengths	• Requirements per components (ceramics, metals, polymers) • Shape and dimensions of other phases • Bond strength between phases

[a] Includes anorganic bone and other naturally occurring inorganic substances.

[b] Includes natural materials made of proteins, nucleic acids, or polysaccharides.

surface modification. Polymers require stating the unreacted monomer content, synthesis method, source (if harvested), viscosity, use of additives/fillers/contaminants, use of curing agents/catalysts/initiators/accelerators, co-polymer ratio, extractables, degradation products (including mechanism and kinetics), residual moisture or solvent content, and contact angle/surface tension. Depending on the type of materials used for composites, the respective chemical requirements are specified. In addition, the phase content, characterization of the bonding process between phases, and the chemical content at the interface are recommended for composites.

Physical and mechanical requirements are also specified in the ASTM standard by class of material (Table 9.1). For ceramics, particle and crystal size distributions, density, specific surface area, crystallinity, and particle porosity are typically specified. The specifications for metals include material microstructure (grain size and orientation), condition (hot-worked, annealed, or cold-worked), melting point, hardness, elastic modulus, and yield/ultimate tensile/compressive strengths. Primary/secondary structures, powder size distribution, water absorption or swelling percent, glass transition temperature/melting point, crystallinity, density, elastic modulus, and ultimate tensile/compressive strengths are typically specified for polymers. The specifications for composites include the shape and dimensions of other phases and bond strength between phases, as well as all other properties described previously for the type of materials used in the composite material.

Additional discussion of standards is included in Chapter 10.

Future and challenges

Tissue engineering, regenerative medicine, and genetic engineering hold the prospects for custom-made medical solutions for injured or diseased patients. Thus, there is a growing need for tissue-engineered products to have more complex functionality. The use of tissue engineering to repair bone defects in humans remains a challenge owing to an inadequate vascular supply, leading to cell death of implanted cells. There have also been concerns raised by the poor resorbability of the scaffolds and instability of the scaffold fixation. Additional research and development is needed to improve the key factor of cell survival in human models, such as improving nutrient and oxygen supply.

Angiogenic control and stem cell biology, cell sourcing, cell/tissue interaction, immunologic understanding and control, manufacturing, and scale-up are additional issues that will be at the forefront of this field for the near and immediate future. Further proof of clinical usage of such therapies over time will need to be strengthened before widespread commercial adoption can be considered.

Tissue engineering must not only overcome the technical and commercial challenges of developing viable and efficacious products but also face daunting regulatory challenges. The regulatory environment for cell-containing products is complex and may impose a substantial financial burden on the product development process due to fulfillment of efficacy standards and clinical trials, as well as indirectly through the financial effects of delayed market introduction. In addition, the health-care reimbursement landscape must also be taken into account as even the most efficacious product may not be approved for widespread use if it cannot ascertain its cost-effectiveness.

It is unclear if there is a viable "business model" for such materials and the probable long-term need for conventional biomaterial-based approaches to provide therapy during the fabrication periods, in much the same way the left ventricular assist devices are bridges to heart transplantation. The costs involved in developing tissue-engineered products can also prove to be an impediment to the growth of this field, particularly in light of pressure to contain medical expenses.

Although there is the potential for regenerative medicine to provide revolutionary clinical therapies that will address unmet patient needs, the community (industry, scientists, patients, and surgeons) must be careful not to overstate what is possible or underestimate timelines necessary for these therapies to reach the patient bedside. One must temper the expectations for the development process, along with the regulatory and reimbursement pathways.

Finally, some ethical concerns have been raised about tissue engineering. The main ethical issues stem from the complexity and continuity that is unique to the tissue-engineering process. The dynamic interaction between the tissue-engineered construct and the human body creates risks and safety issues that may have not yet been encountered in other medical applications, and which have to be observed and treated with great care. There are also potential ethics issues regarding the donation of cells for tissue engineering. These cells carry considerable value, in terms of material value and as an informational resource. Because of the continuity of the process, all participants in the tissue-engineering field, from the cell donor to the tissue engineer to the recipient of the therapeutic tissue-engineered product, may have conflicting interests with regard to the value of these cells. Thus, the ownership and exchange of cells need to be fleshed out in terms of the development of guidance for the informed consent process and for its contents in the specific context of tissue engineering. As the potential value (material and informational) of the donated cells increases because of new scientific insights, technical advances, and economic changes, the demand for clear informed consent documents and a clear informed consent process will also increase.

Problems

PROBLEM 9.1

Match the cell types by their descriptions:
Allogenic, autologous, xenogenic, stem cells, syngenic

A. From a different species

B. Undifferentiated cells

C. From the same species

D. From genetically identical donors

E. From the same individual in which the cells will be reimplanted

ANSWER:

Allogenic, *C*; autologous, *E*; xenogenic, *A*; stem cells, *B*; syngenic, *D*.

PROBLEM 9.2

Which of these are not ethical concerns regarding tissue-engineered products?

A. Patient consent for cell donation

B. Cost/value of the cells

C. Ownership of the cells

D. Safety and efficacy

E. Scaleability

ANSWER:

E—scaleability refers to questions regarding the practicality and commercializability of tissue-engineered products.

PROBLEM 9.3

How is the regulatory pathway for a tissue-engineered product determined?

A. Types of cells used in the product

B. Manufacturing method

C. Intended use/application

D. Primary mode of action

E. Level of biocompatibility

ANSWER:

D—the PMOA is the mode through which the product achieves its therapeutic effect. Since there are three primary centers at the FDA that regulate medical products, the center that is responsible for leading the review process is based on the PMOA.

Annotated bibliography

1. AMERICAN ACADEMY OF ORTHOPAEDIC SURGEONS: Information Statement—Tissue-Engineered and Cell-Based Medical Products, 2008.
   This provides perspective on the use of tissue-engineered and cell-based products in orthopaedics.
2. ASTM F2027: Standard Guide for Characterization and Testing of Raw or Starting Biomaterials for Tissue-Engineered Medical Products. American Society for Testing and Materials, West Conshohocken, PA.

Guidance on writing materials specification for raw or starting biomaterials, which are intended for use in tissue engineering scaffolds for growth, support, or delivery of cells and/or biomolecules.

3. ASTM F2150: Standard Guide for Characterization and Testing of Biomaterial Scaffolds Used in Tissue-Engineered Medical Products. American Society for Testing and Materials, West Conshohocken, PA.

   Guidance for the characterization and testing of biomaterials after they have been formed into three-dimensional scaffolds.

4. KHAN WS, RAYAN F, DHINSA BS, MARSH D: An osteoconductive, osteoinductive, and osteogenic tissue-engineered product for trauma and orthopaedic surgery: how far are we? *Stem Cells Int*, article ID 236231, 2012.

   Describes the principles of tissue engineering of bone and its clinical application in reconstructive surgery.

5. KHAN WS, LONGO UG, ADESIDA A, DENARO V: Stem cell and tissue engineering applications in orthopaedics and musculoskeletal medicine. *Stem Cells Int*, article ID 403170, 2012.

   Brief summary of the use of stem cells.

6. LEE MH, ARCIDIACONO JA, BILEK AM, WILLE JJ, HAMILL CA, WONNACOTT KM, WELLS MA, OH SS: Considerations for tissue-engineered and regenerative medicine product development prior to clinical trials in the United States. *Tissue Eng Part B Rev* 16:41–54, 2010.

   Provides product developers in the early stages of product development with insight into the Food and Drug Administration process.

7. MEYER U: The history of tissue engineering and regenerative medicine in perspective. In Meyer U, Meyer Th, Handschel J, Wiesmann HP (eds): *Fundamentals of Tissue Engineering and Regenerative Medicine*. Springer Berlin Heidelberg, Leipzig, Germany, 2009.

   History of tissue engineering and perspectives on its future.

8. ONG KL, VILLARRAGA ML, LAU E, CARREON LY, KURTZ SM, GLASS SD: Off-label use of bone morphogenetic proteins in the United States using administrative data. *Spine* 35: 1794–1800, 2010.

   Background on the historical on-label and off-label utilization of BMP in the United States.

9. TRICE ME, BUGBEE WD, GREENWALD AS, HEIM CS: Articular cartilage restoration: a review of currently available methods. Committee on Biological Implants Scientific Exhibit. American Academy of Orthopaedic Surgeons, 77th Annual Meeting, Mar 9–13, 2010, New Orleans, LA.

   A review on four most commonly employed cartilage repair techniques with rational, basic science, and indications.

10. 21 CFR Part 1270: Human tissue intended for transplantation.

    Regulations related to banked human tissue.

11. 21 CFR Part 1271: Human cells, tissues, and cellular and tissue-based products.

    Regulations to establish donor-eligibility, current good tissue practice, and other procedures to prevent the introduction, transmission, and spread of communicable diseases by human cells, tissues, and cellular and tissue-based products.

CHAPTER TEN

Hybrid, combination, and replant materials

As described in Chapter 9, the field of tissue engineering has proliferated over the past few decades. The confluence of engineering, biology, and medical devices has led to the development of many so-called tissue-engineered products, some of which are now considered to be standard of care. *Tissue engineering*, as understood most generally, is the use of a combination of cells, engineering and materials methods, and suitable biochemical and physiochemical factors to improve or replace biological functions. A major component of tissue engineering is the development of substrates or scaffolds for cell adhesion. The ultimate goal of this development is to allow controlled degradation of the substrate so that the engineered tissue can support itself. These degradable materials that are used as substrates can be categorized as natural, synthetic, or hybrid materials. Natural materials may include collagen and other naturally derived polymers. However, natural substrates in their current form suffer from the lack of necessary mechanical integrity for fabrication into scaffolds. Natural materials also tend to be limited by supply and suffer from variation based on the source. Naturally derived polymers may also be immunogenic.

Synthetic materials include poly(glycolic acid), poly(lactic acid), and poly(D,L-lactide-co-glycolide) copolymer. The benefit of synthetic materials is the ability to adjust their physical properties so that they can be constructed to a specified size, shape, and morphology. There is also more control over their degradation characteristics.

The use of such cell or tissue scaffolds, either seeded with cells before implantation or attractive to cells after implantation, produces a new class of biomaterials: *hybrid* (sometimes *biohybrid*) *materials*. Although some scaffolds are not resorbable, the overall goal of the engineering designer is to produce hybrid materials that will eventually be remodeled and replaced by normal host tissue. However, the host response between the synthetic scaffold and seeded cells presents a great challenge. Therefore, multiphase materials, which combine the characteristics of both natural and synthetic materials, are commonly used. Multiphase polymers can be designed to provide the desirable physical properties of synthetic polymers and the biocompatibility of natural biopolymers. Two examples include the chemical coupling of the bioactive components of natural substrates with synthetic polymers and chemically modifying natural biopolymers to achieve certain physical properties.

Significance

Although many biomaterials are able to perform their intended function, few biomaterials possess all the necessary characteristics to perform ideally, thus there has been considerable effort to develop biomaterial scaffolds to synergize the beneficial properties of multiple materials into a superior matrix. The combination of natural and synthetic polymers with various other materials has demonstrated the ability to enhance cellular interaction, encourage integration into host tissue, and provide adjustable material properties and degradation characteristics.

The development of complex scaffolds can aid in better controlling the degradation rate, as well as degrading the material congruently as one material, without releasing particulate debris. For example, silica/gelatin scaffolds are used for bone regeneration because it can bond with bone and degrade in the body, releasing ions to stimulate cells for healthy bone production. The degradation rate of silica/gelatin scaffolds can be adjusted based on the control of covalent coupling. On the other hand, synthetic polymers can be blended with calcium for bioactivity by introducing inorganic (e.g., calcium alkoxides) or organic components. These bioactive hybrids can have high strength and resistance to cyclic loads.

Scaffolds can be composed of other synthetic materials such as ceramics, metals, and glasses (Figure 10.1). Alumina, silicon carbide, and zirconia have been used as ceramic components, while soda glass,

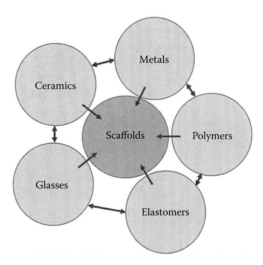

FIGURE 10.1 (See color insert.) Combination of materials to form multiphase scaffolds.

Pyrex, glass ceramics, and silica glass have been used as glass components. Elastomeric components have included neoprene, butyl rubber, natural rubber, and silicones, while polyethylene, polypropylene, nylon, epoxy, and polyester are examples of polymeric components. Steels, cast irons, aluminum alloys, copper alloys, and titanium alloys have been considered as metallic components for constructing hybrid materials.

Combination products

The term *combination product* describes materials or devices composed of two or more components such as drug–device, device–biologic, drug–biologic, and drug–device–biologic couplings, in which the effect of the drug or biologic component is not the primary intended therapeutic goal. Examples include devices coated or impregnated with a drug or biologic, such as drug-eluting stents or catheters with antimicrobial coating. Insulin injector pens and transdermal patches are also widely available combination products. Combination products may also include two or more separate products packaged together in a single package or as a unit and composed of drug and device products, device and biological products, or biological and drug products. An example of this type of combination product is a surgical tray with surgical instruments, drapes, and lidocaine or alcohol swabs.

Regulation
The US Food and Drug Administration's (FDA's) regulation of combination products has been continuously evolving. In late 2002, the Office of Combination Products was established with regulatory and oversight responsibilities during the collaborative review process of combination products. As described briefly in Chapter 9, the jurisdiction of combination products is based on the determination of the primary mode of action (PMOA) through which the product achieves its therapeutic effect. In products where the mode of action is derived through multiple methods, the single PMOA that provides the most important therapeutic action or provides the greatest contribution to the overall therapeutic effect is scientifically identified. The PMOA analysis is then used to determine which center at the FDA will take the lead in regulating the product. The three centers are the Center for Biologics Evaluation and Research for biologics, Center for Drug Evaluation and Research for drugs, and Center for Devices and Radiological Health for medical devices. Even during this process, the combination products are typically reviewed using a team of reviewers from all necessary centers with the expertise to ensure product safety and efficacy.

The FDA typically requires *in vivo* pharmacokinetic studies to quantify the duration of drug exposure, in terms of drug concentrations at the tissue, organ, and systemic levels. For devices with very small drug doses, time-release profiles may be used to demonstrate safety. This will include *in vitro* evaluation of the rates of dissolution. Toxicity studies are also important for evaluating local, regional, and systemic effects but have to keep in mind the method of administration of the combination product. Bench tests are also expected to examine the integrity of the device component of the combination product. These may include assessing that the drug/biologic and device do not chemically or physically interact with each other, as well as determining if the drug or biologic may affect the device's fatigue and corrosion properties, coating integrity, and durability. Depending on the device and availability of predicate or clinical data, biocompatibility testing must also be performed to assess any cytotoxicity, sensitization, acute toxicity, genotoxicity, and hemocompatibility responses, but may also require testing chronic toxicity and carcinogenicity, generally in line with the provisions of ISO 10993 (see ISO 10993: Biological Evaluation of Medical Devices). Given that FDA's testing requirements for drugs/biologics are much more complex than its requirements for devices, it is important to understand the expectations of the regulatory process to avoid setbacks that can ultimately interfere with successful release of a newly approved combination product.

Although the tissue engineering and combination product field is slowly maturing, the regulation of combination products is complex and challenging owing to the large number of possible product types and the multitude of regulations and guidance principles that could potentially be applicable. The hurdles are to determine when to apply existing regulations and guidances originally intended for a combination product's constituent parts to the combined product itself. There will likely be greater clarity in the regulatory framework for combination products as the field matures.

Bone substitutes

Autografts and allografts are used for treating nonunion bone defects and critical sized fractures. However, autografts are challenged by a limited supply of viable donor tissue, the need for additional surgeries, increased risk of infection, and donor site pain and morbidity. Allografts also face similar challenges in terms of limited donor supply, but there are also concerns with disease transmission and inadequate physiologic and biomechanical responses.

As an alternative, two or more materials can be combined to develop an ideal tissue-engineered construct with osteoconductive, osteoinductive, and osseointegrative properties. These characteristics may be achieved using a porous interconnected structure to allow cells to migrate and function within its confines (osteoconductive). Although soft tissue has been reported to be permitted in pores of 500 to 600 microns and neovascularization is favored in pore sizes in the range of 200 to 300 microns, others have noted that pore sizes greater than 100 microns can better facilitate rapid ingrowth of vascularized connective tissue. Others have also shown that 30-micron pores can produce minimal foreign body capsule formation. Pores should allow leukocytes (9–15 microns) and macrophages (16–20 microns) to penetrate in sufficient quantities; host proteinaceous and fibrinous material is then able to penetrate into the pores, having the effect of eliminating dead space and minimizing the chance for seroma formation.

These provide factors to stimulate the proliferation and differentiation of progenitor or osteogenic cells (osteoinductive) and are also able to assimilate into the surrounding tissue (osseointegrative). In essence, osteoinductivity is the ability of a substance to initiate bone formation in a non-bony site. Osteoconduction involves the facilitation of blood vessel incursion and new bone formation into a defined trellis structure, while osseointegration involves cellular elements, either from the host or from the tissue-engineered product, which survive transplantation and synthesize new bone at the recipient site. For example, ceramic–polymer composites have been developed to serve as bone defect fillers. Combinations such as calcium phosphate ceramics and tricalcium phosphate/hydroxyapatite have been the focus of current research efforts. Polymers have also been combined with ceramics to create bioactive scaffolds for enhancing tissue formation with greater initial strength.

As described in Chapter 9, bone morphogenetic proteins or BMPs have been developed as a natural alternative to bone graft. The device or carrier of the product is the osteoconductive collagen sponge, which is soaked in a solution of BMP, and allows local delivery and containment of the protein.

At this time, two recombinant BMPs (rhBMPs) have received FDA approval for use in the United States. In 2001, the first FDA approval of BMP was granted to OP-1 (rhBMP-7, Stryker Biotech, Hopkinton, Massachusetts), under a humanitarian device exemption (HDE), for use as an alternative to autograft in recalcitrant long bone nonunions. The following year, the FDA granted premarket approval of InFUSE (rhBMP-2, Medtronic Sofamor Danek, Memphis, Tennessee) for spinal fusion procedures with the LT-CAGE Lumbar Tapered Fusion Device (Medtronic Sofamor Danek) via the anterior approach in patients with degenerative disc disease at one level from L4-S1. Subsequently, the FDA approved the expanded indications for OP-1 in 2004, under an HDE, for revision posterolateral (intertransverse) lumbar spine fusions. Similarly, InFUSE also received approval (HDE) in 2008 for the repair of symptomatic, posterolateral lumbar spine pseudarthrosis. Other approved indications for InFUSE also include treating open tibial shaft fractures that have been stabilized with intramedullary nail fixation and sinus or localized alveolar ridge augmentations.

Although BMP demonstrated extensive popularity, growing substantially in use after its clinical introduction, in recent years there has been controversy with its use. Concerns with its use in anterior cervical fusion led to the FDA publishing a Public Health Notification in 2007 to alert the public to the possible "life-threatening" complications from compression of the airway and neurological structures in the neck. Then, in 2011, more controversy arose with increasing questions about the complications associated with rhBMP-2 use during off-label applications, including concerns with potential neuroinflammatory reactions of retrograded ejaculation and radiculitis, infection and wound problems, and uncertainty with carcinogenicity. This led to an independent evaluation of all clinical studies of rhBMP-2, which found that the indications for use in spinal fusion were difficult to identify based on the available evidence.

Cartilage

In contrast to bone, articular cartilage has extremely limited capacity to regenerate itself, largely by chrondrocyte mitosis and replacement; therefore, relatively minor lesions or injuries to articulating surfaces of joints may lead to progressive damage and subsequent joint degeneration. As described in Chapter 9, cartilage repair using autologous chondrocyte implantation was first performed in the late 1980s. This method uses the growth of autologous chondrocytes in a biodegradable matrix, which is then transplanted in place of the damaged tissue. The basic biological principle behind the use of this technique is that perichondrial and periosteal tissues contain cells that possess a lifelong chondrogenic potential. A pool of precursor or adult-type stem cells is expected to be present in these tissues with self-renewable capacity and the ability to induce tissue healing. A disadvantage of autologous chondrocyte implantation is that the donor site may experience severe morbidity because the explantation site will lose as much chondral or osteochondral tissue as the diseased implantation site will receive. Patches from porcine collagen bilayer membranes instead of periosteum are also being developed as alternative defect fillers. Numerous studies have shown that repairs achieved with autologous chondrocyte implantation can yield increased type II collagen content, which is "hyaline-like" cartilage. Thus, the grafted areas tend to show heterogeneity rather than the typical zones of hyaline cartilage, elastic cartilage, and fibrocartilage in natural cartilage. Mesenchymal stem cell transplants also show promise in inducing bone and connective tissue growth. However, some concerns with the formation of fibrocartilage and progression of degenerative changes in the joint have been raised. To overcome this limitation, further developments have focused on the *ex vivo* growth of a three-dimensional cartilage-like tissue, which integrates intimately in the defect site after being implanted. Other areas of research have also focused on the use of specific chondrocyte populations rather than an unselected source of cartilage. This is to provide improved cartilaginous structure to mimic the distinct phenotypic and functional properties of chondrocytes across zones of cartilage. A continuing problem has been the inability to encourage healing between the regenerated and host cartilage. Cartilage repair and restoration is a relatively new advancement and is becoming an increasingly important part of orthopaedic care. Knowledge and understanding of the available surgical techniques are critical to the appropriate use of these interventions.

Carticel (Genzyme Corporation, Cambridge, Massachusetts) is the first and only FDA-approved cell therapy product used to repair articular cartilage injuries in the knee of adults who have not responded to a prior arthroscopic or other surgical repair procedure. The product was first released as an unregulated device in 1995, largely owing to the FDA not having a protocol for evaluating human autologous tissue and cell therapy products. After working closely with the FDA to set quality standards for cellular products, the FDA approved the product in

1997. It uses a patient's own cells to repair cartilage injuries in the knee and is implanted in a surgical procedure called autologous chondrocyte implantation. Autologous cultured chondrocytes are derived from *in vitro* expansion of chondrocytes harvested from the patient's normal, femoral articular cartilage. The source of chondrocytes are biopsies from a lesser-weight bearing area, which are isolated, expanded through cell culture, and implanted into articular cartilage defects beneath an autologous periosteal flap. Prior to final packaging, cell viability is assessed to be at least 80%. The implanted cells can form new hyaline-like cartilage, with properties similar to normal cartilage, which may reduce pain and improve knee function. It has been reported that the most common complications include arthrofibrosis/joint adhesions, graft overgrowth, chondromalacia or chondrosis, cartilage injury, graft complication, meniscal lesion, and graft delamination.

Blood vessels

Autologous blood vessels, such as the internal mammary vein and the saphenous vein, have been used for grafting bypass procedures. However, because of vascular disease, amputation, age, or limited allograft supplies, patients may not possess appropriate vessels for grafting purposes. Therefore, there has been interest in developing engineered blood vessel substitutes that can meet the mechanical, biological, and hemocompatibility demands of the vascular system. Some of the key characteristics for tissue-engineered biohybrid vessels include elasticity and compliance, as well as exhibiting a luminal surface that can prevent thrombus formation and leakage to mimic the function of the endothelial lining in native vessels.

Engineered vessels using expanded polytetrafluoroethylene (ePTFE) have been used clinically for almost three decades. These possess the benefit of low thrombogenicity potential, scaffold porosity, and high strength. However, they are relatively noncompliant, leading to a stiffness mismatch with the native vessel, which could lead to intimal hyperplasia, activation of coagulation and complement cascades, thrombus formation from turbulent flow, and graft malfunction. Synthetic molecules and extracellular matrix materials have been added to the ePTFE constructs to limit their thrombogenicity. These promote endothelial cell adhesion and decrease turbulence. A key issue continues to be provision of appropriate wall porosity to enable healing without excessive loss of non-cellular vessel contents.

As an alternative to synthetic scaffolds, natural materials have also been used to construct composite scaffolds. For example, collagen and fibrin scaffolds have been found to have improved mechanical properties over scaffolds that have been constructed using solely the pure component. Although biologically based composite scaffolds have improved properties, questions still persist over their relative strength compared to synthetic scaffolds. Engineered constructs also often require weeks of mechanical conditioning or growth in an *ex vivo* phase to gain the necessary properties of an adequate vessel. However, there has to be sufficient initial strength to exist *in vivo* to allow the construct to remodel and the tissue elements to grow and mature.

Standards

Several tissue-engineering specific standards already exist (Table 10.1). As the tissue-engineering field continues to mature and the clinical applications and indications become clearer, there will certainly be further development of more guidance documents and international standards. Some of the core standards include ASTM (American Society for Testing and Materials) F2150 (Standard Guide for Characterization and Testing of Biomaterial Scaffolds in Tissue-Engineered Medical Products) and ASTM F2212 (Standard Guide for Characterization of Type I Collagen as Starting Material for Surgical Implants and Substrates for Tissue-Engineered Medical Products). ASTM F2150 helps guide the characterization of the bulk physical, chemical, mechanical, and surface properties of a scaffold construct, with the aim to evaluate if they affect cell retention, activity, and organization; the delivery of bioactive agents; or the biocompatibility and bioactivity within the final product. According to ASTM F2150, important characteristics include the identification of impurities, an understanding of the dissolution properties, porosity, surface properties, and degradation properties, as well as compressive, tensile, flexural, and creep behavior. Biocompatibility of the selected materials also need to be evaluated using ISO 10993 (Biological Evaluation of Medical Devices). Because collagen-based medical products are becoming more prevalent, especially in the area of soft tissue augmentation, ASTM F2212 seeks to provide some guidance for evaluating specific attributes of purified Type I collagen as a starting material for surgical implants and substrates for tissue-engineered medical products.

Viscosupplement use in orthopaedics is one prominent example of the use of naturally occurring biopolymers for biomedical and pharmaceutical applications and in tissue-engineered medical products.* Viscosupplements are partly covered by ASTM F2347 (Standard Guide for Characterization and Testing of Hyaluronan as Starting Materials Intended for Use in Biomedical and Tissue-Engineered Medical Product Applications). Hyaluronan is also used as a matrix material in bone repair/bond graft products.

---

* For example, this involves single or repeated injections of hyaluronic acid into the knee joint to relieve pain. Hyaluronic acid is a naturally occurring substance found in the synovial (joint) fluid. It acts as a lubricant to enable bones to move smoothly over each other and as a shock absorber for joint load. The first approval by the FDA was issued in 1997, which at the time was only for treating osteoarthritis of the knee. However, the long-term efficacy of viscosupplementation is not yet known and research continues in this area.

Table 10.1 Examples of standards relevant to tissue-engineered products

Standard	Title
ASTM F2027	Standard Guide for Characterization and Testing of Raw or Starting Biomaterials for Tissue-Engineered Medical Products
ASTM F2064	Standard Guide for Characterization and Testing of Alginates as Starting Materials Intended for Use in Biomedical and Tissue-Engineered Products Application
ASTM F2150	Standard Guide for Characterization and Testing of Biomaterial Scaffolds Used in Tissue-Engineered Medical Products
ASTM F2211	Standard Classification for Tissue-Engineered Medical Products
ASTM F2212	Standard Guide for Characterization of Type I Collagen as Starting Material for Surgical Implants and Substrates for Tissue-Engineered Medical Products
ASTM F2312	Standard Terminology Relating to Tissue-Engineered Medical Products
ASTM F2315	Standard Guide for Immobilization or Encapsulation of Living Cells or Tissue in Alginate Gels
ASTM F2347	Standard Guide for Characterization and Testing of Hyaluronan as Starting Materials Intended for Use in Biomedical and Tissue-Engineered Medical Product Applications
ASTM F2603	Standard Guide for Interpreting Images of Polymeric Tissue Scaffolds
ASTM F2383	Standard Guide for Assessment of Adventitious Agents in Tissue-Engineered Medical Products
ASTM F2386	Standard Guide for Preservation of Tissue-Engineered Medical Products
ASTM F2450	Standard Guide for Assessing Microstructure of Polymeric Scaffolds for Use in Tissue-Engineered Medical Products
AAMI/ISO 13022	Tissue-Engineered Medical Products—Application of Risk Management to Viable Materials of Human Origin Used for the Production of Medical Products
ASTM F2103	Standard Guide for Characterization and Testing of Chitosan Salts as Starting Materials Intended for Use in Biomedical and Tissue-Engineered Medical Product Applications
ASTM F2451	Standard Guide for *In Vivo* Assessment of Implantable Devices Intended to Repair or Regenerate Articular Cartilage
ASTM F2149	Standard Test Method for Automated Analyses of Cells—The Electrical Sensing Zone Method of Enumerating and Sizing Single-Cell Suspension
ASTM F2739	Standard Guide for Quantitating Cell Viability within Biomaterial Scaffolds
ASTM F1983	Standard Practice for Assessment of Compatibility of Absorbable/Resorbable Biomaterials for Implant Applications

Replant materials

A *replant material* consists of viable cells or formed tissue elements that are either genetically identical to or immunologically acceptable to the patient or are from some universal donor, such that it can be incorporated without initial remodeling, thus replacing absent or diseased tissue in both structure and function. A surgical example, not usually considered to be the product of tissue engineering, is the practice of transplantation of a lobe of the liver between genetically matched individuals, leading to organ regeneration in both donor and recipient. However, it is not a great stretch to imagine a liver biopsy, perhaps obtained percutaneously, grown up in a suitable tissue reactor and then replanted—this would now be considered tissue engineering.

The best current musculoskeletal research example is the use of an immune-suppressed mouse to serve as a host for the regrowth of ear cartilage, utilizing the patient's own stem cells in a suitable supporting mold, followed by replantation, with appropriate skin coverage. This is an energetic field of research and clinical investigation, where the fields of tissue engineering and regenerative medicine meet. The appropriate clinical goal is a therapeutic future in which most biomaterials and devices need only serve as bridges to replantation, supporting structure and function until live tissue is available.

Conclusions

The use of hybrid, combination, and replant materials is both diverse and promising. New technologies are being developed to revolutionize the treatment for many debilitating diseases and conditions. However, many hurdles need to be overcome for full acceptance into the medical community, including addressing the many material interactions in a tissue-engineered product along with regulatory obstacles as the field matures. Although not addressed in this book, market adoption issues, reimbursement questions, and viability of business models for such products will also need to be overcome.

Annotated bibliography

1. ASTM F2150: Standard Guide for Characterization and Testing of Biomaterial Scaffolds Used in Tissue-Engineered Medical Products. American Society for Testing and Materials, West Conshohocken, PA.

    Guidance for the characterization and testing of biomaterials after they have been formed into three-dimensional scaffolds.
2. ASTM F2212: Standard Guide for Characterization of Type I Collagen as Starting Material for Surgical Implants and Substrates for Tissue-Engineered Medical Products. American Society for Testing and Materials, West Conshohocken, PA.

    Guidance for evaluating specific attributes of purified Type I collagen as a starting material for surgical implants and substrates for tissue-engineered medical products.

3. ASTM F2347: Standard Guide for Characterization and Testing of Hyaluronan as Starting Materials Intended for Use in Biomedical and Tissue-Engineered Medical Product Applications. American Society for Testing and Materials, West Conshohocken, PA.

   Guidance for use of hyaluronan as a matrix material in bone repair/bond graft products

4. DAVIS HE, LEACH JK: Hybrid and composite biomaterials in tissue engineering. In Ashammakhi N (ed): *Topics in Multifunctional Biomaterials and Devices*, 2008.

   Overview of composites in bone tissue engineering.

5. LEE MH, ARCIDIACONO JA, BILEK AM, WILLE JJ, HAMILL CA, WONNACOTT KM, WELLS MA, OH SS: Considerations for tissue-engineered and regenerative medicine product development prior to clinical trials in the United States. *Tissue Eng Part B Rev* 16:41–54, 2010.

   Provides product developers in the early stages of product development with insight into the Food and Drug Administration process.

CHAPTER ELEVEN

Friction and wear

When two bodies are placed in contact and then caused to move relative to each other, we find that a force is required to maintain a constant velocity. This is contrary to our ideas of equilibrium: we expect that, once set in motion, the bodies will continue to move with respect to each other at a constant velocity. To preserve this idea, a new force concept, called the *frictional resultant* or *restraining* force, was created. As we will see, this force results from interactions between the bodies.

Friction dissipates energy, primarily as heat but sometimes as noise ("squeaking"), and the deficit must be made up continually to maintain motion. Sometimes friction is desirable, as in producing "traction" during walking or retention of bone screws. Sometimes it is necessary to regulate frictional forces, as in braking an automobile when too large a force would result in a precipitous stop, whereas too small a force would produce inefficient stopping and perhaps result in a collision. In other cases, as in designing total joint replacements, it is necessary to reduce friction to as low a value as possible, since such forces might contribute to bearing surface damage and loosening.

Accompanying the presence of frictional forces between two sliding surfaces are the processes of *wear*. Material interactions between contacting surfaces may produce transfer of matter from one body to another or create small particles called *wear debris*. It is usually desirable to keep wear at an absolute minimum, both to preserve the properties of the surfaces involved and to minimize the production of wear debris. This is the case in total joint prostheses. However, there are isolated examples in which controlled wear acts to preserve properties, as in the self-sharpening of teeth of the beaver.

Friction and wear may be controlled by introducing additional materials to change the nature of the interface between sliding bodies. These materials, which may be solids, liquids, or gases, are collectively termed *lubricants*. In the natural joint, components of synovial fluid act as lubricants. The exact nature of the effects of lubricants on friction and on wear is not clear and remains an active target of research in biologic and engineering systems.

Friction

Coefficients of friction

If two bodies are placed in contact under a normal force W, both chemical and mechanical interactions may occur. This produces a net attraction between the surfaces. If we now try to slide one surface over the other, we find that there is an initial force, F_i, needed to start motion, and then to maintain a constant velocity, a smaller steady-state force, F_s, is required.

Both of these forces are related to the interfacial load:

$$F_i = \mu_S \cdot W$$

$$F_s = \mu_D \cdot W$$

where μ_S and μ_D are called the static and dynamic coefficients of friction. It is usual for $\mu_D < \mu_S$; thus, it is easier to maintain motion in the presence of friction than to initiate it.

PROBLEM 11.1

Find the values of μ_S and μ_D from Figure 11.1.

ANSWER:

The force perpendicular to the interface is the gravitational force acting on 5 kg of mass, which equals 9.8×5 or 49 N. Thus, $\mu_S = 15/49$ or 0.31, whereas $\mu_D = 10/49$ or 0.20.

Thorough investigations of frictional phenomena have resulted in the recognition of more or less two universal rules:

1. The frictional coefficients depend on *load*, W, rather than upon *stress*; that is, they are independent of the area of the interface (this statement is sometimes referred to as the "law of friction").

2. Over broad ranges of interfacial loads, the coefficients of friction are linear; that is, they are independent of W.

Origin of frictional forces

Frictional forces depend on both the roughness of the opposed surfaces and their chemical composition. Of these two effects, the role of roughness is the easier to understand. Surfaces show a wide range of roughnesses, defined as the average height of local elevations or "asperities"

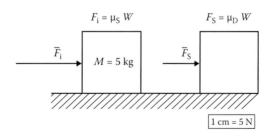

FIGURE 11.1   Production of frictional resultant force.

Table 11.1 Surface roughness

Type of surface	Surface roughness maximum asperity height (μm)
Saw cut	3–25
Inside of drilled hole	1–12
Lathe turned surface	0.4–3
Reamed	0.75–3
Lapped (150 grit)	0.5
Lapped (600 grit)	0.1
Optically polished	0.005–0.1
Articular cartilage	0.02–0.2
Alumina[a]	0.004
Polyethylene[a]	1
Metal[a]	0.02

[a] From Stewart, T.D., *Orthop and Trauma* 26: 435–440, 2010.

above the average level. Table 11.1 gives some typical ranges of values for surfaces of manufactured parts, in comparison with a natural bearing surface, normal articular cartilage.

Frictional forces in everyday applications arise directly from surface roughness. The existence of these asperities prevents surfaces from actually coming into contact. When it is believed that contact has occurred, what has actually happened is that only some asperities on each surface have come into contact (Figure 11.2). The true contact area, A_T, is between 0.001% and 1% of the overall surface of the interface (A) (this percentage has been exaggerated in Figure 11.2 for clarity of illustration). As a result, modest forces can easily produce at the tips of asperities stresses that exceed yield and ultimate strengths. Bonding, secondary to diffusion, encouraged by high local stresses, occurs at these locations. Thus, the initial force exerted to produce relative motion must act to disrupt physical junctions between the surfaces.

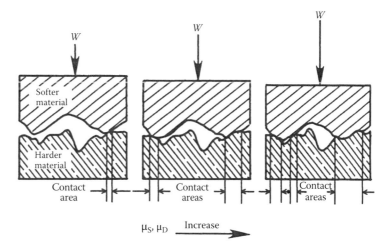

FIGURE 11.2 Effect of load on surface contact.

Chemical reaction between the two materials will tend to promote failure, during motion, through the weaker of the materials. A small increase in surface roughness can have a large effect on wear. Experiments have shown that increasing the surface roughness of a femoral component by a factor of 3 can lead to a 10-fold increase in polyethylene wear in a metal-on-polymer (MOP) total hip replacement (THR).

It can be shown that the value of A_T/A for materials that can undergo plastic deformation is given by the ratio of the load across the interface to the hardness, p, of the softer of the two materials involved. As a result, the force, F_i, required to initiate motion is simply the shear strength of either the interface or the weaker of the two materials, $\sigma_{u(sh)}$, times the area of the true area of the interface. Thus, the static friction coefficient is given by

$$\mu_s = F_i/W = \sigma_{u(sh)}/p$$

The ratio of shear strength to hardness of materials (which depends on $\sigma_{u(t)}$) tends to vary only over a very narrow range; thus, static coefficients lie between 0.1 and 1 for the vast majority of material pairs. Dynamic frictional coefficients are smaller than static ones since less deformation of asperities can take place, thus producing a smaller value of A_T. Table 11.2 gives values for some combinations of materials. Note that frictional coefficients depend on three factors: the two opposing materials and the nature of the lubricant (if present). Since frictional coefficients are ratios of forces, they are dimensionless.

Table 11.2 Frictional coefficients

Material combination	Coefficients	
	μ_S	μ_D
Rubber tire/concrete (dry)	1.0	0.7
Rubber tire/concrete (water)	0.7	0.5
Leather/wood	0.5	0.4
Steel/steel		0.5
Co–Cr/Co–Cr (saline)		0.35
UHMWPE/steel (serum)	0.35	0.07–0.12
UHMWPE/steel (synovial fluid)	0.07	0.04–0.5
UHMWPE/Co–Cr (serum)		0.05–0.11
UHMWPE/Ti6Al4V (serum)		0.05–0.12
Al_2O_3/Al_2O_3 (saline)		0.09
UHMWPE/Al_2O_3 (saline)		0.05
Hip joint (natural) (saline)		0.005–0.01
Hip joint (natural) (synovial fluid)		0.002

Lubrication

Effects of lubricants

In Table 11.2, we see the effects of lubrication. The pattern that can be seen here is that the introduction of a fluid between the sliding surfaces reduces the values of *both* μ_S and μ_D. This is the basic idea of lubrication: to interpose a material between two solids to minimize interaction between them. It is desired that the lubricant have a low shear strength such that the shearing motion will take place within the lubricant film rather than through asperities on either surface. However, fluids with low shear strength (low viscosity) can be squeezed out from between the surfaces, so that lubrication becomes a very complex problem.

Recent research has shed more light on the role of proteins in the lubrication process. Historically, it is thought that lubrication theory is based on an understanding of simple continuum fluids and does not capture important mechanisms of protein film formation, encountered either *in vivo* or *in vitro* with biological lubricants such as serum. Synovial fluid is a viscoelastic shear-thinning fluid that is assumed to be Newtonian (constant viscosity) at physiologic shear rates, though its behavior is actually non-Newtonian over a broader range. In terms of composition, synovial fluid is composed of a mixture of large, surface active molecules, consisting mostly of proteins, hyaluronic acid, and phospholipids. Proteins in synovial fluid are thought to be subjected to shear-induced aggregation and surface deposition at the inlet region of contacting surfaces, participating as an active agent in boundary film formation.

This film is characterized by a multimolecular layer with complex time-dependent behavior. First, protein molecule adsorption is directly responsible for the formation of a thin adherent film of 10 to 20 μm on contacting surfaces. The initial solid film is augmented by a thicker, hydrodynamically generated film of high-viscosity "gel-like" material. Clearly, our understanding of wear is dependent on the nature of synovial fluid lubricant formed during gait process. At the start of gait, the multimolecular film thickness is increased in comparison to that suggested by classic elastrohydrodynamic theory. Film thickness drops at higher speeds, due to some breakdown of the high-viscosity material, though it is unclear at this point why this occurs. Practically, because of the high conformance of mating surfaces in orthopaedic applications such as hip replacement, it is suspected that the escape of protein agglomerations from entrainment will occur less than in laboratory studies. Osteoarthritis and rheumatoid arthritis affect the chemical and physical makeup of synovial fluid, generally decreasing its viscosity and altering the pH and protein content. Protein content may even increase in periprosthetic synovial fluid. The conclusion from these recent findings is that classic lubrication theory may underestimate the thickness of the hydrodynamic film and the subsequent local reduction of wear *in vivo*. It is noted that these films are sensitive to contact pressure, may be disrupted during initiation of motion, and may be destroyed if pressure during motion exceeds a certain tolerance.

Velocity dependence

Fluid entrainment occurs when articulating surfaces drag lubricant into the contact region.

The thickness of the film between the two surfaces, h, is proportional to a parameter ϕ, sometimes referred to as the Sommerfeld number, which is given by

$$\phi = \eta \cdot V/P$$

where η is the viscosity of the lubricant, V is the relative velocity of the two surfaces, and P is the stress across the interface, seen as a pressure in the lubricant phase. (It should be remembered that η may be a function of V; see Chapter 4) This parameter affects the mechanism of lubrication, through its effect on h (see below), and, indirectly, the dynamic coefficient of friction, as seen in Figure 11.3.

Fluid film thickness is also considered in relation to the respective mating surface roughnesses when incorporated into a λ ratio, which is the ratio of the minimum predicted film thickness to the combined surface roughness of the mating surfaces (R_a).

$$\lambda = \frac{h_{\min}}{\sqrt{(R_a)^2_{\text{head}} + (R_a)^2_{\text{cup}}}}$$

While this equation is tailored specifically for hip replacement components, the principle can be adapted for alternate mating surfaces as long as geometric details of the surfaces can be parameterized appropriately.

Figure 11.4 is a key to interpreting the relationship between friction and film thickness. When film is sufficiently thick ($\lambda > 3$), asperity contact will be prevented, whereas a thinner film ($\lambda < 1$) will lead to a boundary lubrication environment.

This analysis assumes that the surfaces remain in contact and only move parallel to each other, thus shearing the lubrication film.

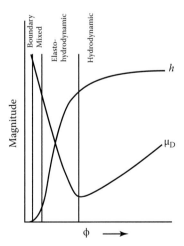

FIGURE 11.3 Dependence of lubricant film thickness and dynamic coefficient of friction on ϕ.

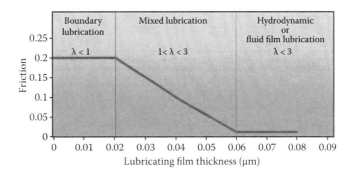

FIGURE 11.4 **(See color insert.)** Mechanisms of lubrication as dependent on film thickness and friction. (Adapted from Stewart, T.D., *Orthop Trauma* 26: 435–440, 2010.)

Displacement perpendicular to the interface of as little as h_{min} as possible in lateralization or microseperation can disrupt the lubricating film and introduce impact and fatigue wear, replacing the normal mechanisms of lubrication (discussed in the next section).

Mechanisms of lubrication

There are four principal lubrication mechanisms or regimes that depend on the nature of the relative motion and on the type of the lubricant used (Figure 11.5).

Hydrodynamic or Fluid Film. This is the lubrication mechanism present in most engineering applications, such as rotating bearings in electric motors, internal combustion engines, and turbines. As motion of the surfaces occurs, sufficient pressure results in the lubricant that the surfaces are completely isolated from each other and all shear deformation occurs in the film between them. If intermediate viscosity lubricants are used with very smooth (lapped, etc.) surfaces, the dynamic coefficient of friction and the wear rate are both

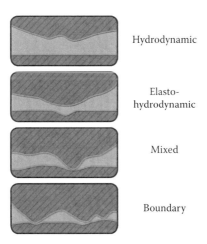

FIGURE 11.5 **(See color insert.)** Principal mechanisms of lubrication.

small. Because of their extreme hardness, ceramic components can be polished to a fine surface finish that will facilitate their potential for fluid film lubrication during walking.

Boundary. The other extreme occurs at low values of ϕ that permit surface–surface contact. Lubricant films are very thin, on the order of the asperity height, and lubrication occurs not by lubricant shear but by modification of surface properties. For a material, either liquid or solid, to be a good boundary lubricant, it is necessary for it to interact with the surface. Long-chain molecules with a chemically active region, such as fatty acids, are highly effective in this respect, reacting with surfaces to form soaps. However, both frictional coefficients and wear rates are relatively high, compared with those in other lubrication regimens. Because of the relatively high roughness of polyethylene, traditional MOP arthroplasty contact articulations fall into the boundary lubrication regime.

Elastohydrodynamic. The transition from hydrodynamic to boundary lubrication is not abrupt but passes through two other regimes. In the first of these regimes, the elastrohydrodynamic, the lubricant prevents the surfaces from interacting directly, but pressure waves conducted through it can produce elastic deformations in one surface opposite asperities in the other. This permits maintenance of a thicker lubricant film than would be otherwise expected. The result is excellent lubrication, with slightly higher μ_D than in pure hydrodynamic lubrication, and with relatively low wear rates.

Mixed. At still lower values of ϕ, the lubricant film becomes discontinuous and a mixed regimen of elastohydrodynamic and boundary lubrication occurs. This regimen is not terribly efficient and is usually accompanied by higher wear rates than the other three. Traditional metal-on-metal bearings typically fall into the mixed lubrication category.

In addition to these four classical lubrication regimes, there are additional important lubrication processes that may occur in special cases (Figure 11.6).

Hydrostatic. In some engineering applications, an external pressure source is provided to maintain h above some critical limit, thus producing lower values of μ_D.

Weeping. If the bearing surfaces are porous and deformable, relative motion may squeeze additional lubricant out of the surfaces into the separating film. This is a highly efficient mechanism and is believed to be a contributing factor to the low coefficients of friction observed in articular cartilage-lined joints.*

---

* The mechanisms of lubrication in natural joints are still a matter of some debate. The present consensus is that it is a combination of boundary, elastohydrodynamic, and weeping lubrication. Lubrication in replaced joints is primarily elastohydrodynamic, with the lubricant, produced by regenerating synovial tissues, resembling normal joint fluid.

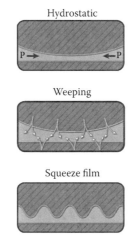

Hydrostatic

Weeping

Squeeze film

FIGURE 11.6 **(See color insert.)** Alternative mechanisms of lubrication.

> *Squeeze film.* Structured surfaces may be used to hinder the lateral flow of lubricant out from the sliding interface under the influence of the applied pressure. This produces a dynamic version of hydrostatic lubrication, without the need for an external pressure source. Squeeze film lubrication may be assisted in the natural joint by deformation of the cartilage, which will restrict fluid movement out of the contact region.

Wear

Normal wear Because of the contact of surface asperities during relative motion, it is usual for one or more of the materials to be eroded or worn away. This has unfortunate consequences both to the material, since its original shape and size are changed, and to the surrounding biologic system through the production of wear debris.

Such debris are produced by all material pairs used in total joint replacement (TJR) articulations; they may also be produced in other multipart devices. After an initial high wear rate period, called the *wearing in (or running in)* period, the quantity of wear debris produced, usually measured as a volume, is given by the relationship (Figure 11.7)

$$V = k \cdot F \cdot x$$

where k is a constant characteristic of the material pair making up the articulation and its local environment, F is the force across the articulation, and x is the distance of relative travel between the articulating faces. It should be noted with care that wear depends on interfacial *force*, not on interfacial *stress*; this is a result of the true contact area increasing with load while the true stress (greater than the geometric stress) actually stays nearly constant ($\approx \sigma_y$).

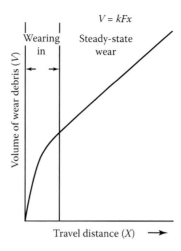

FIGURE 11.7 Wear rate curve.

PROBLEM 11.2

If a Co–Cr coupled with ultrahigh-molecular-weight polyethylene (UHMWPE) THR (28 mm head diameter) retrieved after 5 years *in vivo* shows a total surface recession of 0.75 mm (Figure 11.8), find (A) the annual volume of wear debris, (B) the number of wear particles produced per year (assume spherical particles 5 μm in diameter), and (C) the appropriate value of the wear constant (*k*). (Neglect creep in this calculation.)

ANSWER:

A. Wear volume

$$V = 2\pi r^2 \times 0.75/5$$

$$= 185 \text{ mm}^3 = 1.85 \times 10^{-7} \text{ m}^3$$

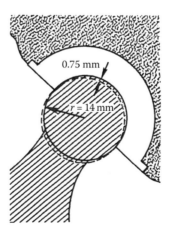

FIGURE 11.8 Polymeric wear in THR (Problem 11.2).

B. Volume of particle

$$V_p = (4/3)\pi r_p^3$$

$$= (4/3)\ \pi\ (2.5 \times 10^{-6})^3$$

$$= 6.54 \times 10^{-17}\ m^3$$

No. of particles

$$V/V_p = 2.8 \times 10^9\ \text{or}\ 2,800,000,000\ (2.8\ \text{billion!})$$

C. Assume: 1 million paces per year, total angular motion per pace (hip extension–flexion–extension) of 80°.

$$x = 10^6 \times (80/360) \times 2\pi r = 1.94 \times 10^4\ m/year$$

$$V = kFx \rightarrow k = V/Fx$$

F: Assume 70 kg body weight, average load (over gait cycle) = 2.5 × body weight = 1715 N

$$k = 1.85 \times 10^{-7}/(1.94 \times 10^4 \times 1715) = 5.56 \times 10^{-15}\ m^2/N$$

Wear mechanisms   Since both coefficients of friction and wear rates depend on interfacial load rather than stress, there is a natural tendency to draw the conclusion that good lubrication implies low wear rates. Unfortunately, that is not the general case, owing to the radical differences between the processes that generate frictional force and those that produce wear debris. For a particular wear process, improved lubrication may radically reduce the wear rate; however, different wear processes have widely different intrinsic rates. Thus, there is no correlation between μ_D and k.

When two surfaces are in contact and in relative motion, there are three primary wear processes that may result (Figure 11.9).

1. In the simplest case, asperities on the harder surface wear groove in the softer surface. This is termed *plowing* or *abrasive wear* and produces the lowest wear rate of these processes. However, resulting stress concentrations may result in accelerated component failure, by single-cycle or fatigue fracture. Chemical bonding between surfaces, especially in the absence of adequate lubrication, may increase abrasive wear. During abrasion, debris size is of a similar size to the roughness of the harder surface.

2. It is possible for the softer material to adhere to the harder surface, filling in the spaces between the asperities, thus forming a smooth *transfer film*. If the film is fairly strong and adherent, a stable intermediate wear rate occurs.

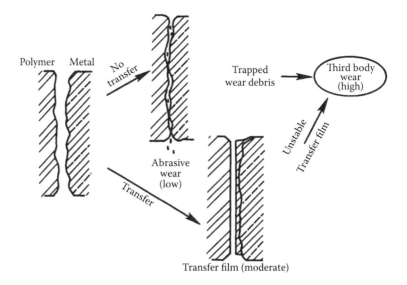

FIGURE 11.9   Primary wear processes.

3. However, it is possible for either abrasive debris or portions of transfer film to be trapped between the surfaces. These debris produce extremely local, very high stresses, resulting in rapid (high-stress, low-cycle) localized fatigue failure. This process, called *third-body wear*, is generally discontinuous, characterized by rapid variations in wear rate even after wearing-in, rather than by the constant rate shown in Figure 11.7.

Fatigue wear

In third-body wear, fatigue plays a major role, especially in the cases of rough initial surfaces. This commonly occurs when surfaces adhere prior to eventual asperity fatigue owing to shear stress at the adhered asperity. In certain cases, delamination can occur when cyclic shear stress from asperity adherence exceeds the fatigue limits of the bulk material. Because fatigue processes depend on stress rather than on load, some consideration must be given to an aspect of design of articulating implants that may produce a more general fatigue wear process.

In a spherical ball-in-socket joint, such as a THR, when the radius of the socket is essentially that of the ball, the interfacial compressive or contact stress is given by

$$\sigma_0 = W/\pi r^2$$

where W is the normal load (assuming that μ_S and μ_D are very small) and r is the common radius ($= r_i = r_0$) (Figure 11.10). This is called a *congruent* design.

However, two factors can contribute to higher surface stresses:

1. If the surfaces are *incongruent*, that is, $r_0/r_i > 1$, there is an increase in contact stress (σ_c) above σ_0. This would be the case in a poorly

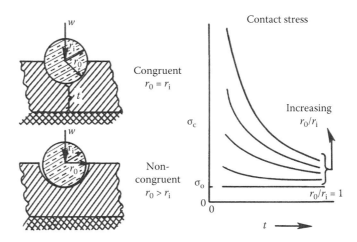

FIGURE 11.10   Effect of congruence on contact stress.

fitting THR combination or in the articulation of a total knee replacement (TKR) or, for that matter, in most natural joints.

2. If the softer material, usually the socket because of creep considerations, is too thin ("t" too small), then the contact stress is additionally increased. This occurs since the "substrate" or supporting material, whether in a natural joint or in an artificial replacement, is much stiffer than either articular cartilage or a typical bearing polymer, respectively. One may easily appreciate this effect by comparing the feeling of standing barefoot on concrete or on soft earth; the relative sensations are a direct consequence of the difference in average contact stress imposed by the metatarsals on the soft tissues of the mid- and forefoot. (This is, unfortunately, not a pure example since contact areas may also differ.)

These effects may combine to produce increases of up to 10 times normal in contact stress in noncongruent thin polymeric components such as thin metal-backed tibial plateaus in TKRs. For the typical radial dimensions encountered in THR and TKR designs, these effects diminish and approach a lower limit for polymer (UHMWPE) thicknesses of 7–10 mm and are unimportant at greater thicknesses.

The consequences of such high local contact stresses in polymers are first a localized surface cracking called "mud-caking" because of the similarity of appearance to the surface of dried mud. As the process progresses, fatigue cracks extend parallel to the surface, releasing fragments and producing accelerated wear, through both material loss and third-body wear (Figure 11.11). This has been observed in late failure of early metal-backed acetabular components with thin polymer shells; evidence of the early stages has also been found in more conventional implants retrieved after long periods (7–10 years). The similarity between these defects in polymeric components and those observed in articular cartilage in osteoarthritis (OA) has led to suggestions that fatigue

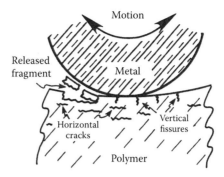

FIGURE 11.11   Fatigue "wear" of polymer.

processes also play a role in OA, secondary to stiffening of subchondral bone (owing to sclerosis or microfracture) and thinning of cartilage.

Small degrees of incongruence in hard-on-hard bearings such as metal-on-ceramic (MOC) (e.g., $CoCr–Al_2O_3$), ceramic-on-ceramic, and metal-on-metal (MOM) bearing pairs can produce extreme elevations of local stress leading to high wear and failure. Thus, very precise tolerances are necessary for successful manufacture of such component pairs.

Other wear phenomena

Wear is a complex process, with many features of specific materials pairs and designs affecting the outcome. Some important additional processes, which may occur independently or together, are as follows:

> *Corrosive wear.* When sliding takes place in a corrosive environment, wear processes may disrupt the passivation layer on the metal part of the pair, producing accelerated material loss. This is discussed further in Chapter 12.

> *Fretting.* When relative motion is possible, but over a very restricted range, such as between screw head and hole in a screw plate internal fracture fixation device, significant localized wear, called *fretting*, can occur. The amount of debris produced is often amazing, producing extensive tissue discoloration *in vivo* even under conditions that do not favor corrosion processes. *In vitro* studies demonstrate that serum proteins act as lubricants, radically reducing the effects seen in saline solutions.

Wear rates

There have been many efforts made to measure the rate of wear debris production in the laboratory. In general, the results depend on the geometry of the test, on the lubricant selected to simulate synovial fluid, and, to some degree, on the experimenter. There have been great difficulties encountered in reproducing *in vitro* experimental results. However, all of these studies agree in that both the size of the individual particle and the number of particles produced in a given situation vary *directly* with the ability of the surfaces to "stick" and *inversely* with the elastic modulus,

E, of the material in question. Since like materials are able to bond easily, the former factor explains why like pairs of materials tend to show higher wear rates than unlike pairs. However, the range of moduli is far greater than the range of surface associations ("stickiness") in the presence of lubrication, so modulus effects dominate production of wear debris.

Thus, *in vivo*, we expect that wear will occur preferentially to the less stiff (possessing lower modulus) member of the articulating pair. In a MOP pair, the polymer wears almost exclusively, and in a MOC pair, the metal will wear but will produce much smaller particles than in the previous case (<0.01–1.0 μm for metal [against ceramic] vs. 1–100 μm for UHMWPE [against metal]).

These general relationships have been verified clinically, at least with respect to typical wear debris particle size, through a number of studies of tissue retrieved from patients during THR arthroplasty revision. However, such studies have failed to provide reasonable estimates of either relative wear rates or total volume of wear debris, owing to the high solubility of fine metallic debris and the increase in phagocytosis and transport rates with decreasing particle size.

The limit on radiographic determination of dimensional changes associated with wear *in vivo* is probably ±0.25 mm/year, although this number has been criticized as being too small. Thus, most reliable data on wear–creep rates are obtained from prosthetic components recovered during revision surgery and, occasionally, at autopsy. The best estimates for *in vivo* volumetric wear rates for typical THR designs are given in Table 11.3. There is general agreement that the rate of 0.15 mm/year (expressed as surface recession rates rather than volume of wear debris) is a fair estimate of the true wear rate of conventional UHMWPE/cobalt-base alloy pair in THRs.

Wear-induced osteolysis continues to be a salient concern in large joint arthroplasty. In general, reducing the volume of wear particles associated with arthroplasty components should reduce the adverse biologic responses to them. Concerns over polyethylene wear-induced osteolysis have spurred interest in alternative bearing surfaces. Volume

Table 11.3 Estimated *in vivo* wear rates

Material combination	Material worn	Rate (mm³/year)
Metal/polymer (Co–Cr/UHMWPE)	Polymer	40.8
Metal/metal (Co–Cr)	Metal	0.023–6.3
Ceramic (alumina)/polymer (Al_2O_3/ UHMWPE)	Polymer	51
Ceramic (alumina)/ceramic (alumina) (Al_2O_3/Al_2O_3)	Ceramic	0.004–0.04
Ceramic (zirconia)/ceramic (alumina) (ZrO_2/Al_2O_3)	Ceramic	0.1

Source: Data adapted from Vassilou K, Scholes SC, Unsworth A. Laboratory studies on the tribology of hard bearing hip prostheses: ceramic on ceramic and metal on metal. *Proc IMechE, 221 Part H*: J. Engineering in Medicine 11–20, 2007.

of wear debris in hard-on-hard joints is one to two orders of magnitude lower than traditional metal-on-polyethylene bearings. (Also of note: dimensions of hard bearing wear particles are also much smaller.) The past 15 years have seen further development of hard-on-hard bearings to directly address the issue of implant wear.

Wear in newer generations of dense, polycrystalline alumina is on the order of a few microns per year, though there are exceptions. Some alumina bearings show a patch of localized surface damage, including loss of grains, commonly termed *striped wear*. The initiation of striped wear is suspected to occur when the femoral head dislocates slightly from the bearing and impinges upon the edge at the beginning of the gait cycle. This process is variously termed lateralization or microseparation. Zirconia has improved fracture toughness properties compared to alumina, but the amount of wear in zirconia ceramic on ceramic bearings is somewhat controversial. Some studies have reported severe wear, while others report wear to be very low. Still, because of the typically low wear rate of ceramic bearings, osteolysis is very rare.

MOM bearings have also gained significant market share, though the tenure of this bearing has been more controversial. MOM bearings exhibit a linear wear rate that is on the order of a few microns per year, though wear tends to be very dependent on finding an optimum clearance. A smaller clearance in MOM bearings increases the capability to generate fluid film thickness. Unfortunately, if the tolerance of the sphericity is larger than that of the clearance, binding or excessive wear may occur. On the other hand, too large a clearance will not facilitate fluid film lubrication, lead to a smaller contact area, and ultimately result in higher contact stresses. Carbon content and heat treatment are also important and can affect this distribution of surface carbides, which directly affect wear. Also notable, it has been proposed that MOM bearings can self-polish, moderating surface scratches *in vivo*.

As a gross approximation, total volume of wear is equal to the wear depth multiplied by the contact area. Increasing the diameter of the head will increase the contact area and the sliding distance. In metal-on-polyethylene total hip arthroplasty articulations, the volume of wear per step has been noted to increase with increasing ball diameter. This relationship does not hold for metal-on-metal bearings. This is likely due to the ability of larger-diameter metal articulations to achieve fluid film lubrication. Because of this, larger-diameter MOM components were considered advantageous in that they could reduce the risk for dislocation, and the thinner acetabular cup component facilitated the conservation of more bone stock in the acetabulum. There have been noted potential biological adverse effects of metal ions, which is discussed in detail in Chapter 14.

Wear rates for any material pair increase with higher patient weight and activity. Larger femoral head sizes tend to result in lower surface recession rates due to the lower contact stress but may be associated with greater volumes of wear debris due to the greater sliding distance. This may be particularly obvious with surface replacement devices for the hip, for which it has been estimated that wear rates (as measured by rate of debris production) are 1.5 to 2 times those for conventional THR designs.

Contribution of creep to wear

Materials subject to creep, such as UHMWPE, may show local deformation that may be mistaken for wear. This is easily appreciated in polymeric prosthetic components for tibial plateau replacement, in which peak stresses may exceed 10 MPa, and has come to be called "cold flow" in the clinical literature. At more moderate stresses, such as the 3–4 MPa experienced by the typical acetabular cup, it may not be obvious but has been estimated to account for as much as one-fourth to one-half of the apparent wear observed in retrieved UHMWPE cups. This type of deformation depends on geometric stress, so that heavier patients or those whose femoral prostheses have relatively smaller heads will experience greater creep. In addition, there is believed to be some slight increase in creep rate over time *in vivo*, owing to absorption of low-molecular-weight species that can act as plasticizers, making creep easier.

The limiting creep rate for a typical patient for an acetabular cup of at least 10 mm wall and 32 mm internal diameter is believed to be between 0.03 and 0.1 mm/year. Composite materials, such as carbon fiber–reinforced UHMWPE, may be expected to show lower creep rates *in vivo*. Metals and structural ceramics essentially do not creep at body temperature.

Examples of wear

Wear produces changes in surface appearance, particularly since bearing surfaces are usually highly polished. The most frequent change in appearance of metals associated with wear is a "frosted" or matte appearance. This is due to an increase in surface roughness, secondary to the inhomogeneous nature of wear. When relative motion is oriented, parallel lines or score marks occur, as seen in the hinge pin of a fully constrained stainless steel TKR retrieved after 7.5 years (Figure 11.12). Evidence of wear of metal components in MOP devices is usually less obvious. However, exceptional cases may occur, as seen in the Ti6A14V femoral head retrieved after 15 months shown in Figure 11.13. The origin of such extreme wear in titanium-base alloy components is not known.

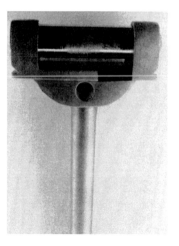

FIGURE 11.12   Wear of hinge pin of TKR (stainless steel).

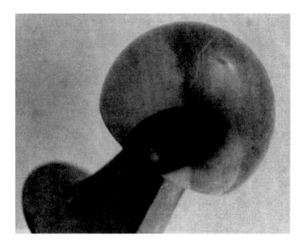

FIGURE 11.13   Wear of femoral head of THR (Ti6Al4V).

Although it apparently occurs quite rarely, it produces sufficient volumes of wear debris to require revision surgery for pain relief.

Polymers wear at much higher rates than metals (see Table 11.3), and large material removal may occur, as seen in the UHMWPE tibial liner shown in Figure 11.14. This damage reflects both wear and creep. Therefore, in such cases of polymeric wear, care must be taken to distinguish between wear and creep; microstructural examination of the material below the surface may be necessary to resolve the relative contributions when such questions arise.

When third-body wear occurs in a joint replacement, it is frequently accompanied by the presence of embedded debris in the polymeric component (metal, poly(methyl methacrylate), bone chips, etc.) and associated score marks on the metal component. Figure 11.15 shows the appearance of a UHMWPE acetabular liner cup removed after 12 years. The darker spot near the top is a fragment of bone, while wear, delamination, and local fatigue breakdown are all visible as well.

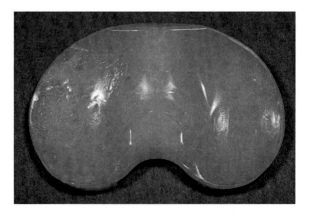

FIGURE 11.14   **(See color insert.)** Wear of tibial plateau (UHMWPE).

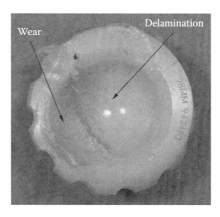

FIGURE 11.15 (See color insert.) Wear and delamination of an acetabular cup (UHMWPE).

Final remarks

Wear continues to be a challenge in implant surgery. As will be discussed at greater length in Chapter 14, the biologic response to wear debris may prove to be a limiting factor in TJR arthroplasty life. Although it will take very long development periods, new materials and possibly newer designs offer future hope of performance improvement in this area.

Additional problems

PROBLEM 11.3

Refer to Figure 11.16 and observe that TKR *A* has bearing surfaces that fit closely, whereas TKR *B* has a distinctly smaller radius of curvature for the femoral component than for the tibial component.

Considering the bearing surfaces, select the true statements from the following:

1. Because type *A* prostheses allow no entrance for lubricating fluids, they wear out faster.

2. The bearing contact stress for prosthesis *B* is greater than that for *A*.

3. Considering the coefficient of friction between Co–Cr alloys and UHMWPE, prosthesis *A* should significantly resist flexion–extension more than *B*.

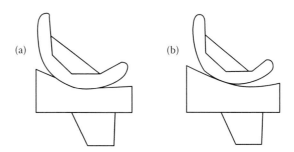

FIGURE 11.16 TKR profiles (Problem 11.3).

4. Little or no cold flow will occur for prosthesis *B* since there is less contact between the parts than for *A*.

5. The greater area of contact for prosthesis *A* will result in a greater volume of wear debris for the same usage period.

ANSWER:

F, T, F, F, F. 1 is incorrect since both designs allow easy entry of knee joint fluids. 2 is true since congruency and contact stress vary inversely. 3 is false since frictional forces are independent of contact area; in either case, such low-congruency designs, using modern materials, produce very low resistance to relative motion. 4 is false since, for a given joint force, "cold flow" (creep) increases with decreasing contact area. 5 is false since the rate of wear debris production is dependent on sliding distance rather than contact area.

PROBLEM 11.4

When two surfaces slide over each other (select the best answer[s]),

A. The surfaces wear

B. A frictional force resists motion

C. The surfaces become smoother

D. Some wear will occur and a friction force occurs

E. The surfaces become rougher

ANSWER:

The best answer is *D*. Wear always occurs; the consequence may be either smoother or rougher surfaces depending on the situation.

PROBLEM 11.5

"Stiction" friction is unimportant and disappears on motion (true or false).

ANSWER:

True. *Stiction* is an older concept that arose from the observation that static frictional coefficients are higher than dynamic ones. In reality, both static and dynamic frictional resultant forces for modern TJR designs are so low that it is not credible that they contribute to loosening of components. The actual effects previously ascribed to stiction were more likely related to deformation of polymeric components producing "pinching" effects and apparently large frictional resistive forces.

PROBLEM 11.6

When a smooth metal slides on a smooth polymer (select the best phrase[s]),

    A. It is necessary to use a lubricant to prevent wear

    B. Frictional forces will be very high

    C. Wear will be abrasive in character

    D. Fatigue wear will likely occur

    E. There will be no wear at all

ANSWER:

D is the best answer.

PROBLEM 11.7

Wear in a metal–polymer total hip prosthesis (true or false)

    1. May be easily detected *in vivo*

    2. May be produced by PMMA and bone fragments

    3. Is confined to the acetabular component

    4. Is confined to the femoral component

    5. Occurs on both femoral and acetabular components, but unequally

ANSWER:

F, T, F, F, T.

PROBLEM 11.8

Hydrodynamic lubrication (select the best phrase[s])

    A. Occurs at high loads and low speeds

    B. Is desirable because it reduces turbulence

    C. Is the lubrication mechanism in THRs

    D. Results in a complete separation of the two surfaces

    E. Can only occur if the surfaces are very smooth

ANSWER:

D is the best answer.

PROBLEM 11.9

Wear debris (true or false)

    1. Are spherical

    2. Differ in size for different materials

    3. May be retained between articulating surfaces

    4. Are a rare occurrence

    5. May produce third-body wear

ANSWER:

F, T, T, F, T.

PROBLEM 11.10

Rank the following wear pairs in *decreasing* order of (1) dynamic frictional coefficient and (2) wear debris production rate (assume saline lubrication):

    A. Co–Cr/Co–Cr

    B. Al$_2$O$_3$/UHMWPE

    C. Co–Cr/UHMWPE

    D. Stainless steel/UHMWPE

    E. Ti6A14V/UHMWPE

ANSWER:

1: A (C, D, E [equivalent]), B; 2: D (C, E [equivalent]), B, A.

Note: In 2, $D > C$ because of relative corrosion rate of stainless steel.

Annotated bibliography

1. BOWDEN FP, TABOR D: *The Friction and Lubrication of Solids.* Clarendon Press, Oxford, 1986.

    Includes the majority of Frank Philip Bowden's extensive contributions to tribology, extended by the work of his student David Tabor. An engineering text but extremely clear and straightforward.

2. CAMPBELL P, SHEN FW, McKELLOP H: Biologic and tribologic considerations of alternative bearing surfaces. *Clin Orthop* 418:98–111, 2004.

    A good synopsis of tribology in polyethelyne, ceramic, and metal bearings.

3. DUMBLETON JH: *Tribology of Natural and Artificial Joints.* Elsevier, Amsterdam, 1981.

    Discusses properties and test methods in great depth. Includes some of Dumbleton's work on modification of properties of ultrahigh-molecular-weight polyethylene (UHMWPE).

4. FAN J, MYANT CW, UNDERWOOD R, CANN PM, HART A: Inlet protein aggregation: a new mechanism for lubricating film formation with model synovial fluids. *Proc. IMechE 225 Part H* 1–14, 2011.

    Research discussing the role of proteins in the lubrication process.

5. GALANTE JO, ROSTOCKER W: Wear in total hip prostheses. *Acta Orthop Scand*, Suppl. 145, 1973.

    Early effort to relate coefficients of friction to wear rates.

6. McKELLOP H, CLARKE I, MARKOFF K, AMSTUTZ H: Friction and wear of polymer, metal and ceramic prosthetic joint materials evaluated on a multichannel screening device. *J Biomed Mater Res* 15:619–653, 1981.

    Often-cited compilation of laboratory studies.

7. MITTELMEIER H: Total hip replacement with the Autophor cement-free ceramic prosthesis. In Morscher E (ed): *The Cementless Fixation of Hip Endoprostheses.* Springer-Verlag, Berlin, 1984.

Review of clinical experience with a THR device including a ceramic–ceramic articulating pair. Includes reports of laboratory wear tests of Al_2O_3/UHMWPE and Al_2O_3/Al_2O_3 wear pairs.

8. RABINOWICZ E: *The Friction and Wear of Materials*. John Wiley & Sons, New York, 1965.

An intermediate level work on friction and wear, with the main emphasis on metals.

9. STEWART TD: Tribology of artificial joints. *Orthop Trauma* 24:435–440, 2010.

A review of basic tribological principles for orthopaedics, including the relationship between lubrication and film thickness.

10. SWANSON SAV: Friction, wear and lubrication. In Freeman MAR (ed): *Adult Articular Cartilage*. 2nd ed. Pitman Medical, Bath, UK, 1979.

This chapter deals with friction, wear, and lubrication in natural joints.

11. WALKER PS, BULLOUGH PG: The effects of friction and wear in artificial joints. *Orthop Clin North Am* 4(2):275–294, 1973.

Early discussion of friction and wear in total joint replacements, with comparison of metal-on-metal with metal-on-polymer devices.

12. WEIGHTMAN B: Friction, wear and lubrication. In Swanson SAV, Freeman MAR (eds): *The Scientific Basis of Joint Replacement*. John Wiley & Sons, New York, 1977.

A concise review of the basic principles, with relevant *in vitro* test results and patient observations, related to wear in total joint replacements.

13. VASSILOU K, SCHOLES SC, UNSWORTH A. Laboratory studies on the tribology of hard bearing prostheses: Ceramic on ceramic and metal on metal. Proc IMechE Part H: 11–20, 2007

CHAPTER TWELVE

Corrosion and degradation

Materials may react chemically with their environment. These reactions may produce changes in the properties of materials as well as alterations in the environment. When the materials are metallic, composed of atoms coupled by metallic bonds, the reaction processes are collectively termed *corrosion*. In exceptional cases, bacteria and cells, such as macrophages, can mediate corrosion processes enzymatically; this phenomenon is properly termed *biocorrosion*. In all other cases, corrosion *in vivo* is identical to that elsewhere, depending on the material involved and the conditions of environmental exposure.

The results of corrosion include release of free metallic or metal-containing ions and production of ionic and covalently bound metallic compounds as well as alteration of pH and of the concentration of other chemical species near the corroding interface. In orthopaedic applications, gross (or bulk) properties of metallic materials are rarely affected, but local attack may produce dramatic consequences.

When the materials are ionically or covalently bound, as in the case of ceramics and polymers, the result of chemical reaction with the environment, when present, is most generally called *material degradation* or sometimes *biodegradation* when the effect is observed *in vivo*. *Biodegradation*, although a term in general use, should be reserved to describe effects that are explicitly cell mediated, that is, degradation produced by cellular enzymatic action that would not occur under the same physiologic conditions in the absence of cells and cellular products. Biodegradation, although rare, may occur occasionally in orthopaedic applications.

The chemical results of nonmetallic degradation of materials include simple release of compounds and molecules by dissolution or bulk diffusion (elution) and reaction with the bulk material to produce rearrangements in bond structure and occasionally in bond type. These processes introduce components of materials into the environment and may result in profound changes in the mechanical, electrical, and optical properties of the bulk materials. In the extreme case, materials may be deliberately designed to dissolve, as in the case of resorbable sutures or resorbable internal fixation devices. Although this process is generally termed *bioresorption*, it is usually physiochemical in nature and not directly affected by the presence of viable cells.

Environments

The confusion produced by the use of the prefix "bio-" to mean "*in vivo*" should be avoided. We usually distinguish between conditions outside and inside the body by the use of the terms *in vitro* and *in vivo*, respectively. However, much of what we know about corrosion and material degradation *in vivo* results from experiments performed *in vitro*, with assumptions being made about true *in vivo* conditions and their effects on observed *in vitro* processes.

In thinking about the effect of environment on corrosion processes, it is useful to distinguish between five different exposure conditions or environments.

Laboratory. The classic *in vitro* environment in which pH, pO_2 (partial pressure of oxygen), and concentrations of other chemical species are varied over broad ranges to examine the mechanisms of inorganic chemical reactions.

Physiologic. A combination of controlled pH, pO_2, osmolarity, and chemical composition, *in vitro*, to simulate presumed or experimentally determined physiochemical conditions in some *in vivo* location, in the absence of cells or cellular products.

Biophysiologic. A physiologic environment with the addition of cell products, such as amino acids, proteins, lipids, and so on, but with the absence of viable cells, used especially in experiments to examine the production of organic-containing corrosion or material degradation products. These conditions are usually produced *in vitro* but may be achieved as well, with some difficulty, *ex vivo* or *in vivo* by the use of special chambers, flow cells, and so on, that prevent material–tissue contact.

Biologic. An environment in which viable cells, tissues, or organs are present, under homeostatic conditions, to produce *in vivo* service conditions. This is the classic *in vivo* condition produced by implantation, considered on a macroscopic scale. However, there is no single defined biologic environment, since there are significant regional differences in any living system and disease states may impose further variations. Differences in response of materials when exposed to biologic conditions as compared with those found under physiologic conditions may properly be described by the prefix *bio-*.

Pericellular. A special type of biologic environment, taking into account the specific local conditions produced by cells, especially those involved in catabolism, such as macrophages and osteoclasts. Such cells can radically alter the local pH as well as release high concentrations of catabolic enzymes. Differences in response of materials very close to or in contact with live cells as compared with responses in other locations are explicitly "bio-" in origin, unless it can be shown that they are dependent on only the physical presence of the cell and not on its active metabolic processes.

The bioengineering literature is still quite inadequate in making distinctions between these environments (as exposure conditions), both in the design of experiments and in reports of experimental and clinical observations. The reader is well advised to presume that exposure to each of these five conditions may produce different effects and that, thus, the results of exposure to any one may not easily predict the results of exposure to another one.

Corrosion

Corrosion means literally to eat or gnaw away and is usually reserved to describe chemical attack on metals. The visual effects of gross corrosion are familiar: changes in color and texture, production of surface films, and gradual disintegration of the base metal. Rusting is a form of corrosion, the reaction of iron with oxygen and water to form a variety of iron oxides and hydroxides; however, it is improper to call all corrosion processes rusting.

Figure 12.1 shows a total hip arthroplasty (THA) femoral stem taper that is corroded, showing color and surface texture changes. However, corrosion of implants producing significant biologic consequences may take place without any visible evidence. Thus, the best operative definition for corrosion is as follows:

> *Corrosion* is the group of processes that produce compounds and free ions from bulk metals.

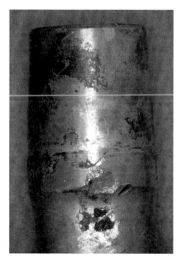

FIGURE 12.1 **(See color insert.)** Corroded hip stem taper.

Corrosion may produce a concentrated attack on metals leading to the initiation of other degradation processes. The stainless steel Kuntscher IM rod shown in Figure 12.2 was retrieved after 4.75 years of implantation. It had been inserted in the femoral medullary canal to stabilize a transverse shaft fracture, and a transcortical screw with its point in the rod groove had been used to limit rotation (Figure 12.2, left). On retrieval, the screw body was missing (completely corroded), but a local form of corrosive attack at its contact point on the rod had served as an initiation site for a nearly complete transverse fatigue crack.

Chemistry of corrosion

Metals as used in implants and surgical instruments are said to be *fully reduced*. That is, they have neutral or zero electronic valence, permitting bulk parts to be made entirely of metal atoms bound together by electron sharing in nondirectional metallic bonds (see Chapter 3). This renders them highly opaque to light and reflective, if smooth, giving the characteristic shiny metallic appearance that we associate with metals.

There are four types of reactions that change the valence of atoms in reduced metals by electron transfer processes and produce metal-containing ions and compounds. These reactions, shown in Table 12.1, are collectively responsible for corrosion. They occur because, in chemical terms, the total energy content of the products (on the right side of each equation) is less than that of the reactants (on the left side of each equation). Thus, they are an expression of the general tendency of the universe to "run down"; of all physical systems to seek their lowest possible energy content (level).

Oxidation and hydroxylation produce surface films of products that may or may not be adherent to the bulk metal. These films may also, themselves, be able to dissolve and release ions into solution, as ionization does, or may be subject to solution reaction, also resulting in ionic release.

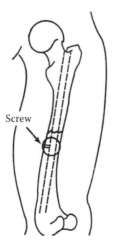
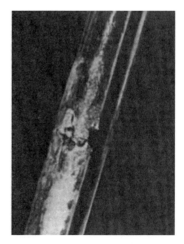

Screw

FIGURE 12.2   Partial failure of IM rod.

Table 12.1 Corrosion reactions

Ionization

$$M \rightarrow M^{n+} + ne^-$$

Valence	$0 \; +n \; -1$
Example	$Co \rightarrow Co^{2+} + 2e^-$

Oxidation

$$M + n/2O_2 \rightarrow MO_n$$

Valence	$0 \; 0 \; +2n, \; -2$
Example	$4Al + 3O_2 \rightarrow 2Al_2O_3$

Hydroxylation

(a)	$M + n/2O_2 + rH_2O \rightarrow MO_n \cdot rH_2O$
Valence	$0 \; 0 \; +1, \; -2 \; +n, \; -1, \; +1. \; -2$
(b)	$M + nH_2O \rightarrow M(OH)_n + n/2H_2$
Valence	$0 \; +1, \; -2 \; +n, \; -2, \; +1 \; 0$
Example	$Cr + 3H_2O \rightarrow Cr(OH)_3 + 3H^+$

Solution reaction

$$M(OH)_n + A^- \rightarrow MAO^- + nH^+$$

Valence	$+n, \; -2, \; +1 \; -1 \; -1 \; +1$
Example	$Cr(OH)_2 + Cl^- \rightarrow CrClO^- + H_2O$

PROBLEM 12.1

What is the valence of aluminum (Al) in the product in the example of oxidation given in Table 12.1?

ANSWER:

The product, aluminum oxide (Al_2O_3), is shown as a neutral or precipitated compound. Thus, the sum of negative and positive charges must be zero. Since oxygen has only one allowable valence state in such a compound (O^{2-}), aluminum must have a valence of +3. Aluminum has lost electrons in the reaction; thus, it is said to be *oxidized*, whereas oxygen, gaining electrons, is said to be *reduced*. Oxygen, or any other reactant that gains electrons, is called an *oxidizing agent*.

Corrosion rates

In conjunction with some related reactions governing acid–base equilibrium in water and the equilibrium between gases and their molecules dissolved in water, the four types of corrosion reactions shown in Table 12.1 are sufficient to describe all of the chemistry associated with corrosion. However, these equations and their related experimentally determined reactant/product ratios only describe equilibrium conditions; conditions under which reactant/product ratios are constant with time. The rates at which equilibria are approached are critical to understanding the consequences of corrosion and are not predicted by equilibrium conditions except in a very general way: it can be assumed that the further away from equilibrium conditions a reaction is (on the basis of the deviation of actual reactant/product ratios from those known to exist at equilibrium), the more rapidly the reaction will proceed. Beyond this, there are no simple general rules, and much of corrosion research has been directed toward determining reaction rates under various conditions.

Consequences of corrosion reactions

All corrosion reactions *will* result in attack on the bulk metal and an increase in the concentration of metallic or metal-containing ions in solution. If any reaction is possible, then there will always be *some* concentration of products in a solution containing the reactants. Thus, if a cobalt-base alloy is placed in physiological saline solution, after the passage of some time, Co^{2+} will always be found in solution, no matter what the physiochemical conditions are. However, the concentration may or may not be sufficient to be of clinical consequence. It is customary in engineering practice to group the equilibrium conditions resulting from corrosion reactions into three generic terms:

Corrosion* is the condition when the sum of the equilibrium concentrations of all ions containing a particular metallic element is equal to or greater than 10^{-6} M.[†]

Passivation is the condition when the sum of the equilibrium concentrations of all ions containing a particular metallic element is less than 10^{-6} M and there is an oxide or hydroxide layer on the surface of the bulk material. This surface layer is called the *passivation layer*.

Immunity is the condition when the sum of the equilibrium concentrations of all ions containing a particular metallic element is less than 10^{-6} M in the absence of an oxide or hydroxide layer on the surface of the bulk material.

Half-cell potentials

Although reaction *kinetics* are hard to predict, examination of reaction *energetics* can provide reasonable assurance as to whether a particular reaction can occur at all and, in the case of several possible reactions, which one is favored.

For any chemical reaction, such as those given in Table 12.1, the difference in energy level between the products and the reactants may be expressed as an electrical potential. This potential can be formally derived from this relationship:

$$\Delta F = -n \cdot E_0 \cdot \mathcal{F}$$

---

* This is a narrower definition of the word *corrosion* than previously given. Both are correct; the latter is used frequently to define the area of a Pourbaix diagram that is associated with neither passive nor immune conditions.

[†] M is the abbreviation for molar, the situation in which one gram-atom/liter equivalent of an element is in solution. Thus, a 10^{-6} M solution of Co^{2+} contains 58.9 µg of Co^{2+} per liter, since the atomic weight of cobalt is 58.9.

where ΔF is the difference in energy (actually, the amount of chemical energy per mole of reactants converted to electrical energy in reactions in which electrons are either released or consumed) between the reactants and products, n is the number of electrons transferred by oxidation per atom of metallic reactant, $\mathscr{F}$ is a constant called the Faraday constant (1 mole of electrons, equal to 96,520 coulombs of charge), and E_0 is the half-cell potential. Values of E_0 have been determined for virtually all chemical reactions under standard conditions (25°C, atmospheric pressure, 1 M concentrations of reactants and products). These electrical potentials, like all potentials, are relative and are referred to a standard reaction taking place at a carbon or platinum electrode:

$$1/2\ H_2\ (\text{dissolved}) \rightarrow H^+ + e^-$$

whose E_0 is set equal to zero. This is often written in shorthand fashion as

$$H/H^+ \quad E_0 = 0$$

Ideal electrochemical series

If we use this notation and rank the most favored ionization reactions by the value of E_0 relative to H/H^+, we obtain a very useful table called an *electrochemical series* (also called "electromotive force" or "galvanic" series, although galvanic series are usually *practical* rather than *ideal* series) (Table 12.2).

The metals with large negative oxidation potentials, such as gold, are called *noble* and are corrosion resistant. Those that have large positive oxidation potentials, such as aluminum, are called *base* and are significantly prone to corrosion. Iron and vanadium each appear twice in this series, since the half-cell potential depends on, among other things, the valence of the resultant ion. Differences in pH and pO_2 affect the valence of the dissolved ions, as will be seen later (other ionic valences are possible but, for simplicity, are not included). The actual values of the half-cell potentials, as given in common reference sources, are small, not exceeding 2 V.

The galvanic cell

Table 12.2 is an *ideal* electrochemical series and predicts the outcome of an experiment as shown in Figure 12.2. Two electrodes of the same shape and size are made from different metals, placed in water containing ions of both metals, and connected externally by an electronic conductor or wire. This arrangement is called a *galvanic cell* in honor of Luigi Galvani's discovery of the electric potential difference produced by a bimetallic pair ("couple") in contact with an electrolyte (moist frog sartorius muscle).

Table 12.2   Electrochemical series (ideal)

E_0 increasingly negative (noble)	Gold	Au/Au^{3+}
	Platinum	Pt/Pt^{2+}
	Silver	Ag/Ag^{+}
	Copper	Cu/Cu^{2+}
$E_0 = 0$	Hydrogen	H/H^{+}
	Iron	Fe/Fe^{3+}
	Lead	Pb/Pb^{2+}
	Molybdenum	Mo/Mo^{3+}
	Nickel	Ni/Ni^{2+}
	Vanadium	V/V^{5+}
	Cobalt	Co/Co^{2+}
	Iron	Fe/Fe^{2+}
	Tantalum	Ta/Ta^{3+}
	Zinc	Zn/Zn^{2+}
	Chromium	Cr/Cr^{3+}
	Manganese	Mn/Mn^{2+}
	Vanadium	V/V^{2+}
	Aluminum	Al/Al^{3+}
	Titanium	Ti/Ti^{2+}
E_0 increasingly positive (base)	Magnesium	Mg/Mg^{2+}

The following observations can be made in such an arrangement:

1. There is a difference in electrical potential between the two metals (*electrodes*), inferred by observing the passage of an electron current through the wire.

2. The metal that is base with respect to the other, that is, below it in the electrochemical series, is negatively charged, is said to be *anodic*,* and undergoes an oxidation process leading to either the release of metal or the formation of a passive layer.

3. The metal that is noble with respect to the other, that is, above it in the electrochemical series, is positively charged, is said to be *cathodic*, and is immune. Such immunity, imposed by electrical coupling to another electrode, is called *cathodic protection*.

---

* There is often confusion about the sign of the potential of the cathode or anode. In a formal way, the cathode is always the electrode at which *reduction* takes place. If the reduction is driven spontaneously by the chemical energetics of the experiment, as in this case, the cathode is *positive* with respect to the anode. If the cathode is polarized by an external power source, as in faradic stimulation of bone growth (see Chapter 5), it is *negative* with respect to the anode.

The appropriate electrode reactions are as follows:

At the anode:

$$M_1 \rightarrow M_1^{n+} + n \cdot e^- \text{ (oxidation)}$$

At the cathode:

$$M_2^{m+} + m \cdot e^- \rightarrow M_2 \text{ (reduction)}$$

However, the more usual cathodic reaction is

$$H^+ + e^- \rightarrow 1/2 \, H_2 \text{ (gas) (reduction)}$$

owing to the high concentration of H^+, especially under acidic conditions. The electrical potential difference measured will be the difference between the half-cell potentials for the reactions occurring at each electrode. When reduction takes place on an externally connected electrode, as in an electrical stimulator, the half-cell potential is equal to but opposite in sign to the oxidation potential.

PROBLEM 12.2

Suppose that, in Figure 12.3, one electrode is silver and the other is chromium. Are the following statements true or false?

1. Silver will be cathodically protected.
2. The anode will release chromium ions.
3. Electrons will flow from chromium to silver.
4. Chromium will be immune.
5. Oxidation will occur at the silver electrode.

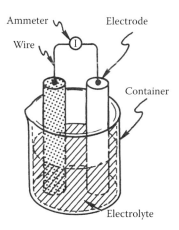

FIGURE 12.3   Galvanic cell.

ANSWER:

Silver is more noble than chromium (Table 12.2); thus, the correct answers are T, T, T, F, F. Chromium is not immune; in this case, it would form chromium hydroxide, the basis of corrosion protection of many alloys, and would be said to be passivated. However, its anodic bias would promote continuing ionic release by surface layer dissolution.

Practical electrochemical (galvanic) series

However, corrosion is dependent on other factors in addition to the differences in half-cell potentials. These include the rate of approach to equilibrium (previously discussed), the physical properties of the reactants and their corrosion products, and the pH, PO_2, and local electrical potentials present in a particular application. These considerations may be combined and expressed in a very general way in a *practical* electrochemical series. Such a series must be derived from experiments under conditions that match the application, using a galvanic cell. No such general series exist for generic or specific biomedical applications, but those obtained in seawater (for marine applications) are a good predictive guide to behavior *in vivo*. A short practical seawater series is given in Table 12.3, together with the relative positions in the ideal series, where they are known.

Changes in position occur in a practical ranking, relative to those in the ideal series, reflecting differences in chemical interaction with the particular environment selected. Thus, platinum is more noble than gold in seawater because it is less reactive with Cl^- ion. Copper and lead react easily with Cl^-, so they are more basic. Aluminum, magnesium, and titanium react easily with oxygen and thus are considered basic in pure water. However, titanium

Table 12.3 Practical versus Ideal Electrochemical Series

	Ideal	Practical (Seawater)
Noble	Gold	Platinum
	Platinum	Gold
	Silver	Stainless steel (passive)
	Copper	Titanium
	Lead	Silver
	Nickel	Nickel
	Iron	Stainless steel (nonpassive)
	Chromium	Copper
	Aluminum	Lead
	Titanium	Cast iron
	Magnesium	Aluminum
Base		Magnesium

forms a very stable passive layer that, unlike that which forms on aluminum and magnesium, is highly resistant to attack by Cl⁻ and thus resists dissolution in seawater. As a result, passivated titanium appears relatively noble in seawater and is highly corrosion resistant *in vivo*. For stainless steel alloys, which are less reactive with oxygen, deliberate passivation during manufacture greatly increases their practical nobility in the presence of Cl⁻, rendering many of them useful as implant materials.

However, such practical series should be used with caution, as the actual implant conditions may affect the relative activity of the metals in question. For instance, wear, as in a bearing interface, or fretting, as in a modular junction, may disrupt the passive layer on the metallic surface.

Effects of environmental variation

Beyond the general role of the environment, it is desirable to be able to predict the effects of changes in pH, PO_2, and so on, within a specific environment on the corrosion process that is favored to take place. There are many possible chemical reactions in any system consisting of a metal and its environment; it is necessary to make some order out of them so that we can approach the problem of corrosion prediction in a systematic way.

All the possible chemical reactions in a system can be classified by answering two questions:

1. Does the reaction depend on pH?
2. Does the reaction depend on local electrical potential?

This classification makes it feasible to sort out the possible reactions in a given system and to begin to understand the effects of pH and PO_2 on them.

The Pourbaix diagram

It is possible to plot the outcome of reactions in a given metal–electrolyte (liquid containing [dissolved] ions) system by connecting points of equal ionic product concentrations, on a diagram whose axes are pH and electrical potential (with reference to the H/H⁺ half-cell). Such diagrams are called *pH-potential* or *Pourbaix* diagrams (named for Marcel Pourbaix [1904–1998], a Belgian electrochemist who has been responsible for popularizing their use). They further simplify consideration of competing chemical reactions since it turns out that in any area of such a diagram, a single reaction, among the 20–30 possible in any metal–electrolyte system, dominates and is the major contributor of dissolved ions. Preparation of such diagrams is difficult and time consuming, requiring the assembly of data from many different types of experiment. Thus, despite their utility, they are available only for most elemental metals in water and are not available for alloys and metals in most other solutions.

Figure 12.4a is the Pourbaix diagram for chromium in water. The solid boundaries connect points at which the concentration of all chromium

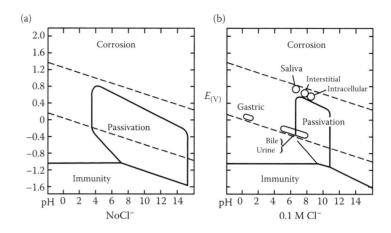

FIGURE 12.4 Pourbaix (pH-potential) diagrams for chromium in water.

ions in solution is 10^{-6} M. They define three areas that correspond to the three fundamental generic processes of corrosion previously discussed.

Corrosion. In this region, a variety of reactions either oxidize chromium (3.9 < pH < 15.2) or promote the solubility of the passive coating (3.9 ≥ pH ≥ 15.2). Throughout this region, the concentration of chromium-bearing ions is greater than 10^{-6} M. Note that the valence of the dissolved species may vary within this corrosion region. Under acidic conditions (pH < 7), the predominant valence is +3, whereas under alkaline conditions (pH > 7), the predominant valence is +6. (This may have a dramatic effect on the biologic effects of corrosion products; see Chapter 14.)

Passivation. In this region, the dominant reactions lead to the formation of oxides and hydroxides of chromium. Since these products are largely insoluble at pH values above 4, they cling to the metal, reducing and eventually preventing further reaction of the base metal with the solution. This renders the chromium passive; it has a similar beneficial effect on any alloy containing chromium and is the basis of the excellent corrosion resistance of stainless steels and chromium-containing cobalt-base alloys. Throughout this region, the solubility of the passive layer is low enough that the concentration of chromium-containing ions in solution is less than 10^{-6} M.

Immunity. In this region, the dominant reaction is ionization. However, throughout this part of the diagram, the resulting equilibrium concentration of chromium in solution is less than 10^{-6} M. The metal remains bright; conditions do not favor formation of a passive layer. If a passive layer is preformed by chemical means, it will disassociate in this region; however, the rate may be slow enough near the passive boundary, as is the case for chromium, to render the passive layer *metastable* and thus effectively to expand the borders of the passive region. Such a process is performed on all chromium-bearing alloy implants during manufacture (see Chapter 7). The resulting chromium oxide–hydroxide passivation layer is extremely thin and colorless and cannot be seen with the naked eye but can be detected instrumentally.

Two additional features of Figure 12.4a are of interest. The upper and lower diagonal dashed lines define the interactions of oxygen and hydrogen, respectively, with water under standard conditions. Between the lines, water is stable; at potentials above the upper line, gaseous oxygen is released, whereas at those below the lower line, gaseous hydrogen is released. These are the familiar anodic and cathodic products of electrolysis; the line separation is constant and equal to 1.228 V, corresponding to the lowest possible inter-electrode electrolysis voltage for water.

On the Pourbaix diagram, dominant reactions that depend on pH produce vertical traces, whereas those that depend on potential (electron availability) produce horizontal traces. Reactions that depend on both pH and potential, such as the equilibrium between oxygen and water, produce diagonal lines that pass from upper left to lower right. Reactions independent of pH and potential do not produce regions of dominance in such a diagram.

In biologic environments, where pH is controlled by buffering, the local oxygen or hydrogen partial pressure can then define an effective local potential. Thus, tissues that are perfused with arterial blood and are maintained at pH 7.37 have an equivalent potential of 0.782 V at 37°C. This characteristic of biologic environments makes it possible to use Pourbaix diagrams directly in predicting the dominant corrosion process (corrosion, passivation, or immunity) for any metal after implantation.

Practical aspects of Pourbaix diagrams

Most environments contain other chemical species in addition to H^+, OH^-, and metal ions released from the bulk. Figure 12.4b is the Pourbaix diagram for chromium in water with a chloride concentration of 0.1 M, to better simulate the typical *in vivo* conditions. The principal difference from Figure 12.4a is a radical shrinkage of the passivation region, owing to Cl^- forming complexes with ions in solution and increasing the solubility of the passive layer.

It is possible to locate conditions present in various body fluids on this diagram through knowledge of their pH and gaseous exposure. In the absence of an applied (external) voltage, the pH and pO_2 at a particular point define an "equivalent" potential. If an electrode possessing this potential is placed at this location, there will be no effect on local chemical reactions. Thus, knowing any two of the triad (pH, pO_2, and electric potential) permits certain knowledge of the third. As a result, fluids exposed directly to air, such as saliva, or present in the upper gastrointestinal (GI) tract may be located near the oxygen equilibrium line (appropriate pH values), whereas endocrine and lower GI fluids lie closer to the hydrogen equilibrium line.

Areas of pH-potential (as defined by pO_2) for various body fluids have been superimposed on the Pourbaix diagram in Figure 12.4b. Note that the areas for interstitial and intracellular fluids actually lie closer to pH 7; they are plotted as slightly more alkaline for clarity. From this, we could predict that pure chromium would likely perform well in neutral conditions in the bile duct or urinary tract but would likely be unsatisfactory in the stomach. General tissue conditions would be marginal since they lie on the boundary between passivation and corrosion, but the slowness in reaching equilibrium (metastability) aids in this case, making pre-passivated chromium-bearing alloys corrosion resistant in such sites.

PROBLEM 12.3

Suppose that a stainless steel stimulating electrode was placed in a medullary space and biased cathodic by 1.5 V with respect to the H/H^+ half cell. What would happen?

ANSWER:

Such a situation presents an environment with a pH near 7.3 and oxygen partial pressures of 40–60 mm Hg (0.05–0.075 atmospheres). The local potential would be approximately 0.8 V (anodic), and a well-passivated electrode would be metastable. Imposing the bias would move the electrode into the immunity region, leading to long-term reduction of the passive film. However, −1.5 V exceeds the electrolysis limit for hydrogen by more than 1 V, and gaseous hydrogen would be released. This is undesirable, and commercial bone growth stimulation devices contain voltage-limiting circuitry to prevent this outcome.

Anodic polarization diagrams

Pourbaix diagrams are difficult and time consuming to prepare. Furthermore, they contain far more data than are required for solving any one engineering problem, such as evaluation of a new metal alloy for fracture fixation plates. Thus, an alternate presentation, the *anodic polarization diagram* (Figure 12.5) is used.

This is produced in an arrangement such as shown in Figure 12.3, with the metal to be studied as one electrode, the solution selected to represent the application environment (usually well-aerated physiological saline, for convenience), and an inert electrical conductor, usually pure carbon, as the other electrode. The important addition is an active device called a *polaristat*, which is connected in series with the ammeter (current-measuring device) in the external circuit. A polaristat is a device that can adjust voltage across its external electrodes, independent of circuit electrical resistance, and change it at a predetermined rate.

The experiment is started by setting the polaristat to make the experimental electrode negative (i.e., cathodic and in the immune region) and

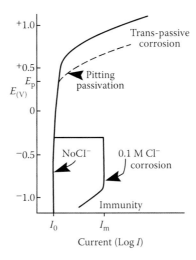

FIGURE 12.5   Anodic polarization curves.

then to reduce the potential (move toward anodic conditions) at a constant rate of 10–50 mV/mm. A continuous plot of the logarithm of current in the external circuit (horizontal scale) versus the external potential of the polaristat (vertical scale) produces the curve seen in Figure 12.5, which represents one that might be obtained for a pure chromium electrode (nonpassivated) at pH 7.2.

The curve has the following (typical) regions:

At large cathodic potentials, a minimum current, I_0, called the *exchange current* flows. This represents the minimum corrosion rate possible and reflects the immune region, if one exists for the metal being examined. In a practical electrochemical series, metals are ordered in increasing I_0 as one moves down (from noble to base).

As positive potential decreases, the current will increase, especially if a complexing ion, such as Cl⁻, is present, reaching a maximum current, I_m. If the metal is passivated or if passivation is very rapid and no complexing ion is present, there will be no current increase.

At a lower potential, the surface can be seen to grow a passive film, current is reduced, often to I_0, and the metal passes into the passive region.

At a still lower potential (more anodic), current starts to rise as active corrosion, called *trans-passive* corrosion, takes place. The potential at which this occurs is often called the *breakdown* potential. If pitting is possible, owing to the presence of Cl⁻ or another suitable ion, the current may begin to rise at a lower anodic potential called the *pitting* potential (E_p).

It should be clear that reference to a generic Pourbaix diagram to determine the pH and pO₂ expected in a particular application combined with performance of an anodic polarization experiment in a suitable medium will provide a reasonably reliable estimate of the corrosion rate to be expected for a particular metal. In fact, a little reflection will show that, allowing for possible errors introduced by the quasi-static conditions (slowly changing potential), an anodic polarization diagram represents a *vertical* cross section of a Pourbaix diagram. This approach to corrosion prediction has proven particularly useful in examining relative changes in corrosion behavior produced by changes in alloy processing and finishing.

Forms of corrosion

Electrochemical series, both ideal and practical, Pourbaix diagrams for selected elements, and anodic polarization diagrams for specific alloys help predict the occurrence of corrosion. However, the study of corrosion in engineering applications has proceeded from recognition of incidents of attack, grouping of these incidents by similarities in their appearance and performance (exposure) conditions, and then by reasoning back to the fundamental aspects underlying the observed phenomena. Such an engineering approach has resulted in classifying corrosive attack phenomena into eight forms.* These forms of corrosion will be discussed in a general way, taking into account aspects specific to orthopaedic applications.

Uniform attack   This is the overall corrosion process that takes place in the corrosion region (by ionization) and the passivation region (by passive film dissolution or reaction) of the Pourbaix diagram (Figure 12.6). It is the most common form of corrosion. In the absence of equilibrium concentrations of constituent ions in the bathing solution or of significant cathodic protection, uniform attack will occur for all metals. Even in the immunity region, uniform attack will result in slow removal of metal from implants, especially if the bathing solution has a very low level of constituent ions. Thus, it is fair to say that, owing to uniform attack, *all* metals have a finite corrosion rate *in vivo* but may not have any clinical consequences.

Figure 12.6 shows the general mechanism. Anodic and cathodic areas exist on the surface of the implant, resulting from small local variations in surface structure and environment. An electron current flows within the metal from anodic to cathodic regions. A characteristic potential, intermediate between the half-cell potentials for each reaction, can be measured with reference to another electrode; this is called the *mixed* or *corrosion* potential.

Uniform attack may not be noticed until or unless a visible amount of metal is lost. Typical corrosion rates for chromium-containing cobalt-base alloys, under normal general tissue conditions, are estimated

---

* This classification was developed by M.G. Fontana and N.D. Greene and is discussed at greater length in Fontana MG (ed): *Corrosion Engineering*, 3rd. Ed. McGraw-Hill, New York, 1986.

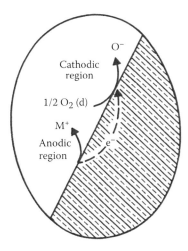

FIGURE 12.6 Uniform corrosion.

from *in vitro* experiments and limited *in vivo* polarization studies to be 40–60 μg/cm² per year. This corresponds to a surface recession rate of no more than 0.1 μm/year. In older (English) units, this equals 0.004 mpy (mils [10^{-3} inch] per year). Put another way, a prosthesis with a surface area of 200 cm² would lose only 0.1–0.2 g in 10 years by uniform attack. Stainless steels have similar corrosion rates, whereas titanium-base alloys, with similar corrosion current densities, have lower release rates owing to lower densities.

However, there is some evidence that serum proteins can complex with chromium and nickel, increasing uniform attack by up to 2- to 10-fold. Furthermore, this complex formation may take place by a process called "charge neutral corrosion" in which protein molecules accept both a positively charged ion and one or more electrons, thus producing no additional current between two electrodes, as in the galvanic arrangement of Figure 12.3.

Galvanic or bimetallic corrosion

This form of corrosion is called *galvanic* or *bimetallic* corrosion. The required physical conditions are (Figure 12.3) as follows:

Two different electrically conducting solids having different half-cell potentials.

An electronic connection between the two solids.

A bathing medium, containing free ions.

The mechanism has been discussed previously in relation to the electrochemical series. In implant applications, it may occur when portions of a single device or two separate devices in contact possess different degrees of nobility (different half-cell potentials for the specific local environment). In this case, the baser metal of the pair may corrode while the more noble metal is protected. The rate of corrosion of the base metal is generally higher than the uniform attack rate, but is very difficult to predict, since it depends on a number of factors including the nature of the direct contact, the relative sizes of the different metals, and so on. Acid pHs favor this process.

The metallic property differences that lead to galvanic corrosion come from a variety of sources. Work-hardening and surface-finishing processes that produce plastic deformation generally make the deformed metal basic with respect to undeformed material of the same composition. Compositional differences, between parts either because of manufacture from different master ingots within the same specification limits or because of deliberate mixing of metals, is the most likely cause of such effects. This latter situation has been investigated *in vitro* with the results shown in Table 12.4.

Thus, although one may choose to avoid mixing or "coupling" metals, the only absolute contraindication appears to be the use of stainless steel as one component. Thus, stainless steel cerclage wire should not be used with cobalt-base or titanium-base alloy implants, unless there is no real likelihood of wire and device coming into contact.

A practical example of galvanic corrosion can be seen in Figure 12.7, which shows an inclusion produced in a portion of a cast prosthesis

Table 12.4   Effects of mixed metals on corrosion rates

Pair	Result
Stainless steel/carbon	Increased stainless steel corrosion
Stainless steel/cobalt-base	Increased stainless steel corrosion
Cobalt-base (cast)/cobalt-base (forged)	No effect
Cobalt-base/titanium-base	No significant effect
Cobalt-base/carbon	No significant effect
Titanium-base/carbon	No effect
Titanium-base/stainless steel	Increased stainless steel corrosion

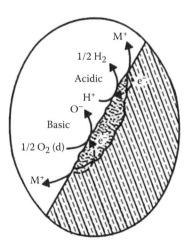

FIGURE 12.7   Galvanic corrosion.

during fabrication. Inclusions may be impurities or may be caused by poor fabrication or heat treatment practices. In general, such inclusions are noble with respect to the bulk metal and produce local corrosion in the underlying metal. This occurs preferentially near the inclusion–metal interface, since the electronic current density is highest there, resulting in concentrated local attack that can physically release the inclusion. Both acidic and basic cathode reactions are shown; *in vivo* conditions (usually slightly alkaline) favor the basic one.

Crevice corrosion   This is one of several forms of corrosion that are related to structural details. The basic feature that initiates this process is a crevice or crack, either between parts of an implanted device, such as between a screw head and a fracture fixation plate (Figure 12.8), or a defect such as an incomplete fatigue crack. The narrower and deeper the crack is, the more likely crevice corrosion is to start. The details of initiation are unclear, but once started, the process is characterized by oxygen depletion within the crevice, anodic corrosion along the crevice faces, and cathodic protective conditions on the metal surface near the defect. Static, non-flow conditions favor progression of crevice corrosion; this is probably associated with the formation of a metallic ion concentration gradient away from the mouth of the defect. The presence of chloride ion, such as *in vivo*, accelerates the process. Since the area of attack is very concentrated, it can be easily seen in the mating areas between screws and plates, and so on, such as shown in Figure 12.9. The design of this direct compression type of plate, with a spherical screw underhead surface in a semicircular "trough" in the plate, produces ideal conditions for crevice corrosion: a line contact between two parts. This degree of attack, seen after 15 months, is exceptional. However, studies of retrieved stainless steel multipart internal fraction fixation devices show visible corrosion in 50%–75% of all devices. Both iron-base and cobalt-base alloys are relatively more susceptible to crevice corrosion, the latter only very modestly, but titanium-base alloys do not demonstrate it to any significant degree.

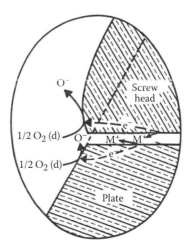

FIGURE 12.8 Crevice corrosion.

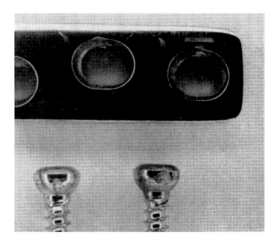

FIGURE 12.9   Fracture fixation plate and screws.

It is not uncommon to observe crevice corrosion in modular devices. In conjunction with stress corrosion processes, it can potentially decrease the life of metals subject to cyclic loading. The possibility of crevice corrosion, either in physical cracks or in crack-like defects in a passivation layer, may lead to the abolition of the fatigue endurance limit for metallic alloys. This is a particular challenge for iron-base alloys, such as the stainless steels. This latter situation is sometimes called *fatigue corrosion*.

Pitting corrosion   This is a special case of crevice corrosion. It is a more isolated, symmetric form of attack (Figure 12.10). Inclusions, scratches, or handling damage may initiate it. It proceeds through processes similar to crevice corrosion, although static (non-flow) conditions and oxygen depletion seem less important. The cathodic reaction shown is the most probable complete one *in vivo* near neutral pH in well-vascularized tissue.

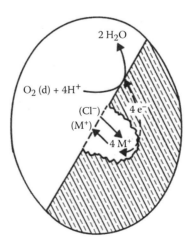

FIGURE 12.10   Pitting corrosion.

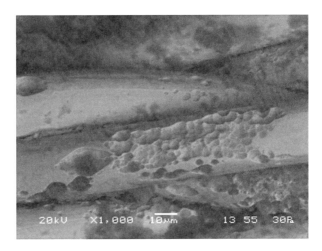

FIGURE 12.11   SEM image showing pitting corrosion.

Concentration gradients of both Cl⁻ (consumed by complexing) and metal-bearing ions (produced by the corrosion process) produce potentials that serve to accelerate the rate of attack. A scanning electron microscope (SEM) image showing clear pitting corrosion in an unidentified material is shown in Figure 12.11.

Pits often occur in large numbers, such as along a scratch, and grow downward in the direction of the gravitational field. They are a hazard in highly stressed devices as they constitute points of stress concentration and may serve as initiation points for fatigue failures. Like the results of crevice corrosion, they are easy to see. When very small, they may change the surface finish, often producing a "frosted" or matte appearance. Larger, more developed pits often contain accumulations of colored corrosion products and show up as brown, green, or black spots against otherwise polished surfaces. However, these products are poorly adhered to the implant and may be lost during too vigorous cleaning after retrieval.

Pitting was frequently observed in older stainless steel fracture fixation hardware, most often on the undersides of screw heads. It also occurs infrequently on the neck or the underside of the flange of proximal femoral endoprostheses. Improved alloy "cleanliness," especially the use of vacuum melting and remelting, has largely eliminated pitting in such hardware; however, it is still seen in older hardware and on the medullary stems of older stainless steel and cobalt-base alloy cast joint replacement components. There continues to be debate over whether pitting occurs in cobalt-base alloys or whether the attack seen is due to corrosion-mediated release of impurity inclusions only. Pitting is rare in titanium-base alloys, but may occur in the presence of very high concentrations of halide ions, which is unlikely to occur *in vivo.*

Intergranular corrosion

As discussed in Chapter 7, cast and forged products both possess regions of continuous structure called *grains.* Between these grains, especially in cast devices, there are disordered regions, the *grain boundaries,*

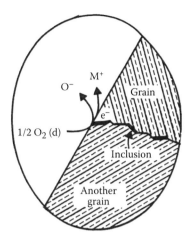

FIGURE 12.12   Intergranular corrosion.

which may contain material of different composition than the adjacent grains. This produces a galvanic cell, usually with the grain boundary inclusions serving as cathodes and producing corrosion of the grain surfaces (Figure 12.12).

Since the grain boundaries in a solid form a very small part of the total volume but possess very high surface areas, they can produce rapid corrosion. Once the process starts, crevice corrosion of the resulting defects can also proceed. The total effect, in an engineering application, is to produce a part that suddenly crumbles into grains under modest mechanical loads, although appearing essentially normal up to the time of failure. Chemical etching used to prepare sections of metallic devices for structural examination utilizes this effect by deliberately introducing an acid corrodant or etchant. The free fragment seen in the previous example of a retrieved stainless steel intramedullary rod (see Figure 12.2) is most probably the product of an intergranular corrosion process, accelerated by the presence of a galvanic current.

This process is obviously more likely in alloys than in pure metals and is favored by high levels of impurities and inclusions. Stainless steels, if improperly heat treated after fabrication, may corrode by this mechanism owing to a relative depletion of chromium from the regions near the grain boundaries. This phenomenon is called *sensitization*. Welding of metals, which produces local melting and solidification, can also lead to a variant of this process, especially in iron-base and cobalt-base alloys, called *knife-edge attack*. The name derives from the appearance of the failure, a straight crack through the metal parallel to and near the weld. Again, proper heat treatment after welding will restore the appropriate compositional distribution and prevent this form of attack.

Leaching

Similar to intergranular corrosion, *leaching* results from chemical differences not within grain boundaries but within the grains themselves. This may occur accidently during fabrication or may be a deliberate effect, produced to meet fabrication or mechanical requirements. The result is that there are wide differences in chemical activity throughout the alloy, with multiple local galvanic cells (Figure 12.13).

Attack of this kind will remove metal with a regular periodic variation of effect at a microscopic level. It is peculiar to certain alloy systems but can be more generally induced by two conditions:

1. The introduction into the solution around the metal of an agent that attacks one component of the alloy selectively. For instance, F^- ion will selectively complex with and remove aluminum from copper–aluminum alloys (alloys not suitable for implantation).

2. The presence of more than one phase in the alloy. Usually, all of the grains of an alloy have the same general composition, within a narrow range. The alloy is said to be single phase. However, it is possible for there to be grains of two or more different discrete compositions and thus chemical activities (see Chapter 7). Heat and mechanical treatment may affect the grain size, but not the composition disparity in such materials, called *multiphase alloys*. For this reason, multiphase alloys are not generally used in corrosion applications. An exception is the 35% Ni-containing cobalt-base alloy, F 582 (see Chapter 7), which is a multiphase alloy. From an engineering standpoint, it performs well *in vivo*, being quite corrosion resistant. However, biologic (local host response) studies suggest that it may release Ni somewhat easily, and thus its application is uncertain.

Leaching produces surface appearances that are similar to those that result from pitting and intergranular attack. It can be verified only by analysis of the corrosion products or the surface concentration of the corroded metal part. Although corrosion products or corroded surfaces of alloys will differ from the alloy composition, there are characteristic ratios that may be established for uniform attack in each system, and leaching produces deviations from these.

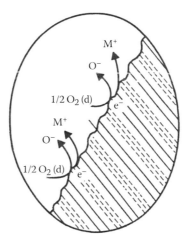

FIGURE 12.13   Leaching.

Erosion and fretting corrosion

In its pure form, *erosion* is a rare form of corrosion. It is an acceleration of attack caused by relative motion between the surrounding electrolyte and the metallic surface. It is not a unique process; it simply serves to increase the rate of attack by several other mechanisms. This occurs since many corrosion processes are self-limiting, that is, inhibited by their reaction products. Flowing solutions will sweep away these products as well as provide new amounts of dissolved reactants, such as Cl^- and oxygen (Figure 12.14). In extreme cases, the solution may actually erode the passive layer in regions of passivity. The continual reformation of this layer and its removal by continued flow processes can produce progressive attack on the metal surface in regions of the Pourbaix diagram where passivation is normally expected.

Fretting corrosion is closely related to erosion corrosion. Fretting is the physical removal of metal, by wear, owing to the relative motion of surfaces. Such a condition may occur between screw head and plate in the case of unstable internal fixation of fractures. However, if the surfaces are passivated and in a corrosive environment, such as *in vivo*, the result will be continued accelerated corrosion as the passive layer is physically removed and reformed. The damage seen in Figure 12.9 is probably partially due to fretting and possibly to fretting corrosion, owing to the intrinsic relative motion in such modular designs. Paradoxically, serum proteins, which increase uniform attack rates, appear to reduce fretting corrosion significantly, at least for stainless steels, *in vitro*.

The physical damage caused by erosion and fretting corrosion resembles pitting, except that the defects are elongated in the direction of flow or relative movement and are generally larger and less symmetric than in true pitting. In true erosion corrosion, especially if the flow pattern is stable, it may be visualized by the resulting etched surface pattern.

Stress corrosion

The final form of corrosion to be considered results from tensile stresses that increase the chemical activity of metals. Thus, a straight fracture plate, when flexed, will experience a tensile stress on its convex surface

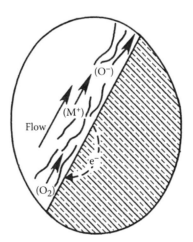

FIGURE 12.14 Erosion corrosion.

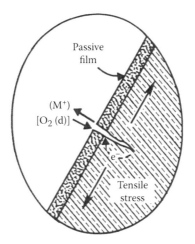

FIGURE 12.15   Stress corrosion.

and a compressive stress on its concave surface. This produces a difference in electrochemical potential, which renders the convex surface anodic with respect to the rest of the plate. Corrosion, as an acceleration of uniform attack, or perhaps secondary to tensile rupture of the passive film, will then attack the convex surface preferentially. The same process will occur at stress risers in loaded devices, such as screw holes in fracture fixation plates or kinks in cerclage wire. In this case, the regions of higher stress, in the immediate vicinity of the stress risers, will corrode at the expense of the surrounding less stressed material.

Since formation of even a small crack in a static or dynamically loaded structure, such as a flexed plate, will concentrate stress, this type of attack tends to initiate cracks that can grow rapidly (Figure 12.15). The cracks extend in between the grains, but this process may be differentiated from intergranular attack owing to the small number and relative isolation of stress corrosion cracks.

Relevance of corrosion to orthopaedic implants

All implant alloys corrode to some extent *in vivo* as they are all constantly bathed in extracellular tissue fluid. Whether this produces an adverse local, systemic, or remote host response depends on a large number of factors and will largely be discussed in Chapter 14, though it will be touched upon briefly here.

Oxide layer   All metals currently used in orthopaedics form continuous, passive nanometer-scale films via reactions with water or fluids *in vivo*, which will limit corrosion rates in the physiological environment. Under ideal conditions, there will be a low level of ion release, though there will always exist some chemical or electrochemical dissolution into the body, as metals are not intrinsically inert. (As an interesting note, the type and amount of ions released are not directly dependent on the quantity of that element in an alloy; i.e., the elements of the released ions should not be expected exclusively from the composition of the alloy.) To be effective, a passive layer must be nonporous, stable, and resistant to mechanical stress, and must have a structure that will impede ion transfer. The stability of passive layer is affected by structure, thickness, presence of defects, and chemical composition. Oxide layer morphology can be affected by surface treatments, electrochemical history, and immersion time.

Because the oxide layer is constantly under attack, there is a potential for the local breakdown of the layer. Most commonly, the integrity of oxide film is breached through mechanical abrasion (fretting, wear), chemical reactions, or biological effects. Consequences of breakdown of the passive layer may lead to increased corrosion rates, possibly causing an inflammatory response in bone or tissue surrounding the implant. Corrosion by-products may also lead to osteolysis.

Beyond the oxide layer, corrosion of a particular material depends on composition, electrode potential, stress, and surface roughness. Stainless steel is relatively more susceptible to pitting and crevice corrosion owing to the inclusion of dissimilar materials (e.g., manganese, included for ease of machining). Impurities may initiate defects at grain boundaries, making them ideal sites for corrosion. Stainless steel is also relatively more vulnerable to high-stress environments via a stress corrosion mechanism. The inclusion of chromium in stainless steel improves corrosion resistance by facilitating a chromium oxide layer on the surface. Co–Cr alloys have good corrosion properties but are relatively more susceptible to crevice and fretting corrosion after scratching or third-body wear. Of the major metals in use, titanium is the most resistant because of the stability of its oxide layer. This layer can be modified through anodization to enhance its corrosion resistance. For a given alloy composition, after preparation and postfabrication heat treatment, the fabrication technique has little effect on uniform corrosion rates. Thus, cast and forged components of the same general alloy type tend to have very similar uniform corrosion rates.

Modular devices

As a general rule, the potential for corrosion is relatively more severe in modular devices, such as plate and screw combinations or hip implants, than in one-part/monoblock devices. Uniform corrosion must be occurring, but the primary physical evidence suggests that crevice, pitting, and fretting corrosion are the most common forms of attack in such situations. Pitting tends to occur on the undersides of screws, whereas crevice corrosion occurs in the crack between screw head and plate, or within the fittings of modular components. The situation in total joint replacement components, such as the femoral portion of a total hip replacement (THR), is far more complex. Restricted environments common in complex orthopaedic designs can increase likelihood for corrosion as discussed above, but there is some concern mechanically assisted corrosion processes such as fretting corrosion, especially owing to the increase in popularity of modular implants. Modular implants are intended to provide surgeons with greater flexibility in adapting implant characteristics to individual patients and to try to obtain more anatomic reconstructions. As a consequence of the modular systems, micromotion between the modular implant surfaces, such as at the head and neck taper junction, may disrupt the passive oxide layer and induce surface fretting and corrosion. In contemporary literature, these effects are sometimes lumped together and referred to as mechanically assisted crevice corrosion. Factors affecting fretting corrosion in modular implants include the time of implantation, flexural rigidity, and the combination of materials used. Surgical factors, such as inappropriate seating of the modular components, may also increase the risk of fretting corrosion. This may allow more fluid to penetrate the interface of the modular components, as well as increase the relative motion and, thus, the risk of fretting corrosion. Blood and urine levels of corrosion by-products have been suggested to be correlated with the severity of corrosion in patients with modular implants. In severe cases, fretting corrosion at the implant surfaces may increase the risk for implant fatigue fracture.

Measuring corrosion

Repeated efforts have been made to measure the uniform corrosion rates of the principal alloys *in vitro*. Corrosion testing is typically performed in Hank's solution, Ringer's solution, phosphate buffered saline, or isotonic saline (0.9% NaCl). Most of these environments are considered to only represent a very simplified version of the biochemical environment to which implants may be exposed. *In vitro* testing is also limited as it does not take into account the protection mechanisms and physiologic response characteristic of the *in vivo* implant. Further, there is still little work done simulating the effect of altered environments. Normal physiological (37°C [98.6°F]) environment is known to have a pH of 7.4 (but may depend on the anatomic site and underlying pathological conditions), whereas tissue surrounding a healing fracture may have a pH of 5.5, while that in the presence of infection may also drop into the acidic range. Organic compounds in blood, synovial fluids, or saliva can also affect the corrosive process.

In vivo measurements of mixed corrosion potential and corrosion resistance (slope of the anodic polarization curve near the mixed corrosion potential), two indicators of corrosion rate, have led to an estimated uniform attack rate of 0.15 $\mu g/cm^2$ per day for cobalt-base alloys and perhaps half as much for titanium-base alloys (owing to lower density). These rates were obtained in animals, using well-passivated materials. Passivation, the formation of a carefully structured oxidized surface coating, is routinely used as a finishing process in the production of metallic implants, since this coating reduces the rate of uniform and other corrosion processes by serving as an electrical insulator.

The uniform attack rate may be a low estimate of the overall corrosion rate for the following reasons:

1. Galvanic, crevice, pitting, and fretting corrosion phenomena may also contribute to corrosive release, especially in the case of modular implants.

2. There is evidence that proteins participate in corrosion, increasing metal release, without affecting externally measurable electrical parameters ("charge-neutral" corrosion).

3. Articulation of bearing surfaces (e.g., THR femoral head) under load is capable of disrupting, and even physically removing, portions of the passive layer, even on titanium-base alloys. The continuing process of passive layer disruption and reformation may result in metal release.

4. The role that the poly(methyl methocrylate) (PMMA) cement layer plays in the corrosion of cemented devices is not clearly understood. Loose devices clearly show signs of fretting on the stem. There are reports of revision THAs demonstrating that the pH of the solution present at the narrow (50–100 μm) crevice between the stem and PMMA cement may be as low as 3, creating an environment for crevice corrosion attack.

5. Porous structures, such as those used for fixation by biologic ingrowth, may have as much as 10-fold-elevated corrosion rates, compared with smooth surfaces. These rates are nearly proportional to the increased specific surface area of the implant. The effect of tissue ingrowth on corrosion rates is unknown.

6. Corrosion of chromium-containing iron-base and cobalt-base alloys is regulated to a large degree by the presence of chromium-oxygen compounds in the passive layer. These compounds are highly insoluble at physiologic pH (see Figure 12.4), but the acidosis associated with local infection is probably sufficient to produce pH values below 6 that will produce significant loss of the passive layer and may interfere with normal repassivation.

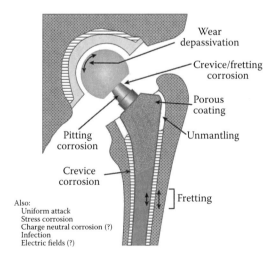

FIGURE 12.16   (See color insert.) Types of corrosive attack on proximal femoral THR component. (Adapted from Semlitsch, M., Willert, H.G., *Med Bio Eng Comput* 18:511–520, 1980.)

7. Concern has been expressed as to whether exogenous electric fields, such as produced by inductive or capacitive stimulation of bone growth, could increase corrosion rates. There is no theoretical reason to believe so, and initial studies on cobalt-base alloys have been equivocal.

These effects are summarized in Figure 12.16. Together, they may produce up to 10- to 20-fold increases in corrosion or metal release rates over those expected from simple electrochemical measurements. Thus, the study of *in vivo* corrosion and related metal release mechanisms remains very active in the field of biomaterials research.

Degradation

Dissolution of inert materials

Materials used today in internal fixation and joint replacement devices do not have appreciable *in vivo* dissolution rates. The exception is the chromium-rich passive layer on stainless steel and cobalt-base alloys, which has been discussed previously.

However, it should not be overlooked that *all* materials will have an equilibrium concentration of dissolved species that is not zero. If the released species are either very scarce in the body or have very high biologic activity, even trace releases may have clinical significance.

Furthermore, selective attack may take place along grain or phase boundaries of nonmetallic materials. Such processes may lead to loss of integrity in polymer matrix composites and are probably responsible for the so-called static fatigue of ceramic materials in fluid environments.

Resorption

There is considerable interest in the use of deliberately dissolvable or resorbable ceramic materials in a number of applications, including coatings to produce tissue adhesion or to promote ingrowth, grouting agents for medullary stems, and as replacements for autologous cortical and cancellous bone grafts. These materials are discussed in Chapter 8 and are primarily based, in so far as their resorbable components, on the calcium–phosphorus system.

In service, primarily in animal models and clinical use, these materials dissolve or resorb since they can take part easily in the normal physiologic inorganic ion control and exchange systems. The released ions are the same as those already present *in vivo*, and there is no evidence that present materials produce release rates high enough to overpower local buffering capacity and thus produce adverse local host response. Materials with similar grain sizes, internal pore volume fraction, and Ca/P ratios tend to have similar dissolution rates, which increase with decreasing grain size or increasing porosity or Ca/P ratio. However, dissolution of such coatings may release particulate debris capable of eliciting a local host response and, in extreme cases, serving as third bodies in wear processes (see Chapter 11).

Fully resorbable polymers are also in use, routinely as sutures and bone anchors, as well as in internal fixation devices. They have well-defined degradation rates, usually characterized by a sigmoidal time-dependent loss of mechanical properties, stretching over days to months, depending on polymer composition and initial molecular weight. A distinction should be drawn between hydrophobic and hydrophilic polymers: the former tend to degrade slowly by surface recession, whereas the latter may fragment catastrophically, in a manner reminiscent of a metal undergoing intergranular corrosion. Further discussion on resorbable polymers can be found in Chapter 6.

Polymer degradation

Permanent and partially degradable polymers may undergo a variety of degradation phenomena *in vivo*. These are summarized below (and in Figure 12.17), and their mechanical consequences are given in Table 12.5.

Mechanical properties may be altered by absorption or desorption (leaching) of low-molecular-weight species. Absorption usually involves water and lipids; its degradative effect may be mediated by local oxygen tension. Desorption is primarily of low-molecular-weight species, either remaining from initial fabrication or produced by chain scission

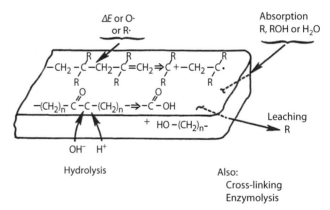

FIGURE 12.17　Degradation mechanisms in polymers.

Table 12.5　Mechanical consequences of polymer degradation

Mechanism	Modulus	Strength
Chain scission	Decrease	Decrease
Cross-linking	Increase	Increase
Absorption	Decrease	Increase[a]
Leaching	Increase	Decrease

Note: Generic effects only; exceptions exist.
[a] Significant absorption may produce crazing and loss of integrity.

processes. The primary mechanical consequences are due to changes in plasticization (see Chapter 6). However, extreme degrees of absorption may produce a local swelling and stress-cracking phenomenon called *crazing*. Polymers that exhibit crazing are generally not suited for implantation, but an exception is the polyamides, which absorb lipids avidly and swell up to 5 volume percent. They are useful as locking inserts for screws in multipart internal fracture fixation devices.

Additionally, several processes actually change the molecular structure of polymers. Chain scission, either by free-radical depolymerization or by hydrolysis, reduces molecular weight and polymer structural integrity. These are the inverses of the two primary polymerization mechanisms: addition and condensation polymerization, respectively. Additionally, a number of agents, including oxygen free radicals and ionizing radiation, can produce cross-linking between molecules.

Most implant-grade polymers are selected for their resistance to these degradation phenomena, in addition to other properties. However, as implantation times increase, relatively low degradation rates may become important. Even a stable material such as ultrahigh-molecular-weight polyethylene (UHMWPE) exhibits molecular weight reduction, primarily associated with the presence of free radicals, after long implantation times. Thus, an increased sensitivity to the possibility of chemically mediated polymer degradation is necessary.

Biodegradation

Biodegradation is a much overused term, frequently applied to any degradation seen *in vivo*. In the limited, more correct use to describe degradation promoted by enzyme systems, it is well recognized in materials science but is a rare phenomenon in the patient. There is evidence for biodegradation of PMMA, which produces naturally occurring catabolic products, but it has not been suggested that this can produce significant degradation of physical properties or any clinical consequences. However, rapid bacterial degradation of resorbable polymers has been reported; this may be secondary to local pH effects, but its true mechanisms or effects are not entirely clear. Apparently, neither metals nor ceramics undergo biodegradation *in vivo*, understood in this limited sense, although metal-binding bacteria are well known and used industrially in ore beneficiation (enrichment).

Additional problems

PROBLEM 12.4

Immunity (select the phrase that best completes the sentence)

A. May be produced by vaccination against stainless steel

B. Is inherent in a metal in a given environment and may provide improved fatigue life

C. Results in the loss of metal from an implant

D. May cause implant rejection

ANSWER:

B. Immunity is the absence of corrosion (as previously defined). Thus, metal loss is trivial, and biologic responses are suppressed. Desensitization to elements present in metal alloys is possible, but it is not called "immunity." The loss of the fatigue endurance limit may not be seen under immune conditions.

PROBLEM 12.5

Crevice corrosion (select the phrase that best completes the sentence)

    A. Only occurs over small areas and so is not important

    B. Is more likely for cobalt-base alloys than for stainless steels

    C. Only occurs if an implant has been in place for a substantial period

    D. Does not occur if a metal has been passivated

    E. May show intense local attack and cause implant failure

ANSWER:

E, since crevice corrosion can produce initiation sites for either single-cycle or fatigue failure. Stainless steels are generally more prone to crevice corrosion than cobalt-base or titanium-base alloys. Crevice corrosion is more likely with longer periods of implantation but may occur at any time. Passivation may be damaged by fretting or reduced by local conditions within a crevice.

PROBLEM 12.6

Passivation of a metal (select the phrase that best completes the sentence)

    A. Is a process intended to increase yield strength

    B. Reduces the tendency to corrode

    C. Is a precautionary measure of little practical use

    D. Reduces the hazard of implant site infection

    E. Occurs after implantation

ANSWER:

B. Although passivation will occur spontaneously *in vivo*, factory treatments are more reliable and provide important protection against corrosion. However, passivation does not affect yield strength nor does it have an apparent effect on implant site infectability.

PROBLEM 12.7

Chromium is placed in a saline solution exposed to air and maintained at $+0.5$ V with respect to an H/H^+ electrode. If corrosive attack is observed, the pH of the solution may be

    A. 7.0

    B. 7.4

C. 2.8

D. 10.3

E. 4.0

ANSWER:

C and *D* (see Figure 12.4). pH values of 7.0, 7.4, and 4.0 are all within the passivated region on the diagram.

PROBLEM 12.8

A metal alloy that might be satisfactory for use in an orthodontic brace might be unsatisfactory as a stomach suture. True or false?

ANSWER:

True. A metal that is passive at near-neutral pH and atmospheric oxygen pressure may lose its passive layer and begin to corrode when exposed to the low-pH, low-PO_2 conditions in the upper GI tract.

PROBLEM 12.9

Match the materials with *in vivo* degradation mechanisms:

1. Stainless steel	A. Enzymolysis
2. Alumina	B. Crevice corrosion
3. Polylactic acid	C. Fretting
4. Ti6A14V	D. Hydrolysis
5. UHMWPE	E. Uniform attack

ANSWER:

1: B, C, and E; 3: D; 4: C and E. No matches for 2, 5, and A.

PROBLEM 12.10

Degradation *in vivo* reduces *both* moduli and strength of polymers. True or false?

ANSWER:

False (see Table 12.5).

PROBLEM 12.11

In a modular hip implant with a stainless steel stem, a titanium neck, and a cobalt chrome head, where would corrosion first be expected to occur?

ANSWER:

It is most likely that corrosion will first occur in the crevice between the stainless steel stem and the titanium neck. Stainless steel is anodic when paired with most other orthopaedic alloys such as cobalt chromium and titanium and is particularly prone to crevice corrosion.

PROBLEM 12.12

Two different implant manufacturers market a stainless steel humeral nail with comparable nail and screw geometries, and which both adhere to ASTM F138 in terms of elemental composition. It is assumed that the corrosion response of both implants will be similar. True or false?

ANSWER:

False. While the final components may, in fact, have the same corrosive potential, there are other variables that can dramatically affect this outcome. For example, if the material is improperly heat treated by the suppliers, intergranular corrosion may be exacerbated if chromium is depleted from regions near the grain boundaries.

PROBLEM 12.13

A modular hip arthroplasty implant is composed of a cobalt chrome stem, a cobalt chrome head, a polyethylene insert, and a titanium acetabular shell. Would the following forms of corrosion be of primary concern?

1. Crevice corrosion
2. Intergranular corrosion
3. Galvanic corrosion
4. Fretting corrosion
5. Stress corrosion

ANSWER:

Yes, No, No, Yes, Yes

Because of the modularity of the cobalt chromium stem/head pair, crevice corrosion and fretting corrosion will be relevant. Stress corrosion is always a concern in a load-bearing implant. Intergranular corrosion is less of a concern with titanium and cobalt chromium implants than those composed of stainless steel. Also, because there is a polyethylene insert separating the titanium shell and the cobalt chromium head, galvanic corrosion will be limited barring significant rim impingement or wear through of the liner, which would present other concerns as well.

Annotated bibliography

1. DRUMMOND JL: Degradation of ceramic materials in physiological media. In Rubin LR (ed): *Biomaterials in Reconstructive Surgery*. CV Mosby, St. Louis, 1983.
   A brief but useful review.

2. FONTANA MG: *Corrosion Engineering*. 3rd ed. McGraw-Hill, New York, 1986.

A standard work on corrosion, written in a clear descriptive style. Chapter 4 on corrosion testing and Chapter 5 on behavior of specific materials are very useful compilations of information otherwise widely scattered in the literature. There is a teachers manual, with worked problems, but it is currently out of print.

3. FRAKER AC, GRIFFIN CD (eds): *Corrosion and Degradation of Implant Materials: Second Symposium*. STP 859. American Society for Testing and Materials, Philadelphia, 1985.

See Ref. 11, below.

4. GILDING DK: Degradation of polymers: Mechanisms and implications for biomedical applications. In Williams DF (ed): *Fundamental Aspects of Biocompatibility*. Vol. I. CRC Press, Boca Raton, FL, 1981.

Discusses both permanent and degradable polymers. Useful bibliography.

5. HOAR TF, MEARS DC: Corrosion-resistant alloys in chloride solutions: Materials for surgical implants. *Proc R Soc Lond (Biol)* A294:486–510, 1966.

Of historical interest; the first modern, systematic examination of the subject.

6. MAREK M: Corrosion testing of implantable medical devices. In Narayan R (ed): *ASM Handbook, Volume 23, Materials for Medical Devices*. ASM International, 2012.

Thorough description of fundamentals of corrosion in the body and the advantages and limitations of common test solutions.

7. POHLER OEM: Degradation of metallic orthopaedic implants. In Rubin LR (ed): *Biomaterials in Reconstructive Surgery*. CV Mosby, St. Louis, 1983.

A comprehensive article on the subject. Exhaustively illustrated with scanning electron microscopic and x-ray images, it includes results of both laboratory and clinical investigations.

8. POURBAIX M: Electrochemical corrosion of metallic biomaterials. *Biomaterials* 5:122–135, 1984.

A discussion of pH–potential diagrams by the one who has been responsible for popularizing their use.

9. SCULLY JC: *The Fundamentals of Corrosion*. 3rd ed. Butterworth-Heinmann, London, 1990.

A historical review of corrosion with excellent examples. Chapters 2 (Aqueous Corrosion) and 4 (Corrosion Attack and Failure) are particularly useful.

10. STEINEMANN SG: Corrosion of surgical implants—*in vivo* and *in vitro* tests. In Winter GD, Leray JL, de Groot K (eds): *Evaluation of Biomaterials*. John Wiley & Sons, Chichester, 1980.

A thorough review. Noteworthy for discussion of the contributions of elemental constituents to corrosion resistance of stainless steels.

11. STEINEMANN SG: Corrosion of titanium and titanium alloys for surgical implants. In Luterjering G, Zwicker U, Bunk W (eds): *Titanium Science and Technology*. Vol. 2. DG fur Metal. e. V. Oberuresel, Berlin, 1985.

A partial updating and extension of Steinemann's previous work (1980).

12. SYRETT BC, ACHARYA A (eds): *Corrosion and Degradation of Implant Materials*. STP 684. American Society for Testing and Materials, Philadelphia, 1979.

This is the first in a series of conference proceedings on the subject of corrosion and degradation of implant materials. Much of the material applies directly to orthopaedic applications.

13. WILLIAMS DF: Electrochemical aspects of corrosion in the physiological environment. In Williams DF (ed): *Fundamental Aspects of Biocompatibility*. Vol. I. CRC Press, Boca Raton, FL, 1981.

A unified discussion of corrosion *in vivo*, with data on the three primary alloy systems.

CHAPTER THIRTEEN

Fixation

This chapter deals with the problems of fixation, that is, the coupling of prosthetic components to the musculoskeletal system so that prosthetic and natural elements may act together in a harmonious manner. It is no exaggeration to say that the failure of fixation is one of the most common causes of failure of partial and total joint replacement arthroplasty and a major contributing element in fracture malunion and nonunion. Solving the problem of long-term fixation is required to extend the present excellent outcome of joint replacement arthroplasty to the younger patient.

Need for fixation

Charnley recognized that the major differences in mechanical properties between bone and the metals used in prostheses were a source of problems in the use of uncemented (press-fitted) femoral endoprostheses such as the Moore or Thompson designs. He demonstrated the problem in a very simple experiment (Charnley and Kettlewell 1965), the results of which are shown schematically in Figure 13.1.

After suitably preparing a cadaver femur, he installed a femoral endoprosthesis, leaving a gap between the flange and the "calcar," and providing a dial indicator so that he could measure the relative motion between prosthesis and bone. (It has become the accepted practice to call the proximal medial femoral cortex, in the vicinity of the lesser trochanter, the calcar, even though it may be anatomically incorrect. For a discussion of this issue, see Harty 1957.) He performed the same procedure in the contralateral femur, but bedded the stem in poly(methyl methacrylate) (PMMA) cement.

When the constructs were loaded, more or less axially (in a constant deformation rate machine), he made the following observations:

> The uncemented stem sank down the medullary shaft, with an occasional decrease in load, until the proximal medial femoral cortex split.

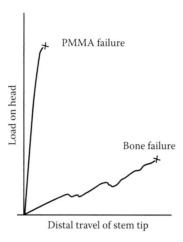

FIGURE 13.1 Role of PMMA in support of proximal femoral total hip replacement component (*in vitro* experiment). (Adapted from Charnley, J., Kettlewell, L., *J Bone Joint Surg* 47B:56–60, 1965.)

However, in the cemented construct, the load rose much more rapidly and smoothly with less distal stem movement, and failure, secondary to PMMA fracture, occurred at a much higher load.

Charnley correctly identified the differences as being related to the ability of the PMMA cement to reduce stress concentrations secondary to stem impingement on the medial cortex and to produce gradual load transmission to the femoral shaft over a long distance, providing both a stiffer construct and, as a result, lower typical stresses. He calculated that the addition of cement increased the "load-bearing capacity" of the femoral prosthesis in the upper end of the femur by 200 times.

Emboldened by this experiment and by earlier work of others showing the biologic acceptance of PMMA cements in bony sites, he began to use cement routinely in his low-friction arthroplasties. The result of this innovation is well known, with greater than 95% excellent or good results expected in average patients at 10 years post-implantation. However, problems have arisen with PMMA fixation, leading to desires for alternate approaches to fixation (see below). It should be noted that in some cases, problems probably are related to surgical technique rather than to intrinsic mechanical or biologic aspects of PMMA fixation. Figure 13.2 shows a cemented UHWMPE cup removed after 3 years and 4 months for loosening and pain. Despite the use of anchoring holes and metallic mesh to reinforce cement over a deep cyst, there had been little cement intrusion into the cancellous bed. In addition, a crack can be seen in the thin cement mantle over the cup. Although such defects are frequently interpreted as evidence of *in vivo* failure, in this case the crack was produced during device removal. Although it is probable that preparations with this appearance may survive for long times in patients, no one would argue today that this presentation represents optimal cementation.

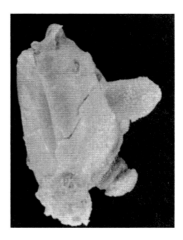

FIGURE 13.2   Inadequate cementation (PMMA).

Types of fixation

The present approaches to fixation, including cementation, can be grouped into four generic types.

Force-fit or press-fit. Fixation began with the so-called force-fit or frictional fit, as used in fracture fixation. A typical screw–plate combination on a long bone (see Figure 3.6) depends on frictional forces to maintain the integrity of the construct. These forces are produced between the plate and the bone fragments as a consequence of axial tensile strains produced in the screws during installation. Creep, stress relaxation, bony (pressure) necrosis, and remodeling around the screw threads may result in loss of these fixation forces. This produces a situation analogous to press-fit fixation of medullary stems of prosthetic devices.

This original (pre-cement) approach to implant fixation has now been updated by redesign of intramedullary stems to reduce local stresses in the supporting bone. Typically, as applied to the hip, these designs feature large, broad (lateral–medial) canal-fitting stems. Although of importance and of increasing interest, force-fit fixation shall not be discussed further in this chapter. (Portions of Chapter 14 dealing with local host response do, however, apply.) Press-fit fixation is also used extensively with acetabular cups to provide initial mechanical stability and resist frictional torque during the initial period of bone healing.

Cemented. Charnley's innovation, involving fixation with PMMA or PMMA variant cements. Designs feature moderate stem cross sections generally with smooth, large radii contours, especially medially, to protect the notch-sensitive cements. Variants include rough or microporous stem surfaces to promote cement adherence; cement precoating (by the manufacturer), often with bonding agents to promote cement adherence and provision of polymeric spacers to regulate and equalize cement mantle thickness; and device design features to produce cement containment and pressurization during insertion. Surgical techniques have matured and emphasize thorough cleaning of the bony bed, mechanical injection

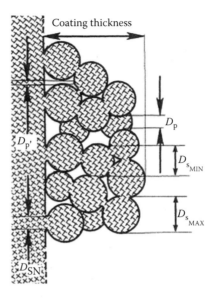

FIGURE 13.3 Characteristic dimensions of beaded surface for fixation by ingrowth.

of cement, and pressurization (before device insertion) to ensure intrusion of cement into bone.

Ingrown. Production of fixation by encouragement of tissue growth into porous portions of implants. For example, stems, as is the case of force-fit or press-fit designs, are large and efforts are made to ensure immediate mechanical stability. There are a number of different surface structures (see Figure 7.10), but a traditional example is a multilayer beaded coating (Figure 13.3). The sphere diameter (D_s) is typically between 250 and 400 μm, producing surface pore diameters (D_p) of 150–250 μm. If the minimal internal interconnect diameter $D_{p'}$ is greater than approximately 50–100 μm, bone will grow in to depths of 3–4 mm, although most coatings are thinner than this. An in-depth discussion of the state of art in porous coatings is given later. Experimental variants of coatings include the use of osteoconductive overcoating of the porous coatings to encourage early ingrowth, or grafting with autologous cancellous bone both to encourage ingrowth and to improve early stability.

Adhered or ongrown. Fixation by direct adhesion of bone to the implant. For example, smooth, broad stems are used, with surfaces consisting of either pure titanium or bioactive ceramics (see Chapter 8). With adequate early stability and limited early loading, direct bony apposition occurs. Implants may also be coated with hydroxyapatite, which provides a nontoxic, biocompatible, and osteoconductive material for promoting bone ingrowth.

Structure of the mature interface

Later, we shall consider the mechanical features of the interface and aspects of its deterioration if it fails. First, however, it is necessary to review the structure of the stable, mature interface, in an area of "accept-able" stresses (Figure 13.4).

Cemented. The cement layer is typically 2–5 mm thick. For a fem-oral stem, unless bonded (precoated stem) to the stem, a 50–100 μm thick fibrous membrane separates stem and cement. At the bone–cement interface, there is also a membrane, which may vary from 50 μm to as thick as 1.5–3 mm, although membranes of greater than 1 mm thick-ness (as estimated by x-ray radiolucency) are generally regarded as evi-dence of impending or actual "loosening." This membrane is fibrous and relatively acellular, but may be more synovial or inflammatory in nature when it becomes thicker or when frank relative cement–bone motion is present. The cement may intrude into bone as far as 1–1.5 cm with no apparent long-term adverse effect on the bone.

There is some discussion on roughening the implant surface and the extent of cementation when used. A roughened implant surface is known to increase the bond between the implant and the cement, the region where cement fragmentation is expected to initiate. It is, how-ever, believed that this bond will eventually fail. At this occurrence, a roughened implant surface has demonstrated an increase in abrasion of the cement mantle, which would lead to increased cement particle generation, inflammation, and resorption. Because of a concern for this outcome, there is some support for the minimization of the cement layer, or a decrease in surface roughness, to limit fragmentation after bond failure. These issues have led to an increase in the use of porous, non-cemented surfaces over the last decade.

Ingrown. The coatings are typically 1–2 mm thick. The pore open-ings cover 25%–40% of the surface in traditional coatings but can be found up to 85% in newer open structured titanium- and tantalum-based "foam" metals. A portion of these pores are ingrown with bone and in some places osteoid and fibrous tissue. Bony tissue will fill most but not all interstices with a D_p greater than approximately 50 μm. Whether in

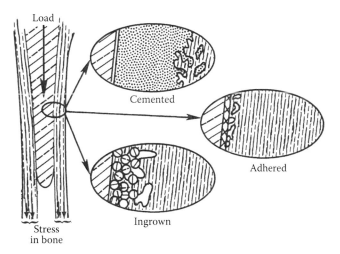

FIGURE 13.4 Structure of the mature interface.

contact with cortical or cancellous bone, ingrowth is focal, varying in degree from place to place in an apparently random fashion. However, portions of the interface within healthy cancellous bone or near to cortical walls tend to be better ingrown. Portions of the surface of the coating in any particular section may show no bone-coating contact or adjacent bone.

When in contact with cortical bone (as shown here), "cancellization" of the bone may be seen near portions of the interface. When in contact with cancellous bone, there is frequently a bony condensation or pseudo-subchondral plate parallel to the interface and 1–2 mm away from it, especially in areas where there has been little ingrowth.

Adhered or ongrowth. Surface coatings are generally very thin, less than 0.5 mm in thickness, owing to their brittleness, except when pure titanium or bulk homogeneous materials are used (in experimental animal models). No fibrous membrane separates coating and bone, although bioactive ceramics show an amorphous layer 1–100 μm thick containing coating elements in a gel as well as collagen and polysaccharides. If placed in cortical bone, as shown here, cancellization may occur, but to a small degree.

Goals of fixation

The presumed goals of fixation are as follows:

1. Limit of relative motion between loaded implant and supporting bone ("micromotion")
2. Production of contact stresses *on* bone within normal (acceptable) limits
3. Maintenance of resultant stresses *in* bone close to normal physiologic preimplantation levels, to minimize bony adaptive remodeling

Micromotion

A few words are in order about "micromotion." Orthopaedic researchers and clinicians have a fundamentally mechanical approach to problem solving, as befits those who deal with repair and restoration of the musculoskeletal system with its primary functions of maintenance of structural integrity and provisions for locomotion.

This naturally leads to seeking a mechanical origin for the loss of continuity between implants and their bony support, that is, "loosening." Most arguments start with an appeal to "micromotion." This appears to be an amount of motion between device and tissue that exceeds acceptable limits, thus leading to loosening.

Charnley, without giving details of the calculation, stated that the motion between the distal tip of a femoral stem and the surrounding bone, during loading, was "only about 25 μm (or the length of three red blood cells)." Others considering the dynamics of tissue ingrowth into porous surfaces have suggested that motion may be unacceptable if it exceeded 0.5 D_p, or 35–50 µm, and maybe even allowable up to 150 µm.

Thus, it is clear that when considering micromotion, we are talking about relative motion that is of the same order of magnitude as cellular dimensions. It is unclear whether it is even appropriate to consider these effects directly as motion (relative strain) or in terms of local increases in stress. This is especially true as detailed mechanical analysis of the cement–bone interface, for instance, is almost impossible, owing to its microstructural complexity. Thus, knowledge of macroscopic movement does not lead easily to certain knowledge of the magnitude or direction of micromotion.

Despite these misgivings, it is clear that the term *micromotion* will continue to be used as shorthand for the mechanical causative aspects of chronic device loosening.

A consideration of fixation

Are these stated goals of fixation credible ones? Or are they chimeric, whose pursuit is foredoomed to failure?

An experiment by Weightman (Figure 13.5) casts a good deal of light on the generic problem (Weightman 1975). In this experiment, a cadaver femur was instrumented with strain-measuring devices (strain gauges) along its lateral and medial faces. It was then secured distally and loaded in a more-or-less anatomic direction. Surface (outer fiber) stresses in the cortical bone were calculated from the strain gauge outputs, assuming

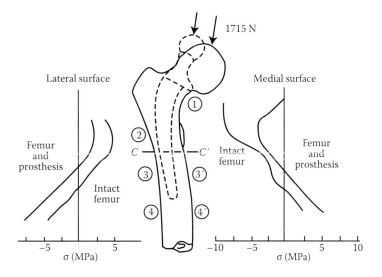

FIGURE 13.5 Femoral cortical stress. (Weightman, B., Stress analysis. In Swanson, S.A.V., Freeman, M.A.R. [eds.]. *The Scientific Basis of Joint Replacement.* p. 18. 1975. Copyright Wiley-VCH Verlag GmbH & Co. KGaA. Reproduced with permission.)

a value for the elastic modulus of bone and using its actual dimensions. Then, a cemented femoral prosthesis was inserted and the experiment was repeated. The results are shown in Figure 13.5. (Weightman performed the experiment with an actual load of 2 kN and calculated results for a 4 kN load. His results have been rescaled for a 1715 N load, corresponding to 2.5 times body weight for a standard 70 kg patient. Other minor adjustments have been made to the figure.)

Several initial points are obvious. The insertion of the cemented stem generally *reduces* outer fiber stresses proximal to the stem tip and *increases* them distal to the stem tip. The reduction of stress in the calcar area is especially noticeable and led to hot debates about the relationship between this reduction and calcar resorption of the role of medial prosthesis collar–calcar contact in load carriage and stress distribution. These are still not fully resolved and are complicated by considerations of the role played by surgical interference with the blood supply to the proximal femur. However, this overall pattern of stress reduction after prosthetic implantation is called *stress protection* or *stress shielding* and is generally appealed to explain postimplantation remodeling leading to osteoporotic or absent cortical and cancellous bone.

However, there are several less obvious points that should be made. At location *1*, the cut edge of the calcar, the integrity of the bone, as a cancellous-supported cortical shell, has been lost and previous normal stresses could not be sustained without either hoop failure (longitudinal fracture) or transverse buckling. The catastrophic consequences of such failure may be appreciated by reference to the differences in areal moment of inertia between a complete and a split cylinder (see Table 2.4). Thus, the goal of restoring normal stresses in this area cannot be safely achieved after partial or total head–neck removal. This will always be the case, independent of fixation techniques, and has led to recent device design proposals that retain the femoral neck. Others have included stem designs with a collared portion in hopes of transmitting more natural stresses to the cut section of the neck. However, in many cases, stress shielding may not be avoided because the collar itself shields the surrounding bone.

At location *2*, within the boundary of the cancellous bed (superior to line *C–C'*), both the stem and the bone are carrying load, with load transfer increasing as one moves distally. A great deal has been said and written about the need to equalize elastic moduli to reduce relative stem–bone motion, that is, to have the stem modulus be as close to that of cortical bone as possible:

$$E_S = E_B$$

where the subscripts S and B refer to the stem material and bone, respectively. However, this proposal is in error. The stem and the bone are both subject to a bending moment at this point. For there to be no relative motion between stem and bone, the appropriate condition is

$$M_{SF}/(E_{SF} \cdot I_{SF}) = M_B/(E_B \cdot I_B)$$

where the subscript SF refers to the stem-fixation construct, M_{SF} and M_B are the bending moments, and I_{SF} and I_B are the areal moments of inertia of the stem-fixation system and the bone, respectively. Thus, it is clear that the condition $E_S = E_B$ is neither a necessary nor a sufficient solution to the problem. Furthermore, since M_{SF} decreases distally and concurrently M_B increases, satisfying the appropriate condition at more than a few points along the shaft is probably impossible.

At locations *3* and *3′*, lateral and medial, respectively, no design can restore normal stresses so long as there is any stem–bone contact. This is the case since, below the limit of the natural cancellous bed (line C–C'), all stress in the intact femur is carried within the cortex. Introduction of stress by intramedullary contact must change either the magnitude or the direction of the stress resultant.

At locations *4* and *4′*, stresses in the implanted femur must always be larger than those in the intact femur. This reflects a greater bending moment, produced as a consequence of the proximal stiffening effect of the stem. For stresses to be normal at this level, (1) there must be no stem–bone contact below C–C' and (2) the stemfixation construct stiffness above C–C' must be near to that of the cancellous bone it replaces; that is,

$$E_{SF} \approx E_{\text{cancellous bone}} \ll E_{\text{cortical bone}}$$

Point 2 is the design consideration leading to the so-called "isoelastic" stems; however, they remain far too stiff to satisfy this condition and extend distal to line C–C', with continuing stem–bone contact.

Similar arguments lead to the same conclusions for intramedullary stem fixation in other skeletal locations.

Role of the interface in fixation

It should be clear from the previous discussion that the three simultaneous conditions of *no* relative motion and normal stresses on and in bone, stated as the goals of fixation, cannot be met by a two-phase (stem–bone) rigidly bonded system. Therefore, the fixation system must act to "decouple" the implant from the adjacent bone while providing for stability and stress distribution and transmission.

Types of bond systems

The bonding of materials with dissimilar mechanical properties is a classical problem in engineering and has been solved in a number of ways. There are three generic approaches, illustrated in Figure 13.6. (In this case, the implant is assumed to be made of a titanium-base alloy [modulus = 100 GPa], but the arguments would be similar for higher-stiffness materials.)

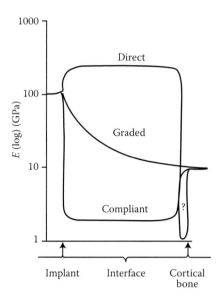

FIGURE 13.6 Types of bonds between materials with different moduli.

Direct. When two brittle materials of different moduli are to be bonded, a layer of a very rigid material may be interposed. In some cases, a low-shear-modulus adhesive will be used at one or the other interface. The presence of this interposed stiff material, often called a "backbone," effectively prevents transmission of bending stress from one brittle material to the other and thus preserves their integrity by limiting their peak flexural strain. In engineering applications, this approach is frequently used to bond glasses together.

Graded. Two materials that are miscible may be formed into a graded "seal." This consists of a continuously varying mixture across the interface, with a concurrently varying elastic modulus. The effect is to "smear" out the stress, greatly reducing the peak circum-interface stress in either material for a given bending moment. An engineering example is the seal between the metal base and the glass envelope of a television tube. In this application, the graded seal also protects the brittle glass envelope from stresses produced by unequal expansion and contraction of base components during heating and cooling.

Compliant. Complete stress relief may be achieved by bonding a very compliant layer, with an elastic modulus well below that of either material, to both of them. Then, stress in one material, whether bending, longitudinal, or shear, is completely taken up within the compliant layer without transmission to the other material. Compressive stresses are still transmitted, as are tensile ones, up to the strength limits of the interfacial layer. This is the design principle for vibration isolation pads for machinery.

Mechanical nature of fixation systems

How do the actual structure and mechanical properties of the various fixation systems compare with these engineering approaches? Are they direct, graded, or compliant interfaces?

We do not know the details of stiffness variation across such implant-fixation interlayer-bone structures, but a good deal may be inferred from their histology and knowledge of the properties of their components. This is shown schematically in Figure 13.7.

Cemented ("C"). This is clearly a fully compliant interface, since the moduli of PMMA cements are far below those of cortical bone and prosthetic implant alloys. The presence of cancellous bone additionally provides a graded interface between cement and cortical bone. Additional "decoupling" may be offered by the presence of the implant–cement and cement–bone fibrous membranes previously described.

Ingrown ("I"). This is a combination of a graded and a compliant interface. Near the implant, the coating is fairly stiff but decreases as the bone is approached, owing to increasing porosity. Near the coating–bone interface, there is an increase in stiffness, owing to ingrowth of bone. However, the adjacent bone is very compliant, being either cancellous bone or a cancellized layer of cortical bone.

Adhered ("A") or ongrown. This is the most difficult case to understand, as it is apparently a direct bond. However, the most likely case is that the bond is a compliant one, resulting from the presence of either a hydrated surface layer ("gel") on the implant or cancellization in the adjacent bone.

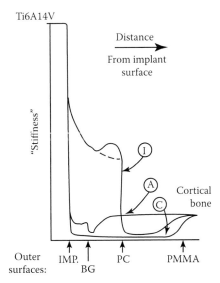

FIGURE 13.7 Variation of "stiffness" across bone–implant interface.

Thus, none of the three major fixation systems achieve the goal of a true graded seal between implant and bone, but probably all rely, to one degree or another, on a compliant interfacial zone. A naturally occurring example of this approach is the periodontal ligament, which forms a compliant interface between a stiff member (alveolar cortical bone) and a stiffer member (the tooth root).

Temporal development of fixation

Another important factor in the success or failure of fixation is the temporal development of the properties of the interface. This is shown schematically in Figure 13.8. Failure to address these temporal features in either device insertion or later clinical management may be a contributing factor to both early and intermediate fixation failures.

Cemented interfaces provide immediate fixation, with stiffness developing during the setting phase and maturing over the next 24 h. This fixation will be maintained indefinitely, unless the cement degrades or the bony support changes. However, since PMMA-type cements produce a narrow region (0.1–0.5 mm) of devitalized bone, owing to chemical and possibly thermal trauma, there may be a period, perhaps years after implantation, when remodeling produces temporary reduction in mechanical properties and integrity.

Ingrown interfaces develop more slowly, with most studies (in animals) reporting little or no mechanical integrity before 2 weeks but nearly complete maturation, in the absence of "significant" motion, in 6–8 weeks. Again, late remodeling, including cancellization, may produce late degradation of mechanical behavior.

Adhered or ingrown fixation is probably the slowest, with little adherence seen before 3 weeks and up to 30 weeks without significant functional loading required, in both animals and patients, to produce a mature interface. Here there is a real concern about late property changes

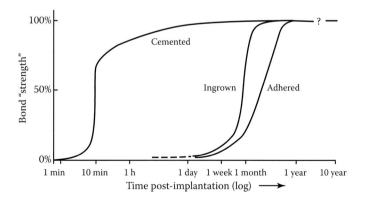

FIGURE 13.8 Temporal development of bond "strength."

resulting from remodeling. All cortical bone will turn over, although the rate in adults is quite low, perhaps 3%–6% per year. However, adaptive remodeling may increase this rate. In any case, the ability of these materials, especially the "bioactive" glasses, to form bonds to bone depends on physical property changes that occur immediately after implantation. There have apparently been no studies done to determine whether implant surfaces released by late remodeling are suitable substrates for bonding of newly formed bone.

Bond strength

Bond strengths are difficult to compare because of the different structures of the interfaces. Cemented interfaces display shear strengths between 0.1 MPa (non-precoated, failure at cement–implant interface) and 10–12 MPa (well intruded, failure at cement–cancellous or cancellous–cortical interface). Mature adhered interfaces appear to exceed the strength of the adhered bone, producing an estimated strength of 5–15 MPa (longitudinal shear, dependent on cortical bone density). Ingrown interfaces produce strengths, which are somewhat dependent on the surface coating structure and anatomic location, of 15–18 MPa (metallic or ceramic coatings, 30% porosity, radial shear, failure in cortical bone). Thus, the peak strengths seem to be limited by properties of the supporting tissue, rather than by their intrinsic structural and compositional differences. Furthermore, these apparent differences in strength of fully mature interfaces may reflect difficulties in testing these different structures. Combined with the absence of any well-documented animal studies comparing all three types contemporaneously, it is safest to assume that all three possess the same ultimate strength, perhaps 10–15 MPa.

It is interesting to compare these values with the peak stresses shown in Figure 13.5. The peak outer fiber tensile stresses, with an implant in place, are calculated to be about 5 MPa (tensile lateral, compressive medial). If it is assumed that the inner fiber cortical stresses are this high (actually, they must be lower for geometric reasons) and the stem is assumed to be infinitely stiff (worst case), then the interfacial shear stress would not exceed about one-third of the single-cycle strength of these interfaces. A more realistic estimate would probably lead to the conclusion that mature, well-formed interfaces of any of the three types are 10 times stronger than the normal peak load carriage requires. Therefore, it is improbable that interfacial failure or "loosening" occurs by a simple mechanical failure, although low-stress, high-cycle fatigue failure remains a possibility.

"Loosening" or failure of fixation

If fixation does not fail by a primarily mechanical process, then its origins are most probably biologic. That is, "loosening" represents an adequate local host response to aspects of the implant rather than a primary materials failure.

There is no agreement as to what actually is meant by "loosening." It is usually diagnosed radiographically, upon complaint of pain. Perhaps the best definition is a functional one:

> A prosthesis is *loose* when it has sufficient associated pain, in the absence of bursa formation, nerve impingement, or infection, to require surgical revision.

The origin of loosening has been addressed by a large number of clinicians and researchers. The resulting literature is too extensive even to summarize here. However, most who have thought about this problem would probably agree with the following propositions:

1. Loosening is somehow associated, both initially and as it progresses, with mechanical aspects of load bearing and transmission.
2. There is a cyclic aspect to the process, with mechanical and biologic factors apparently interacting.
3. Once initiated, loosening progresses at different rates in different patients but is apparently an irreversible process.

Loosening should be defined in terms of the adequacy of the bone–implant interface. An adequate interface, when mature, should produce stability and an absence of pain, whereas an inadequate interface leads to pain and physical (mechanical) degradation of the interface, resulting in loosening.

Mechanism of loosening

Despite real questions about the primacy of mechanical factors in dictating stability or loosening, it seems appropriate to begin with consideration of stresses on either side of the interface (Figure 13.9).

On the bone side of the interface, it is clear that stresses may be acceptable, that is, near to physiologic, or too high or too low. Rubin and Lanyon have demonstrated the continuum of response of bone to stress. Their experiments in turkeys, with 100 cyclic load events per day, suggest that strains of 1000 $\mu\varepsilon$ will maintain normal bony architecture in ulnae that are otherwise essentially unloaded. If this same value of peak strain were to apply to human cortical bone, it would imply that peak stresses of 14 MPa would maintain bone mass. Referring to Figure 13.5, we see that stresses in the isolated (unimplanted) proximal femur reach a peak of 10 MPa and are generally less than this value.

However, the femur experiences closer to 5000 cycles a day, and attached muscles, ligaments, and membranes are additional sources of stress *in vivo*.

Therefore, Rubin and Lanyon's (1984) result seems quite in line with the observed maintenance of bone in the intact skeleton and its waxing

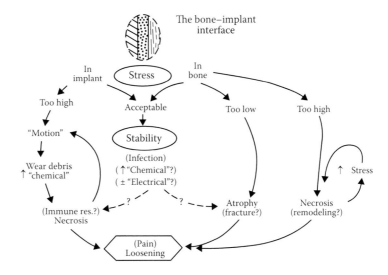

FIGURE 13.9   Degradation of the bone–implant interface.

and waning as functional requirements change. This is expressed in Wolff's law*:

The form being given, bone adapts to the loads applied to it.

When a prosthesis is inserted, local stresses are perturbed from normal (see Figure 13.5). Too high values of stress, applied in times too short to permit adaptive remodeling, may produce local necrosis. This in itself may produce mechanical collapse, or possibly collapse may occur during the resorption phase of remodeling. At this point, a feedback process also may occur: as bone mass decreases, local stresses will rise still further, accelerating the process. However, if stresses are too low, bone atrophy will occur. This may lead to progressive collapse or to fracture in a single overload incident.

Both of these phenomena will degrade the interface and lead to increased relative motion between the implant and bone. This so-called "micromotion" is a matter of much conjecture, as previously discussed. There is no agreement as to how much shear strain any of the three fixation interfaces can sustain before motion is said to take place and the consequences attributed to it occur. Certainly, any reduction in bone mass or quality or both will decrease mechanical coupling between the implant stem and the supporting bone away from the interface.

However, this may occur primarily (Figure 13.9, left side) owing to less-than-optimal device design or inadequate geometry, resulting in unacceptable interfacial stresses and motion, before bony changes occur. This in itself may be enough to constitute loosening. However, it will produce wear debris in the interface, by fretting processes, and may accelerate corrosion processes. Direct biologic responses to these new products

---

* This is a necessary paraphrase. There are many forms of "Wolff's Law" given by various writers, and it is not certain which is the most faithful to his original thesis.

may include both fibrosis, as a classic foreign body immune response, and bony necrosis secondary to chemical toxicity or to local microvascular blockade associated with immune hypersensitivity. Here, again, there is a cyclic effect, with decreased bone quality leading to increased motion and additional wear debris and corrosion product production. (It is necessary to mention several local host responses to implants at this point, for completeness. They are discussed more fully in Chapter 14.)

There are processes that may result in loosening, even in the absence of implant stresses that are, on their face, too high, through an accumulation of wear debris from the articulating interface. Willert and Semlitsch first pointed out that the so-called "cement disease," a dissecting fibrosis at the bone–cement interface, appeared to be related to the production of wear debris. It was originally thought to be produced by macrophages and foreign body giant cells, but more recent studies suggest that activated macrophages secrete an osteoclastactivating factor, thus implicating increased osteoclastic activity in this process. Similarly, with uncemented implants, "particle disease" refers to an enhanced bone resorption response or osteolysis owing to wear particles.

Even if stresses in both bone and implant are acceptable, loosening may result over the long term. Infection with associated increases in corrosion rate may contribute to bone atrophy or necrosis. Immune responses are probably not a contributing local factor in loosening of an initially stable implant. However, the higher surface areas and thus higher intrinsic corrosion rates of noncemented metallic devices anchored by ingrowth may cause this assumption to be questioned in the future. Finally, the presence of an electrically conducting implant may well "short out" or otherwise interfere with the normal electrical polarization pattern (represented by the biopotentials; see Chapter 5), leading to adverse bone remodeling effects.

Porous coatings

In an effort to enhance biologic fixation of metallic implant surfaces and to avoid problems with aseptic loosening of cemented implant surfaces, porous coatings have been developed with very promising clinical results. Porous surfaces are irregular surfaces with substantial surface or bulk porosity, which are intended to encourage the early and increased level of bone ingrowth into the implant. The major functionality provided by a porous surface is twofold: to provide biological anchorage for ingrowth of bony material and to provide a transition between the bone and the load-bearing implant that will limit stress shielding and bone resorption at the implant surface. Mismatch in stiffness between implanted metallic alloys and bone has been identified as the main reason for implant loosening. Coatings not only have been used primarily with joint arthroplasty applications but also are utilized in graft substitutes to fill bony defects in spinal fusion devices.

The ideal structure of a porous surface is an open microstructure resembling cancellous bone in its porosity, stiffness, and frictional behavior. Ingrowth is directly dependent on the coating architecture, including its porosity, pore size, shape, and interconnectivity. Larger pore sizes allow sufficient space for cell migration, adhesion and proliferation, while an interconnected porosity will maintain vascularity by allowing the free movement of body fluids. Pore sizes of approximately 50 μm or greater have been found to be associated with osseointegration, where the optimal pore size has been determined to range between approximately 50 μm and 500 μm. However, these pore sizes have been based primarily on cobalt–chromium surfaces. Instead, these "optimal" pore sizes may be smaller for titanium surfaces, which may be more osteoconductive. The chosen material should further be biocompatible and possibly bioactive. While porosity may aid in facilitating osseointegration, a consideration with porous coatings is the effect of the material porosity on fatigue strength, as the voids in the surface can act as stress concentrations. Further, the increased surface area could potentially lead to higher corrosion rates, increasing concerns with corrosion related fracture and metal ion release. Corrosion concerns explain why stainless steel is not utilized for this purpose. Ceramics, on the other hand, are not used because of their inherent brittleness, while polymers are limited by their poor strength and high failure rates.

Irregular surfaces are realized in a number of embodiments, including wire mesh, sintered beads, grooves, and voids. The first generation of porous coatings included CoCr sintered beads, structured titanium (sintering of pure Ti onto a Ti or CoCr substrate), diffusion-bonded fiber metal mesh (wire lengths can be woven into a mesh and pressure sintered onto a solid substrate), and titanium plasma spray, which is fabricated by casting molten titanium on a substrate surface. Each of these coatings has performed similarly in a clinical setting in terms of bone ingrowth behavior, which has been observed to be heavily dependent on intimate bone contact for long-term biologic fixation. All options in this group are considered to have a relatively low porosity of 30% to 50% and a high interface stiffness, making them relatively limited in their capability for interfacial strength. Further, all traditional porous coatings are theoretically susceptible to mesh shedding and delamination as they are not able to be fabricated into a stand-alone structure (i.e., they must be added to a substrate surface). Specifically, sintered coatings (CoCr and structured Ti) and diffusion bonded mesh have relatively reduced fatigue strengths owing to the high-temperature fabrication process. It is estimated that these coatings will retain less than 50% of their fatigue strength. In comparison, plasma-flame sprayed coating is capable of retaining 90% of its fatigue strength.

In response to these limitations, there is a continued focus of innovations in open-structured metals to replace traditional coated surfaces. Highly porous foam metals in homogenous and non-homogenous open cell pore distributions come closer to the ideal porous coating described above. Current options include titanium- and tantalum-based foams, which are fabricated through deposition onto a vitreous carbon skeleton. These metal foams typically exhibit higher porosities, higher coefficients of friction, and lower stiffnesses in comparison to first-generation coatings. Ranges for these and other properties are provided in Table 13.1.

Table 13.1 Select properties for common materials used as porous coatings for orthopaedic applications

	Cancellous bone	Porous tantalum	Porous titanium	Porous magnesium
Porosity (%)	30–95	75–85	60–72	35–50
Pore size (µm)	20–1000	400–600	150–600	100–400
Modulus of elasticity (GPa)	2.3–20	2.5–3.9	1.6–4.2	0.9–1.8
Compressive strength (MPa)	20–193	50–70	100–200	12–17
Coefficient of friction	—	0.88	0.54 to 1.2	

Marketed titanium-based foams include Biofoam (Wright Medical Technology), Stiktite (Smith and Nephew), Gription (Depuy), Tritanium (Stryker), and Regenerex (Biomet). Zimmer's Trabecular Metal is the only tantalum foam currently available. Porous magnesium coatings are not yet available, but this approach is considered a candidate for future innovations for implant fixation. Further details on the properties and character of these metals are given in Chapter 7.

Hydroxyapatite coatings

As an alternative to porous coatings, hydroxyapatite (HA) was introduced for biological fixation during the 1980s, with the intent of providing strong bone bonding. HA is a nontoxic, biocompatible, and osteoconductive material. In some coatings, the chemical purity of HA can be above 99.99% and have a maximum porosity of 2%. Clinical studies have shown good outcomes following the use of HA coatings, though some have raised concerns about continuous absorption of HA. HA coating can be plasma sprayed onto a porous coating to further enhance the fixation capabilities of the porous coating.

Fixation for bone fractures

When a bone absorbs energy above its ultimate strength, a fracture occurs along line(s) of least resistance. The treatment of bone fractures may include casting, external fixation, or internal fixation, which is currently the preferred method in a majority of cases. Internal fixation makes use of rigid bone plates secured to the endosteal surface with screws or pins, nails implanted into the intramedullary canal, or lag screws and wires that directly secure bone fragments. The aim of treatment is to provide a safe environment for fracture healing, while minimizing the intrusion of the prosthesis on the host region.

Fracture healing is affected by external mechanical stimuli, sex, age, metabolic status, and lifestyle factor. A bone fracture will either undergo primary or secondary fracture healing. Primary healing involves a direct attempt of the cortex to reestablish itself without callus formation. Secondary fracture healing includes an intermediate callus stage. Primary healing is much slower and is considerably more difficult to achieve in most load-bearing bones owing to the requirement of near-complete immobility across the fracture site. Contemporary fracture treatment aims for an uneventful secondary healing process.

A fracture going through uneventful secondary healing will pass through three stages: (1) inflammation, (2) reparation, and (3) remodeling. The inflammation stage will begin immediately, in which a hematoma will form at the fracture site and seal off the region causing the lysis of local osteocytes, contributing minimal mechanical stability, and carrying precursor mesenchymal cells that will eventually generate into osteoblasts, chondrocytes, fibrocartilage, or fibrous tissue. Bone resorption will initiate during this stage as osteoclasts and macrophages are dissolving and removing damaged and necrotic tissue.* During the reparation phase (2 weeks), the repair cells begin to produce proteins that become a soft callus of osteoid, fibroblasts, and chondroblasts, which acts to bridge and stabilize the fracture gap. Over the next 6 to 12 weeks, the callus will harden into woven and lamellar bone. Eventually, trabecular bone will remodel into compact bone and a clinical union will occur at approximately 12 to 16 weeks.

Tissue differentiation is heavily dependent on the amount of vascularization and the mechanical environment of the fracture. The amount of micromotion tolerated at the fracture site has been debated. Carter differentiated fracture strains into dilational and distortional components. In its non-distorted state, a cell has a low-energy natural spherical shape. It is thought that distortional strain alters the cytoskeleton and affects the gene expression and biosynthetic activity of mesenchymal cells, fibroblasts, and chondrocytes. During the early stages of healing, intermittent and moderate shear stress stimulates the proliferation of tissues and the formation of callus. On the other hand, dilational strain is thought to affect gene expression and also inhibit capillary blood flow by decreasing tissue oxygen tension. Too much compression will result in poor vascularity and low oxygen tension owing to inhibited capillary blood flow. Because cartilage has a lesser metabolic demand relative to bone, mesenchymal cells are shunted to a chondrogenic pathway. In a cartilaginous state, cyclical shear will promote ossification while hydrostatic compression will support chondrogenesis and cartilage maintenance. In extreme cases, the fractures may form cartilaginous caps in a pseudarthrosis to accommodate the high compressive strains. In the case that distortional stress or tensile dilational stress are too large, either

---

* Resorption widens the gap and lowers the strain to levels that can be tolerated for the beginning of tissue differentiation. Resorption seems to be strain dependent, as areas of elevated tissue strain have been directly correlated to the spatial distribution of bone resorption in sheep.

fibrocartilage or fibrous tissue is formed owing to fibroblasts increasing the production of collagen oriented in the tensile direction.

In a much more straightforward analysis, Perren theorized that strain between 2% and 10% will lead to the secondary bone formation, while strains below 2% were expected to result in primary bone healing and those between 10% and 100% will lead to a sustained environment of initial connective tissue. According to this theory, strain above 100% will result in nonunion.

Gardner et al. proposed that high octahedral shear stress promotes tissue proliferation and increases the size of the callus in all stages of healing. They proposed that as bone matures, it is able to withstand a higher degree of compressive dilational stress while still undergoing endochondral ossification, limiting concerns about compressive hydrostatic stresses by Carter. Recently, Epari et al. studied the components of fragment movement in osteotomized ovine tibiae that are beneficial for fracture healing. They determined that high shear stability and moderate, not maximal, axial stability are associated with high callus strength and stiffness and a better healing outcome.

Problems

PROBLEM 13.1

Which of these are a characteristic of a porous coating that is NOT expected to directly affect the rate of bone ingrowth?

A. Porosity

B. Fatigue strength

C. Frictional behavior

D. Stiffness

ANSWER:

B. Fatigue strength is important in terms of the failure of the actual coating material but does not have a direct effect on ingrowth.

PROBLEM 13.2

Comment on whether the following interfaces are considered Direct, Graded, Compliant, or a combination of the three.

A. Cemented

B. Ingrown

C. Adhered

ANSWER:

Cemented, fully compliant; ingrown, combination of graded and compliant; adhered, a direct bond with some compliant behavior.

References

CARTER DR, BLENMAN PR, BEAUPRE GS: Correlations between mechanical stress history and tissue differentiation in initial fracture healing. *J Orthop Res* 6(5):736–748, 1988.

CHARNLEY J, KETTLEWELL L: The elimination of slip between prosthesis and femur. *J Bone Joint Surg* 47B:56–60, 1965.

EPARI DR, KASSI JP, SCHELL H, DUDA GN: Timely fracture-healing requires optimization of axial fixation stability. *J Bone Joint Surg Am* 89(7):1575–1585, 2007.

GARDNER TN, MISHRA S, MARKS L: The role of osteogenic index, octahedral shear stress and dilatational stress in the ossification of a fracture callus. *Med Eng Phys* 26(6):493–501, 2004.

HARTY M: The calcar femorale and the femoral neck. *J Bone Joint Surg* 39A:625–630, 1957.

PERREN SM: Evolution of the internal fixation of longbone fractures. The scientific basis of biological internal fixation: Choosing a new balance between stability and biology. *J Bone Joint Surg Br* 84(8):1093–1110, 2002.

WEIGHTMAN B: Stress analysis. p. 34. In Swanson SAY, Freeman MAR (eds): *The Scientific Basis of Joint Replacement*. Wiley, New York, 1975.

Annotated bibliography

1. BAUER TW, SCHILS J: The pathology of total joint arthroplasty—Mechanisms of implant failure. *Skeletal Radiol* 28:483–497, 1999.

   Informative review on common modalities of implant failure in arthroplasty.

2. BOBYN JD, POGGIE RA, KRYGIER JJ, LEWALLEN DG, HANSSEN AD, LEWIS RJ, UNGER AS, O'KEEFE TJ, CHRISTIE MJ, NASSER S, WOOD JE, STULBERG SD, TANZER M: Clinical validations of a structural porous tantalum biomaterial for adult reconstruction. *J Bone Joint Surg* 86-A:123–129, 2004.

   An overview of porous tantalum used in orthopaedic applications.

3. CACHINHO SCP, CORREIA RN: Titanium scaffolds for osteointegration: mechanical, *in vitro* and corrosion behavior. *J Mater Sci: Mater Med* 19:451–457, 2008.

   Mechanical and biological properties for porous titanium.

4. CHARNLEY J: *Acrylic Cement in Orthopaedic Surgery*. Williams & Wilkins, Baltimore, 1970.

   Chapter 2 on the "theory of mechanical fastenings in bone surgery" lays out Charnley's thinking that led to the use of PMMA cement in total joint arthroplasty.

5. DUCHEYNE P: Biological fixation of implants. In Ducheyne P, Hastings GW (eds): *Functional Behavior of Orthopaedic Implants*. Vol. II. CRC Press, Boca Raton, 1984.

   Review, emphasizing fibrous surfaces.

6. FABI DW, LEVINE BR: Porous coatings on metallic implant materials. In Narayan R (ed): *ASM Handbook, Volume 23, Materials for Medical Devices*. ASM International, 2012.

   Descriptions and material characteristics for marketed porous tantalum and titanium forms.

7. HADDAD RJ JR, COOK SD, THOMAS KA: Current concepts review: Biological fixation of porous-coated implants. *J Bone Joint Surg* 69A:1459–1466, 1987.

Review of early clinical experience in the modern era, up to early 1987, including histology associated with retrieved devices.

8. HALAWA H, LEE AJC, LING RSM, VANGALA SS: The shear strength of trabecular bone from the femur and some factors affecting the shear strength of the cement–bone interface. *Arch Orthop Trauma Surg* 92:19–30, 1978.

Laboratory results that support the wisdom of pressurizing PMMA cement into well-cleaned cancellous beds.

9. HENCH LL, ETHRIDGE EC: *Biomaterials: An Interface Approach.* Academic Press, New York, 1982.

A concise discussion of fixation (p. 244–252). Deals with "bioactive" surfaces; Hench invented one of the principle systems of such materials.

10. HOMSY CA: Implant stabilization: Chemical and biomechanical considerations. *Orthop Clin North Am* 4(2):295–312, 1974.

Early proposal for nonrigid stabilization by tissue ingrowth.

11. LEE AJC, LING RSM: Loosening. In Ling RSM (ed): *Complications of Total Hip Replacement.* Churchill Livingstone, Edinburgh, 1984.

A relatively balanced discussion of loosening of PMMA-cemented THRs, by one of the first groups to emphasize the role of technique, including pressurization. Comprehensive bibliography.

12. PILLIAR RM: Powder metal-made orthopaedic implants with porous surface for fixation by tissue ingrowth. *Clin Orthop Rel Res* 176:42–51, 1983.

Unified discussion of fabrication and properties of porous coatings in cobalt-base systems, with reference to earlier basic studies.

13. RUBIN CT, LANYON LE: Osteoregulatory nature of mechanical stimuli: Function as a determinant for adaptive remodeling in bone. *J Orthop Res* 5:300–310, 1987.

An account of practical investigations into Wolff's law.

14. SWANSON SAV: Mechanical aspects of fixation. In Swanson SAV, Freeman MAR (eds): *The Scientific Basis of Joint Replacement.* John Wiley & Sons, New York, 1977.

Descriptive, comparative treatment of fixation by cementation and ingrowth.

15. WILLERT H-G, SEMLITSCH M: Reactions of the articular capsule to wear products of artificial joint prostheses. *J Biomed Mater Res* 11:157–164, 1977.

Useful account by Willert, who originally proposed a model of osteolysis arising from cellular response to wear debris.

CHAPTER FOURTEEN

Host response

In addition to satisfying the physical and functional requirements imposed by implant designs, biomaterials must be easily accepted by the body. In fact, lack of acceptance—adverse host response—is commonly the limiting factor in the application of materials to solve biomedical problems. For this reason, it is extremely important to gauge host response, particularly materials aspects that are not directly dependent on design details but that enlighten us concerning more general relationships between biomaterials and living systems.

Implants must "couple" with the host to produce a host response; this may happen in a variety of ways. The most obvious is through direct chemical effects owing to corrosion, dissolution, or elution of the implant component materials. Implants in particulate form, as in wear debris, produce different tissue responses than they do in bulk form, with the response to a degree independent of the chemical composition of the particles. Mechanical factors, principally seen in remodeling responses to initial changes in stress distribution, are also important to the requirements for biologic ingrowth and to local chemical, thermal, or pressure necrosis. Electrical factors are usually not appreciated, except in the special case of the use of implanted electrodes to stimulate osteogenesis.

The host responses may be classified as structural, physiological, bacteriologic, immunologic, and carcinogenic. The responses are seen most frequently in the immediate vicinity of the implant but may occur systemically or at remote sites, such as the regional lymph nodes. The following discussion will deal with responses primarily by location.

Most of what is known about host response to implanted biomaterials results from animal studies. However, the emphasis will be placed on what can be reliably deduced by comparing these laboratory results to clinical findings.

Local host response

Normal response Implants are placed in intimate contact with soft tissue and bone. The process of placing them (implantation) produces a wound. Thus, the normal response to implantation is that of wound healing, although with some significant differences.

Figure 14.1 shows the cellular progression that is expected in healing of soft tissues (above) and the development of stiffness and strength of the healing tissues (below). The cell progression noted here should be familiar, producing the events of cleanup, repair, and reconstruction of the damaged tissues. Note that stiffness is observed to return before strength, in both soft and hard tissues. This is reasonable if we consider that normal mechanical function requires "all" of stiffness, whereas normal stresses usually do not exceed 10%–20% of ultimate strength. The balance of strength is required to protect against rare overload events; this capability returns late in the healing process.

Even in the absence of an implant, many factors may affect the development shown here. In particular, hard tissue matures more slowly than soft tissue, whereas functional use, promoting remodeling, probably accelerates the later stages of healing of both.

Introduction of an implant assures that events will progress differently. Early protein interactions with the implant surface may activate complement and will produce hapten complexes, which may activate other portions of the immune system. Macrophages will be unable fully to clean up the dead space in the wound, owing to the presence of a physical implant.

Three particular cellular events, not usually seen in healing wounds, occur to one degree or another in the presence of all implants:

1. Macrophages may remain in the vicinity of the implant.

2. Significant numbers of lymphocytes (and even plasma cells) may be seen near the implant.

3. At later times, a population of multinucleated giant cells, called foreign body giant cells, may appear and remain for long periods or chronically.

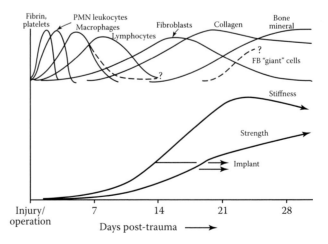

FIGURE 14.1 Cell populations and mechanical properties of a healing wound.

All implants are surrounded with a fibrous capsule. This is a consequence of the classic foreign body response that attempts to degrade all nonself material and, failing that, to sequester it. Such response is to be expected for implanted materials. Direct tissue apposition to pure titanium and tantalum and its alloys is possible, and it appears that the early response to bioactive ceramics is also free of capsule formation. However, these are isolated exceptions to the general rule.

The normal capsule arises through the process of matrix repair and elaboration that accompanies normal wound healing. It is largely collagenous but may resemble fibrocartilage in areas of relative motion, as in the acetabulum in contact with an endoprosthetic head. In areas around loose prostheses, it may even appear synovial in nature. It is usually integral with normal bone or soft tissue and lies directly against the implant.

In its normal presentation, capsular tissue is relatively acellular, containing only small numbers of fibroblasts with rare histiocytes and macrophages. The major matrix protein is type I collagen; thus, the capsule resembles granulation tissue rather than an early stage of fracture healing. However, the capsule is oriented with collagen fibers lying parallel to the implant surface, and cells, when present, are more common in the outer layers.

In occasional cases, there is a volume of serous fluid between the capsule and the implant. Within articular joints, regenerating synovial tissue produces a fluid similar to normal synovial fluid.

When the implant is a source of debris, either from articulating wear, or fretting of multipart or modular devices, particles may be seen in the matrix between the cells and within macrophages. Polymethyl methacrylate (PMMA) is likely present in some instances; however, conventional histologic preparation usually removes some or all of the PMMA debris. Ceramic debris are rarely appreciated since they are generally very small (<0.1 µm) and may be lost from the tissues during histologic processing. Carbon-reinforced ultrahigh-molecular-weight polyethylene (UHMWPE) articulating components shed submicron-sized carbon particles as well as short (10–30 µm), pulled-out sections of fiber, both of which are easily recognized by their opacity, regularity of shape, and black color. Metal wear particles are typically on the order of 1 to 2 µm in size.

The capsular membrane is usually only 20–200 µm thick and thus cannot be seen radiographically. It may be specifically thickened around angles or protruberances of implants, such as at the knots in cerclage wire. More generally, the capsule becomes thickened as a response to increased chemical release from the implant, to stress-concentrating features, and to relative tissue–implant motion. The 1 mm or wider radiolucent line, which may be pathognomonic of incipient or actual loosening, is the result of a more aggressive process, most frequently termed "osteolysis."

In bony tissue, in the presence of acceptable implant stability (as discussed in Chapter 13), bone will grow into close apposition with the implant surface. In PMMA-cemented devices, a zone of "dead" bone, 0.1–0.5 mm thick, is produced secondary to chemical toxicity of the methacrylate monomer (MMA) and to the release of heat during PMMA curing. This is replaced by a new bone with time, but may persist for relatively long periods. If a porous or perforated surface with minimum internal openings of at least approximately 50 μm is provided, bone will grow into the surface down to the solid base. Examination of early post-operative retrievals reveals regions of unmineralized osteoid that should not be confused with the fibrous capsule. If there are large gaps between a porous prosthesis and bone (>1 mm), a bony plate may condense near the implant surface with a volume of more cancellous bone behind it.

Bone ingrowth and maturation are more rapid from a cancellous bone region than from cortical bone, with the tissue–implant interface reaching peak shear strength in dogs in 8 weeks. The process may take longer in patients, with remodeling still possible up to 2 years postoperation. Inadequate device designs, especially those that combine stiff stems with good distal fixation, may produce continued "stress protection" remodeling as long as a decade postoperation.

Host response to implant removal

Soft tissue sites heal in a traditional manner, by elimination of dead spaces and remodeling to a residual local collagenous scar. If wear or other particulate debris remain, a chronic but modest inflammatory response with associated cell types may persist.

Hard tissue, if fully debrided with all particulate material and dead tissue removed, has the ability to heal and regenerate completely, as in normal fracture healing. Defects produced during device removal, such as screw holes after screw removal, when freshly formed, reduce local bone strength and toughness by up to 50%. If dead bone remains, such as a ring sequestrum around a percutaneous traction pin, healing and remodeling may progress without obliteration of the defect. However, animal studies suggest that such defects cease to be regions of stress concentrations within 6 months, whether they persist or not.

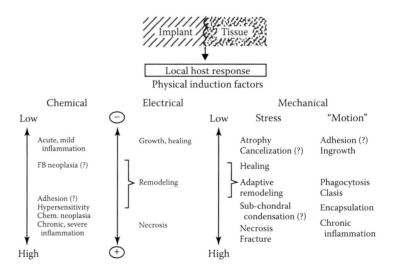

FIGURE 14.2 Physical induction factors in local host response.

Factors in local host response

It is clear that chemical, mechanical, and possibly electrical factors contribute to the maturation of tissue around implants. These factors are summarized in Figure 14.2, with an attempt to relate local responses to the level or "dose" of each factor. It is possible that synergistic or antagonistic interactions take place between these factors, but this question has been largely unexplored to date. On these scales, normal local host response is characterized by *low* chemical activity, *intermediate* electrical activity (near charge neutrality), and *intermediate* stress, combined with *low* to *moderate* motion. Special cases, such as fixation by adherence, require other combinations of levels.

Adverse host reactions

Chronic inflammation

If there is a sustained challenge from the implant, owing perhaps to the accumulation of large amounts of wear debris, to a related delayed hypersensitivity reaction, or to the presence of an implant site infection (all discussed specifically below), a sustained or chronic inflammation may occur. In this case, the capsular membrane will contain significant numbers of monocytes, macrophages, and occasional multinucleated foreign body giant cells. Histiocytes may even be seen condensed into layers or sheets. The presence of plasma cells and lymphocytes is widely believed to reflect some specific hypersensitivity reaction. This chronic inflammatory response has the hallmarks of such incidences in the absence of implants, but is distinguished by the long-term presence of macrophages and of significant numbers of multinucleated giant cells.

Metallosis

Resurgence in the use of metal-on-metal (MOM) hip arthroplasty has brought with it distinguishing presentations of adverse host response in some cases, although such responses have also been observed with other articulations such as metal-on-polyethylene (MOP) hip bearings and other prosthetic joints such as knee replacements. The designation for the body's response to significant metallic wear debris or localized, focal corrosion of metallic implants produced in MOM articulations, and historically, but less prominently, tissue reflected from above the heads of screws in fracture fixation devices has been termed *metallosis*. (Metallosis is distinguished from the body's hypersensitive response to a moderate release of metal debris, which is called "ALVAL" and is discussed in the following sections.) Its presence seems to be associated most prominently with MOM THAs, which have been targeted to a younger, more active patient population. In 2008, it was estimated that approximately 40% of THAs done in the United States were MOM, but this articulation has almost ceased to be used in the general population because of concerns about host response.

Metallosis is characterized as an infiltration of metallic debris in the periprosthetic soft tissue and bone secondary to arthroplasty. At the microscopic level, an extensive collection of metal-stained phagocytic cells can be observed. The term *metallosis* is most often associated with its primary clinical presentation characteristic: discoloration, primarily blackening, of the surrounding tissue. It often results in aseptic fibrosis, local necrosis, or loosening of the device.

The activation of the host response can be thought of as a reaction to the debris particles themselves or to their corrosion products—though response to corrosion products and wear particles is considered the same by some. It has been suggested that metal wear products may have toxic effects on human cells. Upon spreading through the joint space, the immediate response is a histiocytic immune response, resulting in increased levels of macrophages and the release of inflammatory cytokines. When there is metal particulate beyond a patient specific threshold, tissue destruction owing to the inflammatory response will self-perpetuate, as actions to destroy the foreign body will lead to further ion formation. In a normal response, the bacteria and defensive cells will die and the inflammation will eventually subside. When particles remain, the reactive cells will still die, but the tissue response will be repeated and possibly escalated, with the end result being fibrosis, necrosis, and osteolysis.

The biologic response is highly dependent on the size, type, and amount of particles. Transmission electron microscopy analyses have shown that Co–Cr particles are on the order of a submicrometer to a nanometer in size, an order of magnitude smaller than UHMWPE particles. They are majorly round in shape, although there were some that exhibited shard or needlelike morphology. The size and shape are thought to be highly dependent on the processing technique of the implant. Intensity of the reactions depends on the metal type, the particle size and volume, the rate at which the debris is being generated, and exposure time. The level of patient response is undoubtedly affected by the patient's comorbidities.

It has been reported that women, smaller-size patients, and implantations with steep abduction angles are predisposing factors for metallosis. Cases of inappropriate angulation (malpositioning) of the socket in abduction and anteversion will lead to edge loading, cause greater-than-expected wear, and resulting greater metal release. This risk is further increased in small-diameter components. Other drivers of greater particle generation from various material combinations include prosthetic head articulation with the acetabular shell (after polyethylene liner wear-through or fracture), fretting of the acetabular shell with screws, backside wear between the shell and the liner, shedding of porous coatings, or any other femoral prosthesis loosening and motion. Any improper articulation can cause disruption of the passive oxide layer, leading to direct contact and eventually fretting corrosion. The rate of THA revision owing to metallosis is unclear.

Diagnosis of metallosis is done via clinical manifestation and imaging. Aspiration of synovial fluid from the hip can produce dark gray or black fluid. During revision, black fluid in the joint space or grayish tissue surrounding the prosthesis is often noted. This tissue is commonly engulfed by histiocytes in a densely fibrotic background. Clinically, metallosis may present with hip or buttock pain, a palpable lump, nerve irritation, or nerve palsy. Its presentation is often accompanied by radiographic identification of component failure or dislodgement, spontaneous dislocation, or eccentric positioning. Osteolysis associated with MOM wear may occur, but it seems there is a rare occurrence of this activity. Evidence of this includes an absence of multinucleated giant cells in surrounding tissues, while levels of tumor necrosis factor (TNF)-α are observed to be low.

"Sterile abscess"

The sterile abscess phenomenon is reasonably well recognized in association with multipart or modular fracture fixation devices. It presents as a focal tissue lesion at the tissue–implant interface and is associated with highly localizable pain. On exploration, modest tissue discoloration is found, cultures are negative, and curettage with device removal or exchange produces prompt remission of pain.

The sterile abscess is believed to be a local inflammatory response with kinin-induced pain, secondary to elevated local concentrations of corrosion products. These concentrations may be caused by local chemical potential gradients, fretting, or possibly by alloy inclusions, or in the case of fracture fixation devices, crevice, pitting, or galvanic corrosion. Immune responses are also involved in some cases. The sterile abscess may also be a long-term consequence of a minor local infection that resolved but persists as a localized chronic low-grade inflammation owing to inhibition of macrophages by corrosion products.

The presence of the sterile abscess in total joint replacement (TJR) arthroplasty is less well recognized. However, reports of local osteolytic zones, which may occasionally resolve, seen in the patients with PMMA-cemented THRs as well as with uncemented, porous-coated metallic components may be an expression of this process. The sterile abscess is highly focal and less florid than a chronic inflammation. It is frequently misidentified as a local infection, since it is recognized that failure to culture microorganisms from a tissue site is not clear evidence of their absence.

Osteolysis

Wear debris excite a phagocytic macrophage response. If the debris are sufficiently small in quantity and volume, they are successfully phagocytized, transported through the lymphatic drainage, and extruded into the patient's airway through the lung parenchyma. If they are more chemically active, they may lodge in regional lymph nodes, causing a local granuloma, such as the "teflonoma" reported by Charnley secondary to the use of a polymer with poor wear resistance as an acetabular cup material.

Neither of these outcomes is particularly threatening to the patient in the presence of combinations of modern biomaterials. However, the production of large amounts of wear debris as a result of abnormal wear or fretting results in a situation that macrophages derived from monocytes cannot deal with. Succeeding generations become engorged and die, producing a local caseation, and multinuclear giant cells appear. This produces the appearance and symptoms of a chronic inflammatory response, which may be mistaken for local infection. However, it tends to be, at least initially, restricted to one portion of the implant capsule or one side of a replaced joint and to have the appearance of a sterile abscess. As discussed in Chapter 13, causation of this process in TJRs is generally seen as dominated by implant motion ("micromotion"); it is unclear which comes first: the motion producing the debris or the biologic reaction leading to motion and production of debris.

There is substantial *in vitro* evidence that stimulated macrophages can attack bone directly and that, in addition, they release pro-inflammatory cytokines and other mediators of inflammation, which attracts and stimulates osteoclasts. Animal studies suggest that TNF-α is a key cytokine involved in osteolysis. The result may be a quick "dissecting" osteolysis that moves into the interface between normal bone and the implant, leaving a broad (1–5 mm wide) lucent zone and potentially leading to rapid clinical failure. There is an established correlation between number of macrophages, volume of UHWMPE wear debris, and osteolytic regions. Size and volume of particles are determinant of resulting host response. *In vitro* studies of human and murine macrophages have shown that the most biologically active size range is 0.1 to 1.0 μm in terms of macrophages producing cytokines and resulting in bone-resorbing activity. Osteolysis has been demonstrated most graphically in the unfortunate use of a UHMWPE femoral head in the Monk "soft-top" endoprosthesis, which bears directly against bone in the acetabulum, leading to aggressive polyethylene granulomatosis.

Infection

Infection is the great enemy of the surgeon, rendering useless the best reconstruction and hindering its revision. Implant site infections are a major revision risk and can prolong hospital care, although their incidence in previously uninfected sites rarely exceeds 1%. Infections may be separated into early and late occurrence.

Early infections are generally due to the introduction of skin or airborne pathogens during surgery. The role of the implant in the establishment and maintenance of early infection appears to be largely mechanical, in serving as a barrier to easy revascularization of the damaged tissue immediately adjacent to the implant. Pre-existing sensitivity to metal has also been implicated in the related problem of early infection of internal fracture fixation sites. However, animal studies suggest that all commonly used prosthetic materials produce modest increased infectability of the implant site by *Staphylococcus aureus*. However, sites with PMMA polymerized in situ, as is the case in TJR arthroplasty, are particularly sensitive, requiring as few as 1000 colony-forming units of *Staphylococcus epidermidis* and *Escherichia coli* for infection. Any particulate debris can act as a scaffold for bacterial adhesion and biofilm growth and ultimately reduce the minimum number of bacteria needed to cause an infection.

Late infection frequently has a hematogenous source, and thus local vascular insufficiency seems a weak explanation for its tenacity. However, *in vitro* studies demonstrate that stainless steel and cobalt-base alloy constituents, in concentrations present in the immediate vicinity of metallic components, inhibit both macrophage chemotaxis and phagocytosis. Further, corrosion products of CoCr may inhibit release of reactive oxygen species required by neutrophils to kill bacteria. An additional factor may be the residence of bacteria in the glycocalyx, an adherent coating that forms on all foreign materials placed *in vivo*. This glycoprotein-based coating, 5–50 µm or so in thickness, protects bacteria, perhaps through a diffusion limitation process, and serves to decrease their antibiotic sensitivity by 10 to 100 times. Devices retrieved from infected sites frequently show bacterial colonies resident within this film. Finally, some researchers have implicated metal sensitization, also leading to a loss of macrophage chemotactic ability, as a factor in the ease of establishment and persistence of implant site infections. Patient comorbidities have also been implicated as a significant risk factor for periprosthetic infections.

Infection is difficult to address clinically with the implant in place. This is probably due to a number of factors already discussed, including the low vascularity of the implant capsule and the presence of the implant surface glycocalyx. This is particularly a problem in TJR, in which the device is intended to remain in place chronically. Most surgeons now favor revision with immediate or delayed replacement, as the only way to stop infection is to remove the infected device. Bacteria form a biofilm mode of growth on the implant surface, which can increase the antibiotic resistance, complicating treatment of implant site infections. A common procedure is removal and insertion of an antibiotic impregnated "preform" as a bridge to later re-implantation.

When PMMA cement is used, the addition of an antibiotic to which the principal infecting organism has been shown to be sensitive has become common and is apparently successful in a good proportion of both types of procedures. Addition of appropriate dry-form antibiotics to PMMA cements appears to degrade their initial properties only slightly. Broad-spectrum antibiotics, in powder form, added to PMMA have also been used, apparently successfully, as a prophylactic measure in primary TJR arthroplasty. Also, surface coatings with antimicrobial agents can be used inhibit to bacterial attachment and growth.

Neoplasia

Biomaterials researchers have long been concerned about the possibility of implant materials producing neoplastic transformation or promoting neoplastic growth. Two primary mechanisms have been proposed and explored in animal models: foreign body and chemical transformation.

Foreign body neoplasia is a transformation process associated with the shape of implants, independent of their composition, so long as they are sufficiently chemically inert. It is characterized by a single transformation event and a long resting or latent period, during which the presence of the implant is still required, before clonal expression occurs. This type of transformation is well known in animals, especially as a response to implantation of impermeable materials in the subdermal space in rodents. However, gathering evidence suggests that this effect, sometimes called the Oppenheimer effect, is related to the relatively primitive immune system of rodents. Retrospective clinical studies suggest either that it does not occur in humans or that it has a very long latency period, probably greater than 40 years.

Questions have been raised over the possibility of foreign body neoplasia arising from release of needlelike particles from composites. This mechanism is believed to be contributory in the etiology of asbestos-related mesothelioma. However, animal experiments suggest that particles require very high length-to-diameter ratios (>100) to produce this effect. Such particles are highly unlikely to arise from orthopaedic implants.

Chemical transformation appears to be a more real concern. Metals and metallic compounds have long been recognized among the narrow range of presumptive chemical oncogenic agents in humans. Our knowledge of the risks posed by chemical oncogenes comes from animal injection and exposure experiments and from human epidemiologic studies, primarily involving industrial exposure.

Applying strict criteria to try to eliminate false-positive conclusions, it appears that chromium and some of its compounds, nickel and some of its compounds, and cobalt are potent carcinogens in animals. The concern about chromium has recently increased owing to suggestions that corrosion of chromium-bearing alloys under physiologic conditions releases Cr^{6+}, rather than Cr^{3+}, the normal dietary form, as previously assumed. Hexavalent chromium easily penetrates cell membranes (as Cr^{3+} cannot) and thus has far more biologic activity, including carcinogenicity, than the dietary form. The presence of Cr^{3+} in non-phagocytic cells, such as erythrocytes, is often interpreted as evidence of the prior presence of Cr^{6+}. Once inside a cell, Cr^{6+} is reduced to Cr^{3+} through reactions, by-products of which are highly reactive species with the potential to damage the cell's organelles, or DNA. Also, Cr^{3+} within the cell may form complexes that can cause mutagenesis. Typically, cells with Cr^{3+} will enter apoptosis. In the case this is prevented, they may survive and replicate, and potentially lead to a neoplastic formation. Titanium and aluminum are not known to be oncogenic in animals, whereas the evidence concerning vanadium is inconclusive.

Implants of metallic nickel and cobalt foils as well as cobalt-base alloy wear debris are oncogenic in rodents, producing fibrosarcomas and rhabdomyosarcomas in soft tissue sites. Hard tissue responses are poorly documented. Small, nonfunctional solid implants tend not to produce tumors, probably owing to low release rates, although high-nickel-content cobalt-base alloys, such as MP35N, do produce small numbers of tumors in such models in less than 3 years. Cobalt-base alloys have not been used frequently in veterinary clinical practice, but stainless steel has seen wide application in fracture fixation devices. There are a significant number of reports of implant site tumors in dogs and cats, primarily osteosarcomas and fibrosarcomas, associated with stainless steel devices. These tumors occur with 3–5 years latency and may be associated with infection, perhaps reflecting increased metal release, secondary to local acidosis. A summary of typical cases is given in Table 14.1.

Table 14.1   Implant site tumors in animals

Tumor	Time of diagnosis (years postimplantation)
Chondroblastic osteosarcoma	3.5
Osteosarcoma[a,b]	3.8
Chondroblastic osteosarcoma[a]	4.0
Chondroblastic osteosarcoma[a,b]	6.0
Telangiectatic osteosarcoma	6.0
Undifferentiated sarcoma[b]	6.8
Chondroblastic osteosarcoma	8.5
Average	5.2

Note: All dogs, with F 55 plate–screw fixation.
[a] With metastases.
[b] *S. aureus* infection.

Until 1984, there were only six reports of implant site tumors in human orthopaedic patients. Most of these were associated with stainless steel fracture fixation devices, whereas only two were definitely associated with cast cobalt-base implants. More recently, there have been reports of a number of cases associated with cobalt-base alloy TJRs (Table 14.2). By 2003, there were 46 cases of implant-related malignant tumors reported at the site of a total hip arthroplasty. Overall, this is a remarkably low occurrence. However, these may represent a very small proportion of the clinical TJR arthroplasty population and the tumors were discovered generally 2–5.25 years after implantation, whereas minimum latency periods for chemical oncogenesis in humans may be 5–10 years and average 20 years. The report of Bauer et al. (1987) of a primary osteosarcoma at the site of an F 75/UHMWPE THR was perhaps the first case that should have been taken seriously. In addition to this case, there are anecdotal reports of others with similar characteristics; it is to be hoped that reports appear in the literature so that they may be evaluated. The reader is guided to Visuri et al. (2006) for a recent review of known cases of malignant tumors.

However, these findings of implant site tumors must in general be regarded with concern for several reasons. The TJR cases diagnosed as malignant fibrous histiocytomas may reflect oncogenic transformation in the histiocyte sheets frequently observed at THR arthroplasty revision. Additionally, Weber specifically shows possible transformation of a previously identified histiocytoma (Weber 1986). The parallel to malignant histiocytic transformation of bony infarcts is striking; perhaps the general suppression of macrophage activity by metallic ions further hinders host defenses and increases the possibility of such a transformation in the presence of a metallic implant. Introduction of higher-surface-area implants, designed for biologic fixation, into younger, more active patients may also increase risk through both higher metal ion concentrations and longer expected exposure time. Neoplastic transformation

Table 14.2 Implant site tumors in humans

Author and year	Device	Tumor[a]	Time of diagnosis (years postimplantation)
Fracture fixation devices			
McDougall (1956)	Plate–screws (F 55?)	EW (?)	30
Delgado et al. (1958)	Plate–screws (F 55?)	OS	3
Dube et al. (1972)	Plate–screws (F 55?)	HE	30
Tayton (1980)	Plate–screws (F 75?)	EW	6
MacDonald (1981)	IM rod (F 75)	L	17
Dodison et al. (1983)	Plate–screws (F 75)	L	7
Ward et al. (1987)	Smith–Petersen (F 55)	OS	9
Total joint replacement			
Bagó-Granell et al. (1984)	Charnley–Mueller THR (F 75?/UHMWPE)	MFH	2
Swann (1984)[b]	McKee–Farrar THR (F 75?/F 75?)	MFH	3.3
Penman et al. (1984)	Ring THR (F 75/F 75)	OS	5.25
Weber (1986)	Variable axis TKR (F 75/ UHMWPE)	ES[c]	3.7
Ryu et al. (1987)	Mittlemeier THR (F 75/ Al_2O_3)	STS	1.25
Bauer et al. (1987)	Charnley–Mueller THR (F 75/UHMWPE)	OS[d]	10
Albert et al. (2009)	Insall Burstein TKA (CoCrMo)	AS	10
Iglesias et al. (1994)	? TKA (CoCrMo)	MFH	10
Lucas et al. (2001)	Long-stem THA (?)	MFH	2
Lucas et al. (2001)	Osteonics Omnifit (CoCrMo)	MFH	8
Mallick et al. (2009)	Burch Schneider reinforcement cage (Ti, broken)	AS	30 (original THA), 10 (revision)

Sources: Bagó-Granell, J. et al., *J Bone Joint Surg* 66B:38–40, 1984. Bauer, T.W. et al., *Trans Soc Biomater* 10:36, 1987. Delgado, E.R., *Clin Orthop Rel Res* 12:315–318, 1958. Dodion, P. et al., *Histopathology* 6:807–813, 1983. Dube, V.E., Fischer, D.E., *Cancer* 30:1260–1266, 1972. McDonald, I., *Cancer* 48:1009–1011, 1980. McDougall, A., *J Bone Joint Surg* 38B:709–713, 1956. Penman, H.G., Ring, P.A., *J Bone Joint Surg* 66B:632–634, 1984. Ryu, R.K.N. et al., *Clin Orthop Rel Res* 216:207–212, 1987. Swann, M., *J Bone Joint Surg* 66B:629–631, 1984. Tayton, K.J.J., *Cancer* 45:413–415, 1980. Ward, J.J. et al., *Trans Soc Biomater* 10:106, 1987. Weber, P.C., *J Bone Joint Surg* 68B:824–826, 1986. Iglesias, M.E. et al., *J Dermatol Surg Oncol* 20:848–849, 1994. Albert, A. et al., *Acta Orthop Belg* 75:549–553, 2009. Lucas, D.R. et al., *Histopathology* 39:620–628, 2001. Mallick, A. et al., *J Arthroplasty* 24: 323e17–323e20, 2009.

[a] Tumor types: AS, angiosarcoma; ES, epithelioid sarcoma; EW, Ewing's sarcoma; HE, hemangioendothelioma; L, lymphoma; MFH, malignant fibrous histiocytoma; OS, osteosarcoma; STS, soft tissue sarcoma.

[b] Anecdotal reports of three additional cases, including one metastatic osteosarcoma.

[c] Previous histiocytoma.

[d] Previous enchondroma.

is far more probable in remote organs such as the liver, pancreas, and lungs, where tissues are capable of concentrating corrosion products, than in the relatively insensitive primary tissue for most orthopaedic procedures, including bone. These remote site concerns will be discussed below.

Systemic and remote host response

Acute effects

Introduction of implants may produce marked transitory systemic effects. Perhaps the best known of these is central hypotension after PMMA insertion. The mechanism is poorly understood but animal studies suggest that it is potentiated by hypovolemia. It is well controlled in modern clinical practice by normovolemic (replacement) management of blood volume. Some researchers have suggested that it is an embolic phenomenon, since insertion of cement into a closed medullary space, as in the femur, may produce transient pressures up to more than five times venous blood pressure. Although there was a brief vogue of venting the femoral canal by a distal drill hole or by a later withdrawn catheter before PMMA insertion, these practices have fallen out of favor. It is hoped that the current interest in pressurizing PMMA after insertion into both the acetabulum and femur will not produce a return of this phenomenon.

There are also short-term changes in chemical composition and blood coagulation parameters, unrelated to deep venous thrombosis, secondary perhaps to operative stress, to medications used intraoperatively, or perhaps to the rapidly resolving high levels of metal release seen immediately postoperatively.

Chronic effects

Corrosion and wear, produce longer-term changes in blood composition, primarily in its metal content. Table 14.3 summarizes currently accepted normal values for implant-contained metals in blood, serum and urine.

As discussed in Chapter 12, it is extremely difficult to estimate the true rates of metal release *in vivo* because of the combination of the processes possible. Traditional methods of radiologically assessing wear are not practical for MOM bearings. While serving an important role in product evaluations, simulator studies are only somewhat useful, as there is no free exchange with blood and synovial fluid. Further, it is difficult to isolate and characterize Co–Cr particles from lubricant fluid. The alkaline digestion method (used to isolate UHMWPE particles) may alter the size and can reduce the amount of chromium. Isolation with enzymatic digestion of periprosthetic tissues has been more successful, although to understand the potential systemic implications of metal release, detection of metal ions circulating peripherally is required. Of the available methods, measuring serum is the simplest and most common, though circulating levels may not accurately represent total body ion level. Further, chromium concentrates in erythrocytes, so measuring serum may not be sufficient in some cases.

Table 14.3   Metal content of human blood, serum, and urine

Metal	Blood (ng/ml)	Serum (or plasma) (ng/ml)	Urine (ng/mg creatinine)
Al	?	<10	?
Co	<0.3	<0.3	<2.5
Cr	<1	<0.3	<0.6
Fe	445 (mg/ml)	1090	65
Mn	?	<0.7	?
Mo	<1	<1	?
Ni	<1	<1	<5
Ti	?	<2	?
V	?	<1	?

Sources: Lyengar, G.V. et al., *The Elemental Composition of Human Tissues and Body Fluids*, Verlag-Chemie, New York, 1978. Versieck, J., Cornelis, R., *Acta Analyt Chim* 116:217–254, 1980; Cornelis, R., Trace element studies in the biosphere with neutron activation analysis, *Proc. Conf. on Frontiers in Nuclear Methods of Analysis*, College Station, TX, 1984. Michel, R., *CRC Crit Rev Biocompatibility* 3:235–317, 1987; plus author's data.

Note: ?: no reliable normal (control) data. ng/ml, p/pb.

With any method, interpretation of metal ion levels must be done cautiously. There is a wide variability according to method, laboratory, and patient.

The established release rates are sufficient, in animals and patients with either stainless steel and cobalt-base components, to produce elevations of metallic content in tissue (at both local and remote sites) and of metal-bearing ion concentrations in serum and urine. In TJR patients, large elevations of chromium and cobalt concentration levels in serum occur in the early postoperative period, significant elevations may persist for more than a decade, and accumulations of 10 to 100 times normal of chromium and nickel in tissues remote from the implanted hip are possible. It has been reported that elevated ion levels will decrease over time. Typically, measured elevated levels are still within limits imposed on employees in industrial settings exposed to pertinent chemicals. Levels measured clinically are also reported to be lower than those that are shown to cause toxicity *in vitro*. After revision of large-diameter MOM implants, metal ions have been reported to decrease to near-normal levels within 1 year. Long-term animal studies with titanium base alloy implants suggest significant release of both titanium and aluminum and concentration in remote tissues, including the lung. Of particular interest is the apparent failure of these animals (baboons) to excrete more serum aluminum, secondary to a presumed protein-binding process. Vanadium release from the Ti6A14V alloy is a concern because of its potential high *in vitro* cytotoxicity, but longitudinal concentration patterns have not yet been studied.

Role of metals in biologic activity

It is reasonable that there be an emphasis on the examination of metal release and distribution in the consideration of systemic and remote site effects. Metals play a central role in metabolic and catabolic activity, with metals involved to some degree in all enzymatic processes. For this reason, when metals are metabolically active, they are seen to have an effect far out of proportion to their prevalence. Two examples of this "multiplier" effect have been given by Mertz (1981) and are shown in Figure 14.3.

Immune response

"Metal allergy" is a well-recognized, everyday phenomenon frequently associated in women with the use of cheap, high-nickel alloy costume jewelry or earrings. Metal ions, by themselves, lack the structure and complexity required to challenge the immune system. However, when combined with proteins, such as those available in the skin, connective tissues, and blood, a wide variety of metals produce immune responses and thus must be considered haptens. Cobalt, chromium, and nickel are included in this category, with nickel perhaps the most potent. Aluminum, titanium, molybdenum, and manganese are not believed to be haptens, whereas the immune role played by vanadium remains unclear.

As a rule of thumb, it may be considered that at least 10% of a normal population will be sensitive by epicutaneous (skin) test to one or more of these metals, at some threshold level. Nickel sensitivity is probably the

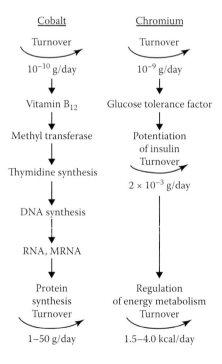

FIGURE 14.3 Magnification of effect of trace metals. (Adapted from Mertz, W., *Science* 213:1332–1338, 1981.)

most common, and metal sensitivity is three to four times more common in women than in men, perhaps reflecting cultural practices, especially ear piercing. Industrial exposure is often correlated with sensitivity to metals; workers in tanning, heavy-metal finishing, printing, and construction industries have a two to five times higher risk of sensitivity to chromium and nickel. Cross-sensitivities, especially between nickel and cobalt, are also recognized. Sensitivity to cobalt without environmental exposure is rare. The results of several studies of sensitivity to metals in normal individuals are summarized in Table 14.4. There is currently some controversy on whether metal hypersensitivity is dose dependent or a threshold phenomenon.

The most typical response of a metal-sensitized individual to a challenge is a type IV delayed hypersensitivity. This is a T-cell-mediated inflammatory response that peaks in 48–72 h after challenge, but that may continue in the presence of a continuing source of hapten–protein complex. It is primarily local, particularly if the antigen complex is tissue bound, involving pain, swelling, and tenderness, but systemic features including remote site eczema, urticaria, pruritus, and bronchospasm have been reported in orthopaedic patients.

Table 14.4   Immune response to metals (epicutaneous testing)

Subject description	% Sensitive to		
	Ni	Co	Cr
THR candidates (212)[a] (6.6%)[b]	5.2	3.3	<1
Normal controls (173) (5.6%)	4.6	3.5	1.1
(Deutman et al. 1977)			
Veterinary students			
Male (233)	0.4	nt	nt
Female (154)	5.4	nt	nt
(Kieffer 1979)			
Healthy adults			
Male (410)	nt	nt	2.0
Female (412)	nt	nt	1.5
(Peltonen et al. 1983)			
Adults presenting at dermatological clinic			
Male (2329) (11.2%)	2.4	4.2	9.8
Female (3087) (9.0%)	6.7	4.8	2.3
(Fregert et al. 1966)			

Sources: Deutman, R. et al., *J Bone Joint Surg* 59A:862–865, 1977. Fregert, S., Rorsman, H., *Acta Dermatol Venereol* 46:144–148, 1966. Kieffer, M., *Contact Dermatitis* 5:398–401, 1979. Peltonen, L., Fraki, J., *Contact Dermatitis* 9:190–194 1983.

Note: nt, Not tested.

[a] Total number of individuals.

[b] Overall percent sensitive.

Concern was first raised about immune response to metals with regard to THR arthroplasty when it was proposed that, by producing local microvascular blockade and bone necrosis, it might play a role in loosening of high-release-rate MOM prostheses. Several studies have supported this view, whereas others show either a modest degree or an absence of association between preoperative sensitization and loosening. However, of greater interest is the finding that postoperative sensitization could occur, owing to the continued release of metal, the formation of hapten complexes, and the possibility, increasing with postoperative (implantation) time, of the patient encountering a sensitizing episode (exposure to various drugs, heat stress, etc.). This has been seen in studies of sensitivity in patients with metal-on-polymer prostheses, but with no apparent association to loosening yet demonstrated. Some clinical series are summarized in Table 14.5. One specific reaction, termed aseptic lymphocyte-dominated vascular associated lesion (ALVAL) has seen continued presentation with, most commonly, MOM THA components, and is described in more detail below.

Table 14.5 Sensitivity to implantation or other exposure (epicutaneous testing)

Subject description	% Sensitive to			
	Ni	Co	Cr	PMMA
THR patients (metal-on-polymer) (42)				
No symptoms (29)	6.9	3.5	nt	21
"Loose" (13)	0	0	nt	100
(Clementi et al. 1980)				
THR patients (metal-on-polymer) (64)				
No symptoms (28)	3.6	0	0	nt
"Loose" (36)	2.3	5.6	13.9	nt
(Grosshoff et al. 1984)				
Schoolgirls (960)				
Pierced ears (687)	13	nt	nt	nt
Unpierced ears (273)	1	nt	nt	nt
(Larsson-Stymie et al. 1985)				
Cobalt-alloy metal workers (853)				
Male (485)	0	1.9	0	nt
Female (368)	2.7	8.2	0.8	nt
(Fischer et al. 1983)				

Sources: Clementi, D. et al., *Ital J Orthop Traumatol* 6:97–104, 1980. Fischer, T., Rystedt, I., *Contact Dermatitis* 9:115–121, 1983. von Grasshoff, H. et al., *Beitr Orthop Tramatol* 31:299–304, 1984. Larsson-Styme, B., Widstrom, L., *Contact Dermatitis* 13:289–293, 1985.

Note: nt, Not tested.

The majority of these studies depend on a simple epicutaneous test for sensitivity. These tests are notorious for lack of sensitivity and, in particular, may produce false negatives if the test subject is already responding to a challenge agent. A more recent study using skin patch testing of patients with well-functioning implants found positive reactions to metal ions at about twice that of the general population (25%). In patients with a failed or poorly functioning implant, this number increases to 60%. This sensitivity still has room for improvement. Using a much more sensitive *in vitro* test of leukocyte chemotactic ability (the leucocyte migration inhibition or LIF test), one study suggests that a high proportion, perhaps as high as 75%, of patients having cobalt-base implants removed may have developed a sensitivity to metal and that as many as 50% of these may show signs of active response, suggesting a continuing challenge above the sensitivity threshold. The results of these studies are shown schematically in Figure 14.4. Although common, skin testing is not considered an accurate preoperative predictor of the potential for metallic implant hypersensitivity and is still not routine part of the patient selection process. There are currently no known definitive tests to confirm metal hypersensitivity, although considerable progress has occurred (Hallab and Jacobs 2009).

A parallel study by Merritt and Brown provided a rare opportunity to examine 32 patients presenting for internal fixation of fractures and then to retest them at removal (both tests were LIF). The results are shown in Figure 14.5. Despite the unusually high level of sensitivity seen preoperatively (59%), the same pattern emerges. Patients who have

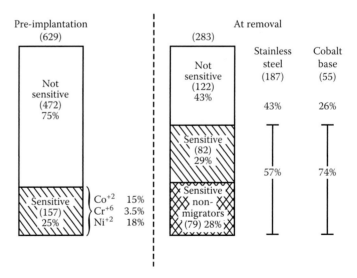

FIGURE 14.4 Preimplantation and postremoval hypersensitivity to metallic implants. (Adapted from Merritt, K., Brown, S.A., Biological effects of corrosion products from metals. In Fraker, A.C., Griffin, C.D. (eds): *Corrosion and Degradation of Implant Materials*. ASTM STP 859. American Society for Testing and Materials, Philadelphia, pp. 195–206, 1985.)

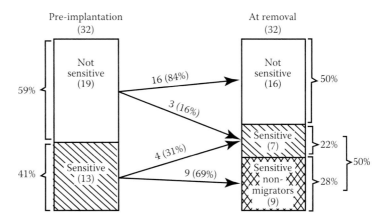

FIGURE 14.5 Development of hypersensitivity during fracture treatment by internal fixation (From K. Merritt, personal communication.)

preoperative metal sensitivity run the risk of activation by implantation, whereas those who are insensitive preoperatively have a real probability (in this case 3 of 19 or 16%) of becoming sensitized.

Delayed hypersensitivity (and rare anaphylactic responses) to methyl methacrylate monomer has been reported, but seems to be an important problem only for persons with repetitive exposure to uncured PMMA, such as dentists and orthopaedic surgeons (Figure 14.5). One study (Clementi et al. 1980; see Table 14.5) suggests a relationship between sensitivity to PMMA and TJR device loosening. Immune responses to other polymers in orthopaedic clinical use have not been reliably reported, although there is growing evidence for such a response to silicones. Immune responses to ceramics are highly unlikely owing to the extremely low solubility of these materials; they have not been reported in an orthopaedic context.

Aseptic lymphocyte-dominated vascular-associated lesion

ALVAL is an inflammatory reaction caused by a delayed hypersensitivity response to metallic wear debris and corrosion products. Metal debris degradation products complex with local proteins and begin an allergic response through the formation of haptens, which initiate an antibody reaction. The reaction is similar to delayed type (Type IV) hypersensitivity response to repeated exposure to, in this case, metallic debris.

Histopathologic descriptions of ALVAL are somewhat nondescript and similar to failed arthroplasty soft tissues generally. ALVAL is characterized by areas of coagulated necrosis, subsurface band-like infiltrate of macrophages and giant cell granulomas, and perivascular aggregates of lymphocytes (predominantly B cell). There will also potentially be synovial inflammation and hyperplasia. Unique and distinguishing features of ALVAL are the presence of dense perivascular inflammatory infiltrate, along with the overall magnitude of chronic inflammation. Although there is little consensus on the differences between ALVAL and metallosis, and patients often show a mixture of different reactions, there is some distinguishing the responses. Metallosis is thought to be a toxic reaction to excessive amount of metal particulate, while ALVAL is a hypersensitive reaction to a normal amount of metal particulate.

The most common radiographic finding associated with ALVAL and one of its flagship symptoms is a cystic mass, located either posterolateral to the joint or anterior to the joint. This mass, termed *pseudotumor*, is an enlarged, fluid-filled soft tissue mass that is neither malignant nor infective. Some common features of pseudotumors include extensive necrosis of the dense connective tissue, sometimes associated with cystic degeneration, macrophage, and lympocytic infiltrate. In some cases, necrosis is so rampant as to prevent histological characterization. Ultrasonography can be utilized to differentiate solid from cystic lesions. Most pseudotumors will contain metal ion particles. Pseudotumors, like other signs of ALVAL and metallosis, are most commonly reported in association with malpositioning of MOM hips, though these reactions have also occurred in patients with no evidence of excessive wear or hypersensitivity and have further occurred in non-MOM hips as well. Consequently, some of these could be possibly related to patient factors. It is expected that there are an appreciable number of unrecognized and asymptomatic pseudotumors.

Campbell et al. (2010) created a 10-point histological scoring system to distinguish ALVAL in patients with pseudotumor-like tissue responses in MOM hip arthroplasty and ranked cases with signs of higher wear as having a lower ALVAL score, as they were also associated with fewer lymphocytes, more macrophages, and more metal particles. While macrophages and lymphocytes present in all cases, there were two distinct groups. Those scoring lower on the ALVAL scale had more infiltrates of macrophages and were associated with smaller lymphocyte aggregates. They also displayed less disruption of the synovial surface and greater preservation of normal tissue architecture. Those with a higher ALVAL score exhibited large, dense lymphocyte aggregates, usually distal to the surface, will fewer macrophages. These patients, with suspected metal sensitivity, also described more pain. While there was focal to moderate necrosis in all tissues, including few intact synovial linings, the most extensive damage to tissues was in the high-score ALVAL group.

ALVAL should be considered in cases of chronic aching pain with evidence of synovitis and in the absence of infection or implant fixation issues. Because of a similarity in histology between ALVAL and that of, for example, rheumatoid arthritis, diagnosis can be difficult. Postoperatively, there is often radiographic evidence showing solid and cystic peri-implant masses. Serology testing may indicate elevated quantities of Co and Cr, though this is not definitive. Ultimately, intraoperative histologic assessment of frozen section of tissue for infection and acute inflammation is necessary. Unfortunately, this is also not definitive. Mechanical causes of failure can cause similar histology, including inflammation, fibrosis, and repair, though loosening will likely have a greater amount of foreign metal and cement debris. Because implant loosening can accelerate the generation of wear particles, it is difficult to know whether hypersensitivity to particles is the cause or the result of the implant loosening.

Current incidence of ALVAL is speculated to be approximately 1% in MOM patients, but is expected to increase over time. Clinical confirmation of ALVAL will necessitate a replacement of the implant. Despite its nonspecific nature, this is a well-recognized cause of MOM joint replacement failure.

Implications of immune response

It should be emphasized that the observation of sensitization and even sensitization with accompanying response to challenge ("nonmigration" in LIF test) does not establish that immune responses to implant materials play an important role in the clinical outcome of device implantation. However, the finding of significantly higher levels of sensitivity in implant populations (than in comparative nonimplant ones) combined with evidence of ongoing increases in sensitivity and isolated case reports of frank immune response to implants raises significant questions. Much research will be required to resolve these issues.

Until then, it seems appropriate to enquire about "metal allergy" during preoperative examination. Additionally, patients who display the stigmata of immune response to metals at the time of device removal or revision (in the case of TJR arthroplasty) should be investigated for evidence of metal sensitivity. The most likely sensitizer is nickel; patients with documented nickel sensitivity with modest to low thresholds should probably not receive implants of nickel-bearing alloys.

Particulate transport

Transport of particulates by macrophages to regional lymph nodes and to the lungs has been previously noted and must be considered a systemic and remote effect, but one that has few if any clinical consequences in modern device designs.

Passive mechanical transport of small, asymmetric metallic objects, such as sewing needles and bullet fragments, is well recognized clinically, and thus small fragments of cerclage wire should be viewed with some caution to determine whether they stay in place or migrate with time. Long-distance transport of such objects to remote vital organs is not unknown. Symmetric particles, such as microspheres released from porous coatings, are unlikely to move far from their site of origin.

Evidence for remote site effects

Transport of corrosion products may lead to systemic effects from leaching of metal ions, including potential effects on metabolic processes, cell mutation, and allergic sensitization, as reported above. The body controls levels of essential metals through ingestion and excretion. Most implant-related metals exist naturally in the body at low levels owing to their role in metabolic processes. At high enough concentrations, essential metals can lead to toxic reactions. Essential metals include iron, cobalt, molybdenum, chromium, manganese, vanadium, and nickel. Those that are nonessential include aluminum, titanium, zirconium, niobium, and tantalum. Any of the essential or nonessential metal ions may bind to proteins and transport to organs via the bloodstream or lymph. There is evidence that ion products from corrosion are circulated and concentrated in erythrocytes. These particles can eventually travel to and accumulate in distant lymph nodes, bone marrow, liver, kidney, and spleen. It has been proposed that there is some potential for DNA damage and genotoxic effects systematically.

In a study of THA revision patients investigating blood and bone marrow, there was a twofold increase in asymmetrical chromosomal aberrations in bone marrow cells near the implants compared to bone marrow in the iliac crest (Brown et al. 2005). Visuri et al. (2006) found an increased incidence of leukemia in MOM hip patients, although there was no observed increase in incidence with other forms of cancer and the authors ended up concluding that metal wear particles were not a concern. Tharani et al. (2001) reviewed all available data and concluded that there was no supported causal link between joint arthroplasty and development of cancer. Ong et al. conducted a matched cohort analysis using the Medicare 100% data set to assess the risk of bladder, kidney, and liver cancer in THA patients with different bearing types (Ong et al. 2013). They observed that the MOM patients had a 30% lower adjusted risk when compared to MOP THA patients, though only 5 years of follow-up was available. Despite this evidence, there is still no long-term systematic study evaluating immunological or carcinogenic reactions to metallic implants, which can have long-term latency.

Stress shielding

In the late 19th century, Wolff reported alterations in the structural properties of bone in response to mechanical stress. Simply put, an increase in load up to a limit will lead to a gain in bone mass, while a decreased load leads to a loss. Any implant in a total joint arthroplasty will alter the magnitude and direction of load transmission through the joint, and accordingly, there are observed changes in bone density surrounding implants. The direction and magnitude of load transferred from the implant to the host bone are thus of paramount importance and the subject of continuing research. Of particular importance is the stiffness mismatch between common implant materials and the host bone. To give some perspective on this mismatch, cobalt chromium and titanium have 100 times and 50 times the stiffness of cancellous bone in the intramedullary canal, respectively. Although the stiffness mismatch is critical, the result is multifactorial as the magnitude of the stress shielding effect is dependent on aging, stress redistribution, implant shape and stiffness, and load-transfer mechanisms.

Most of the understanding of stress shielding in orthopaedics is based around hip arthroplasty. In a standard hip stem, the load applied to the proximal cortical and cancellous bone is reduced and transmitted further distally to the diaphyseal cortex at the end of the stem. Bone will be resorbed to a degree directly related to the magnitude of change in the mechanical load seen by that section of bone. The reduction in load proximally is shown to reduce proximal bone density, which may lead to implant subsidence, while the stress concentration created distally often results in a periprosthetic fracture. Hypertrophy or medullary canal bone stimulation may even occur distally as a result of load transmission through the stem to the canal. The greatest bone loss is in the femoral

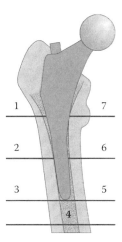

FIGURE 14.6   (See color insert.) Gruen zones for sectionalizing bone resorption in the proximal femur.

metaphysis, proximal to the lesser trochanter, and seems to affect the cortex more severely than the cancellous bone. Bone loss assessed with dual-energy x-ray absorptiometry has been used to estimate the bone loss around porous coated, uncemented stems in the proximal femur to be 7% to 50% primarily in Gruen zones 1 and 7, though this is dependent on cemented versus cementless fixation (Bauer and Schils 1999). (See Figure 14.6 for a graphical description of Gruen zones.) In a study using DEXA comparing cemented and cementless stems, it was shown that bone loss in cemented stems was isolated to the calcar region while loss in the uncemented stem was much more significant (Pandit et al. 2006). Coating in general is often associated with less bone resorption— radiographic investigation has shown that hydroxyapatite (HA)-coated stems have better bone remodeling and implant fixation when compared to porous coated implants. Prevalence of radiographic osteolysis in HA-coated stems has been demonstrated to be 27% lower.

Periprosthetic bone loss seems to stabilize after about 2 years. Some studies on cementless stems have shown an initial postoperative bone loss, followed by a recovery of density somewhere near 2 to 3 years postoperatively, possibly owing to osseointegration of the implant and better resulting load transfer. Reduced physical activity may also play a role in the initial bone loss. Despite it being a significant risk factor, stress shielding is rarely the sole cause of aseptic loosening.

A goal of implant design is to ensure that the quality and integrity of the host bone are sufficient for providing long-term structural support of any implant. Methods undertaken have been to reduce the stiffness of the stem material (e.g., by using Ti instead of CoCr or steel) or to modify the fit and fill of the stem to better conform to bone morphology. Below is a brief discussion on clinical outcomes for four alterations to traditional hip stems: tapered stems, hip resurfacing, isoelastic implants, and short stems. Understanding differences in bone resorption response to implant type has implications for decisions for patients known to have poor bone quality.

Total hip resurfacing

For hip resurfacing, clinical studies have observed that remodeling is focused primarily on narrowing of the femoral neck, possibly exacerbated or driven by necrosis. In some studies, thinning beyond 10% has been observed in select cases. The most frequent reason for early revision in hip resurfacing is neck fracture, possibly the result of the combination of notching owing to suboptimal positioning and a narrowing of the neck. In some resurfacing implants, there is a pronounced stress concentration (up to 5× strain in some cases) on the anterior and posterior head–neck region, which is the known region correlating with clinical fractures (Cristofolini et al. 2009). Remodeling is thought to depend heavily on proper placement of the prosthesis—*in vitro* studies have reported lower stress shielding if the implant is appropriately placed.

Computational models predict initial stress shielding/bone resorption directly beneath the prosthetic head, along with density increases near the distal stem section (Ong et al. 2008). The bone resorption region extends distally and peripherally toward the middle of the neck, likely the driver for clinically observed neck narrowing from a mechanistic standpoint. Similar to remodeling in other devices, resorption stabilizes at about 3 years, though these patients are still considered at potentially higher risk for loosening complications in the long term, along with a continued risk for femoral neck fracture.

Isoelastic implants

Isoelastic implants are intended to match the stiffness of the femur in an effort to reduce stress shielding and bone resorption around the implant. Isoelastic implants may include any of the following: a composite of a metallic core coated with a polymer or porous polymer, a laminated metal core, or a carbon fiber–reinforced polymer with or without a metal core. Historically, there have been numerous setbacks in bringing isoelastic THA prostheses to the market. Higher debris production and poor primary fixation are believed to be the main reason for the high failure rates in early generations.

Studies on bone remodeling in isoelastic stems support the conclusion that reducing stiffness mismatch can reduce bone resorption around the implant. Nagi et al. (2006) used DEXA to evaluate periprosthetic bone remodeling in 92 patients implanted with isoelastic stems and found a change in BMD averaging 15% for all Gruen zones. They concluded that the isoleastic prostheses preserved bone better than cemented or uncemented metallic implants. In a randomized control trial comparing the three-part macrocomposite Epoch stem (including a layer of polyaryletherketone resin) to an HA tricalcium phosphate–coated Ti stem of a similar geometry, Karrholm et al. (2002) confirmed the isoelastic Epoch stem to have lost as little as half the bone mineral in four Gruen regions. A study of the Bradley stem, which has a proximal HA coating, a tapered metallic core, and a CFR-PEEK outer layer, has also shown increased bone mineral density medially (Kurtz et al. 2012).

Tapered stems

Tapered stems aim to transfer loads to the metaphysis and prevent proximal femoral stress shielding. A study of tapered cementless stems by Pandit et al. (2006) using quantitative computed tomography to map bone density found bone resorption from 17% to 28% in the cancellous bone and 5% to 8% in the cortical bone. At 3 years after surgery, Schmidt et al. (2004) found, using quantitative computed tomography, a decrease in density of 14.3% in the femoral metaphysis along with a 17.3% decrease in cortical bone in 24 patients with a Multicone uncemented tapered stem. The same authors saw a slight decrease in resorption (14.2% and 15.5%, respectively), around the same stem with an HA-coated surface.

Short stems

Neck-conserving, short-stem implants are intended to address issues of proximal–distal mismatch, reduce stress shielding and overload, stimulate increased bone formation around the device, encourage bony ingrowth, and limit periprosthetic fractures. Lerch et al. (2012) analyzed bone mineral density around the Metha short-stem implant in 25 consecutive patients. In comparison to immediate postoperative baseline values, BMD at 2 years decreased in the greater trochanter from 0.78 g/cm^2 to 0.72 g/cm^2. BMD actually increased in the lesser trochanter by 12.9% and increased in the calcar region by 6.1%. Most remodeling occured in the distal calcar and lesser trochanter region (zone 6), along with the proximal calcar (zone 7). The authors concluded that this unique result was the achievement of proximal load transfer with the Metha stem. Briem et al. (2011) retrospectively examined radiographs of 155 patients treated with the CFP (collum femoris preserving) prosthesis and observed a relative loss of bone in the proximal region (osteopenic) with bone formation at the distal stem. There were no signs of significant bone loss or osteolysis. Similar to other stems, maximum bone remodeling typically occurs at 6 months after surgery and levels out after 1 year. Additional adaptation will occur over the next 1 to 2 years. While short stems are bone conserving both from the surgical preservation and stress shielding standpoints, this also implies that there may be less surface area in contact (and hence frictional resistance) between the stem and adjacent bone. Therefore, consideration should be given regarding relative motion of the stems.

Stress shielding in TKA

The focus of stress shielding has been around the proximal femur, but it is also known to occur anywhere in the presence of a stiff, foreign implant, including behind the acetabular component and underneath the metal tray of a tibial TKA component. Much less is known about density response in these regions as bone density is more difficult to assess here radiographically.

Electrical stimulation, growth, and repair

All organisms are electrodynamic systems with large and stable gradients. The relationship between mechanical forces and endogenous currents has been well known since research on piezoelectric forces in bone were published in 1953 by Yazuda, who had an interest in manipulation of electromagnetism in bone. Deformed bone is electronegative relative to its undeformed state, and thus an electric current is produced. The amplitude of the electrical potential is dependent on both the rate and magnitude of bone deformation, whereas polarity is driven by the directionality of deformation. It has been shown that deformed rabbit tibias were capable of generating bioelectric potentials up to 6 mV, while *in vivo* measurement of potentials in the ambulating human has been recorded up to 300 mV. Piezoelectricity is considered to be driven by collagen, and potential is decreased with increasing water content. It is useful to consider that structure and chemical composition of bone will vary by age, gender, region, nutrition, and especially hydration.

Electromechanical properties of bone are the biophysical basis for Wolff's law. Bone formation is driven by upregulation and downregulation of cellular signaling molecules, which can be directed by chemical and electrical cues. Any alteration to mechanical stress and electric signals increases secretion of growth factors, cell proliferation, intercellular calcium, and, resultantly, bone remodeling. This is accomplished through affecting the cell membrane. In their natural state, osteoblasts are asymmetric, secreting extracellular matrix only on one side of the cell. During electric stimulation, there is a high voltage drop across the cellular membrane and enzymatic activity is increased on the electrode side, encouraging galvanotaxis, or cellular movement. The change in cellular homeostasis also encourages the free movement of calcium ions through the cell membrane. Increased calcium levels regulate hormones that inhibit signals that prevent the formation of new bone. Meanwhile, mesenchymal cells translate to the cathode via galvanotaxis, before deriving into osteoblasts. Electrical stimulation is also thought to have an angiogenic effect, stimulating tissue healing by affecting vascular growth.

Although the use of electrical stimulation for bone growth therapy is recorded back into the middle of the 19th century, its efficacy was considered controversial well into the 20th century, and there still remains some controversy today. Two areas of interest in orthopaedics include using electrical stimulation as an adjuvant therapy to stimulate bone regeneration during fracture healing and early bone ingrowth and anchorage of arthroplasty components. It has also found some use in spinal fusion treatment. Even moderate success with each of these applications could provide a great benefit to treatment. For example, between 5% and 10% of long bone fractures result in delayed or nonunion, while THA patients may lose up to 14% of their bone mass in the first 3 months after a THA.

The most prominent mechanisms for electric stimulation include pulsed electromagnetic fields (PEMFs), direct current applied either percutaneously or via an implantable device, or a capacitive coupled electric field through conductive plates attached through the skin. All methods use low-level electric currents and are indicated for treatment of fracture nonunion and spinal fusion.

Inductive coupling: pulsed electromagnetic fields

PEMFs use magnetic coils to convert electric current into a series of pulses transmitted through the affected region to induce electric signals. A rapid sequence of pulses results in a magnetic flux density anywhere between 0.1 to 18 G (Gauss: unit of electromagnetic flux to create a low level magnetic field, typically below 1 kHz on the frequency spectrum). *In vitro* studies suggest that PEMFs encourage mineralization and angiogenesis, increase DNA synthesis, accelerate apoptosis of osteoclasts, and alter the cellular calcium content in osteoblasts and their eventual proliferation and differentiation. Calcium ion activity in osteoblasts is known to be driven by the frequency and duration of pulse waveforms.

PEMF has been applied to stimulate osteogenesis in patients with nonunion of bone fractures, foot and ankle arthrodesis, and spinal fusion, all with limited success. It has also found some success in encouraging callus formation and maturation in bone distraction procedures and for the treatment of osteonecrosis of the femoral head. It is important to get a daily dosage for successful treatment, and compliance can be a challenge. More information is necessary in order to optimize the magnetic intensity and dosage. Clinical success in treating fracture nonunion has been reported from 64% to 87%.

PEMF has been less well studied in orthopaedic applications. Similar to other modalities, PEMF studies have shown inconsistent results owing to varied treatments (pulse frequency, duration, size), but at least one study has shown an effect of PEMF in reducing osteolysis after THA. It has been suggested that PEMF is effective in treating patients with aseptic loosening of THA, but not necessarily in severe cases.

Capacitive coupling

Capacitive coupling utilizes two surface electrodes applied on the skin across a region of interest, for example, a fracture site. A battery is used to generate a 60 kHz sinusoidal wave signal that creates an internal field of 0.1 to 20 mV/cm, with a current density in the region of 300 $\mu A/cm^2$. Outside of the application mechanism, there are many similarities between capacitive coupling and inductive coupling treatments, such as PEMF. Like PEMF, capacitive coupling is noninvasive, but there are issues with patient compliance. Also, it is thought that the molecular mechanisms and the pathways by which bone responds to electric stimulus are similar for the two methods. Reported clinical success in healing delayed and nonunion fractures is reported from 70% to 77% for capacitive coupling use.

Direct electrical stimulation

Direct electrical stimulation, approved by the FDA in 1979 for the treatment of established nonunions, utilizes an implanted cathode near the area of interest with a battery-based anode located subcutaneously to administer a constant current to the affected region. Current is often in the range of 20 μA. This method is thought to affect healing differently from capacitive or inductive coupling because of the simulative effect of electrochemical reactions at the electrode sites. Localized pH is altered at the electrode sites owing to reduction oxidation reactions that generate hydrogen and hydroxide ions. The environment near the cathode becomes slightly alkaline, which has been shown to be favorable for bone growth. Oxygen tension in the vicinity is also lowered, which is thought to stimulate mesenchymal stem cells and encourage osteoinduction.

Clinically, there are challenges with using direct stimulation. Electrode implantation and removal has device and infection risks associated with the transcutaneous leads, such as device failure and infection risks. There is often the formation of a fibrous capsule at the electrodes, which can progress to encapsulation under chronic stimulation treatment, potentially leading to increased electric resistance and resulting in reduced power and efficiency. Heat and pain at the treatment sight could be unbearable for some patients, while infection at electrodes has also been reported. Despite the risks, patient compliance is naturally improved with this method. Success rates treating fracture nonunion are between 63% and 86%.

Continuing challenges with electric stimulation

Reported clinical results for any of the above methods are considered controversial owing to lack of homogeneity in trial design and dosage. Resulting from inconsistent information, it is thought by some researchers that treatments have been incorrectly focused on electric current, as opposed to current density. Early literature in the 1970s concluded that a range of 5 to 20 μA was an appropriate current dosage, where any pulse above 20 μA would cause necrosis. Over the next decade, other important factors were proposed to govern efficacy and safety, including the spatial positioning of the electrodes, the current density, and the electric field. Current density can affect the local pH, and substantial changes can lead to degradation of the host bone owing to excessive heating and blood vessel damage. Above a certain threshold, hydroxide ions generated by electrochemical reactions cannot be buffered appropriately. Currently, it is thought that densities above $1–2$ mA/cm^2 can cause tissue degeneration as a result of excessive heating, while blood vessel damage will occur at densities above 5 mA/cm^2. As a result findings showing the effect of current density, electrode placement is now considered an important variable to monitor and control during treatment. Outside of treatment metrics, injury specifics also confound our understanding of treatment effects. For example, there can be extensive variability in fracture healing results owing to extent of trauma, including the effect of the fracture gap size. Despite this, researchers are continuing to collect important information that may help improve the efficacy of stimulation therapy. One critical recommendation is that fracture gap size should not exceed half of the diameter of the healing bone. For orthopaedic applications, conductivity decreases with increasing implant porosity, putting the original intention of porosity somewhat at odds with electrical stimulation therapy. With this understanding, treating a porous stem in the same manner as treating a grit blasted stem is not appropriate.

Some of the difficulties in understanding treatments stem from difficulties in characterizing the dielectric constants and conductivity of tissue in a dynamic *in vivo* environment, which are highly dependent on ion concentrations, temperature, hydration, and fiber orientation. Thus, we are incapable of accurately measuring field strengths and understanding interactions in terms of biophysical principles. Finite element modeling is one avenue being investigated to better understand these interactions and the resulting current density *in vivo*.

Conclusion and summary

Modern biomaterials produce a very low level of acute local or systemic host response in patients. However, mechanisms are known for a variety of immunologic responses, including neoplastic transformation. Increasing periods of implantation, secondary to earlier surgical intervention, and increased surface areas of implants, as required for fixation by biologic ingrowth, may be placing patients at relatively increasing risk. It is to be hoped that as orthopaedic researchers and clinicians become more sensitive to the biologic response implications of the biomaterials that they use. "Whole patient" analyses, as well as reliable longer-term follow-up studies, will clarify the situation and provide upper bounds on the prevalence of such effects.

References

BAUER TW, SCHILS J: The pathology of total joint arthroplasty—Mechanisms of implant failure. *Skeletal Radiol* 28:483–497, 1999.

BAUER TW, MANLEY MT, STERN LS ET AL: Osteosarcoma at the site of total hip replacement. *Trans Soc Biomater* 10:36, 1987.

BRIEM D, SCHNEIDER M, BOGNER N, BOTHA N, GEBAUER M, GEHRKE T, SCHWANTES B: Mid-term results of 155 patients treated with a collum femoris preserving (CFP) short stem prosthesis. *Int Orthop* 35:655–660, 2011.

BROWN C, FISHER J, INGHAM E: Biological effects of clinically relevant wear particles from metal-on-metal hip prostheses. *Proc IMechE Part H: J Eng Med* 220:355–369, 2005.

CRISTOFOLINI L, JUSZCZYK M, TADDEI F, FIELD RE, RUSHTON N, VICECONTI M: Stress shielding and stress concentration of contemporary epiphyseal hip prostheses. *Proc IMechE Part H: J Eng Med* 223:27–44, 2009.

HALLAB NJ, JACOBS, JJ. *Bull NYU Hosp Jt Dis* 67(2):182–188, 2009.

KARRHOLM J, ANDERBERG C, SNORRASON F, THANNER J, LANGELAND N, MALCHAU H ET AL: Evaluation of a femoral stem with reduced stiffness. A randomized study with use of radiostereometry and bone densitometry. *J Bone Joint Surg* 84-A:1651–1658, 2002.

KURTZ S, DAY J, ONG K. Isoelastic polyaryletheretherketone implants for total joint replacement. In *PEEK Biomaterials Handbook*, pp. 221–242. Elsevier, Boston, 2012.

LERCH M, VON DER HAAR-TRAN A, WINDHAGEN H, BEHRENS BA, WEFSTAEDT P, STUKENBORG-COLSMAN CM: Bone remodeling around the Metha short stem in total hip arthroplasty: A prospective dual-energy X-ray absorptiometry study. *Int Ortho* 36:533–538, 2012.

MERRITT K, BROWN SA: Hypersensitivity to metallic biomaterials. In Williams DF (ed.): *Systemic Aspects of Biocampatability.* Vol. 2, 1981.

MERTZ W: The essential trace elements. *Science* 213:1332–1338, 1981.

NAGI ON, KUMAR S, AGGARWAL S: The uncemented isoelastic/isotitan total hip arthroplasty. A 10–15 years follow-up with bone mineral density evaluation. *Acta Orthop Belg* 72:55–64, 2006.

ONG K, LAU E, KURTZ S: Risk of complications, revision, and cancer for metal-on-metal patients in the Medicare population. Metal-on-Metal Total Hip Replacement Devices on May 8, 2012 in Phoenix, AZ; STP 1560, Steven M. Kurtz, A. Seth Greenwald, William H. Mihalko, and Jack E. Lemons, Guest Editors, pp. 1–17, doi:10.1520/STP20120029, ASTM International, West Conshohocken, PA 2012.

ONG K, MANLEY M, KURTZ SM: Have contemporary hip resurfacing designs reached maturity? A review. *J Bone Joint Surg Am* 90:81–88, 2008.

PANDIT S, GRAYDON A, BRADLEY L, WALKER C, PITTO R: Computed tomography assisted osteodensitometry in total hip arthroplasty. *ANZ J Surg* 76:778–781, 2006.

SCHMIDT R, NOWAK TE, MUELLER L, PITTO R: Osteodensitometry after total hip replacement with uncemented taper-design stem. *Int Ortho* 28:74–77, 2004.

THARANI R, DOREY FJ, SCHMALZRIED TP: The risk of cancer following total hip or knee arthroplasty. *J Bone Joint Surg* 83-A:774–780, 2001.

VISURI T, PULKKINEN P, PAAVOLAINEN P: Malignant tumors at the site of total hip prosthesis: Analytic review of 46 cases. *J Arthroplasty* 21:311–323, 2006.

VISURI T, PULKKINEN P, PAAVOLAINEN P: Malignant tumors at the site of total hip prosthesis. Analytic review of 46 cases. *J Arthtroplasty* 21(3):311–323, 2006.

WEBER PC: Epithelioid sarcoma in association with total knee replacement. A case report. *J Bone Joint Surg* 68B:824–825, 1986.

Annotated bibliography

1. BRAND KG: Solid state tumorigenesis. In Becker FF (ed): *Cancer: A Comprehensive Treatise*. Vol. 1. Plenum, New York, 1975.

    Discussion of foreign body–mediated neoplastic transformation by a principal researcher.

2. BROWN C, FISHER J, INGHAM E: Biological effects of clinically relevant wear particles from metal-on-metal hip prostheses. *Proc IMechE Vol. 220 Part H: J Eng Med* 355–369, 2006.

    Detailed discussion on the effect of CoCr particles on the host system.

3. CAMPBELL P, EBRAMZADEH E, NELSON S, TAKAMURA K, DE SMET K, AMSTUTZ HC: Histological features of pseudotumor-like tissues from metal-on-metal hips. *Clin Orthop Relat Res* 468:2321–2327, 2010.

    The histology and clinical presentation of pseudotumors.

4. COBB AG, SCHMALZREID TP: The clinical significance of metal ion release from cobalt–chromium metal-on-metal hip joint arthroplasty. *Proc IMechE Vol. 220 Part H: J Eng Med* 385–398, 2006.

    Discussion of measurement of ion levels, toxicology of chromium particles.

5. FISHER AA: Contact dermatitis due to metals and their salts. In Fisher AA (ed): *Contact Dermatitis*. Lea & Febiger, Philadelphia, 1967.

    The standard reference on "metal allergy," based on patch testing.

6. GRIFFIN XL, WARNER F, COSTA M: The role of electromagnetic stimulation in the management of established non-union of long bone fractures: What is the evidence? *Injury Int J Care Injured* 39:419–429, 2008.

    A comprehensive review on clinical results after electrical stimulation of long bone nonunion.

7. GRISTINA AG, COSTERTON JW: Bacterial adherence to biomaterials and tissue. The significance of its role in clinical sepsis. *J Bone Joint Surg* 67A:264–273, 1985.

    The title tells it all.

8. HOSMAN AH, VAN DER MEI HC, BULSTRA SK, BUSSCHER HJ, NEUT D: Effects of metal-on-metal wear on the host immune system and infection of hip arthroplasty. *Acta Orthopaedica* 81:526–534, 2010.

    Review and discussion on the systemic effects of MOM debris.

9. IYENGAR GV, KOLLMER WE, BOWEN HJM: *The Elemental Composition of Human Tissues and Body Fluids.* Verlag-Chemie, New York, 1978.

A historical source.

10. ISAACSON BM, BLOEBAUM RD: Bone bioelectricity: What have we learned in the past 160 years? *J Biomed Mater Res* 95A:1270–1279, 2010.

Discussion of bone piezoelectricity, cellular response to electrical stimulation, and clinical results of electrical stimulation for fracture healing.

11. KOSSOVSKY N, HEGGERS JP, ROBSON MC: The bioreactivity of silicone. *CRC Crit Rev Biocompat* 3(1):53–85, 1987.

Even supposedly inert silicones produce biologic responses including delayed hypersensitivity.

12. LUCKEY TD, VENUGOPAL B: *Metal Toxicity in Mammals.* Plenum, New York, 1977.

Compilation of physiological function and toxicity of metals and their compounds.

13. MERRITT K, BROWN SA: Hypersensitivity to metallic biomaterials. In Williams DF (ed): *Systemic Aspects of Biocompatibility.* Vol. II. CRC Press, Boca Raton, FL, 1981.

Review of field, with reference to clinical results. Includes critique of Fisher's chapter on metal dermatitis (see above).

14. NELSON FRT, BRIGHTON CT, RYABY J, SIMON BJ, NIELSON JH, LORICH DG, BOLANDER M, SEELIG J: Use of physical forces in bone healing. *J Am Acad Orthop Surg* 11:344–354, 2003. *J Arthroplasty* 21:311–323, 2006.

Discussion of practical applications and clinical results for differing methods of electrical stimulation.

15. PANDIT S, GRAYDON A, BRADLEY L, WALKER C, PITTO R: Computed tomography assisted osteodensitometry in total hip arthroplasty. *ANZ J Surg* 76:778–781.

16. SALVATI EA, SMALL RD, BRAUSE BD, PELLICCI PM: Infections associated with orthopaedic devices. In Sugarman B, Young EJ (eds): *Infections Associated with Prosthetic Devices.* CRC Press, Boca Raton, FL, 1984.

Brief review of etiology and treatment of implant site infections.

17. SCHMIDT R, NOWAK TE, MUELLER L, PITTO R: Osteodensitometry after total hip replacement with uncemented taper-design stem. *Int Ortho* 28:74–77, 2004.

18. THARANI R, DOREY FJ, SCHMALZRIED TP: The risk of cancer following total hip or knee arthroplasty. *J Bone Joint Surg* 83-A:774–780.

19. WATERS TS, CARDONA DM, MENON KS, VINSON EN, BOLOGNESI MP, DODD LG: Aseptic lymphocyte-dominated vasculitis-associated lesion: A clinicopathologic review of an unrecognized cause of prosthetic failure. *Am J Clin Pathol* 134:886–893, 2010.

Case studies with histopathologic descriptions of ALVAL.

20. WILLIAMS DF (ed): *Biocompatibility of Orthopaedic Implants.* Vol. I and II. CRC Press, Boca Raton, FL, 1982.

Part of a large series of works on "biocompatibility" edited by DF Williams, these volumes provide information on biologic performance of manmade biomaterials in orthopaedic applications.

CHAPTER FIFTEEN

Testing and introduction of new materials

The selection of materials for incorporation into medical and surgical devices and implants is not an arbitrary process. The role of the properties of materials in dictating which designs will work and which will fail is critical. How did the materials in use today come to be?

As a general rule, they represent the survivors of a trial-and-error process of the application of existing materials in engineering use to the solution of medical problems. The most common engineering fields have been aviation and marine engineering, since the high demands of these applications have led to the production of strong, highly corrosion-resistant materials. In some cases, specific materials have been selected for particular properties, as in the initial, unsuccessful use of "slippery" polytetrafluoroethylene as an acetabular cup material in Charnley's low-friction arthroplasty.

The vast majority of materials in use in orthopaedic devices now have clinical histories exceeding 10 and, in some cases, 35–50 years, in at least one application. They have proven satisfactory in many applications, but new concerns and design concepts are acting to call forth new materials. However, there are few "candidate" materials remaining for adaptation; thus, these new materials must be designed rather than converted to new uses. Furthermore, the medical–legal environment has changed radically from that present in the 1960s when orthopaedic implantology began to stride forward.

Therefore, this chapter will review the design process, as it applies to prosthetic materials, and lay out the course that a new material must take from concept to routine clinical use. It may be expected that the full process will require up to a decade, particularly for novel materials. This seems like a long period but, depending on the material, may be too short to answer some concerns raised by new materials.

Design process

What is it?

In the simplest form, engineering design is what engineers do. Despite the use of mathematical tools, testing apparatus, and the other technical accouterments of engineering, it is at its heart a creative process, no different from painting a picture or composing a modern dance. It differs from these processes only in its goals and in the perception that these goals may be set prospectively and their attainment measured retrospectively.

Although the creative aspects of design are critical, the word *process* is used with great emphasis. There is a tremendous need in design to define a process that will be followed to complete a task and then to rely on it, step by step, in achieving one's aim. The artistic ideal, embodied in Mozart's alleged remark that he "did not compose music but simply wrote it down," is a romantic illusion. Design is a difficult, painstaking process of drawing inspiration from initial objectives and husbanding creative ideas as they are reduced to practice and confirmed in operation.

Design cycle

A structured design process consists of the consecutive execution of a repetitive design cycle. The design of a simple device, such as a tongue depressor, may be achieved in as little as three or four such cycles, whereas a complex design, such as a powered hospital bed, may require many more such cycles, some in parallel and others in series.

Materials, by their nature, are simpler in design aspects and tend more to be designed in a single cycle. A cycle, with general applicability, that may be used for design of materials has seven steps:

1. Define objectives
2. Set goals
3. Set specifications
4. Develop concepts
5. Select an approach
6. Complete the design
7. Test the design

Figure 15.1 shows how these steps fit together. The concept of consecutive use of such a cycle is clear if the objectives are thought to come from issues raised by the result of a previous cycle and the output is used to start another cycle. Thus, a materials design cycle may arise from a previous device design that was unsuccessful owing to the lack of appropriate materials and may lead to a further cycle whose objectives might be to improve some property of the designed material, to reduce its cost, and so on.

Step 1: Define objectives   A design cycle, like a journey, cannot begin unless there is some reason for its existence. Thus, at the beginning, an objective or objectives must be selected. The process of stating these in

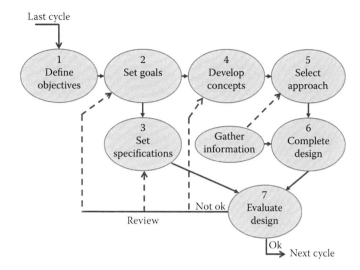

FIGURE 15.1 **(See color insert.)** The design cycle.

writing is an important step, as it focuses the attention of the designer or design team on the design process.

Let us suppose that a materials design cycle is to be undertaken at the request of an engineering design group that is working on a novel total hip replacement (THR) prosthesis. The group reports that none of the materials in their handbooks provide the appropriate combination of stiffness, strength, and fatigue life that they require.

Thus, the design objective may be stated as

> The objective is the design of a new material suitable for use in fabrication of THR prostheses that combines optimum stiffness (modulus) with greater strength and a higher endurance limit than those presently available.

Step 2: Define goals Design is not a simple process that leads to a unique output. Thus, objectives must be refined to limit the number of choices at each step and to guide the design cycle. This is achieved by selecting goals whose attainment either (1) is necessary to attain the desired objective or (2) represents generally recognized "good" attributes of engineering design. The first type is called *specific* goals, while the second is called *general* goals. An initial list of specific and general goals that might follow from the previously stated objective is given in Table 15.1.*

The initial list of objectives arises from a discussion with the "customer," in this case the device design group, and represents the true starting point of the design cycle. It embodies the customer's concept

---

* These are sometimes referred to as "must have" and "should have," respectively. The design process often turns up a third category: "like to have." If all of the first two types can be met, then this latter type is a bonus!

Table 15.1   Hypothetical design goals: new THR material

Initial

Specific

    Modulus <0.5 times Ti6AI4V

    Strength as high as possible

    Endurance limit as high as possible

    Corrosion/release rate "low"

    No wear against ultrahigh-molecular-weight polyethylene (UHMWPE)

    Color: yellow

General

    Minimum cost

    No limit on source of supply

    Simplicity in fabrication

Refined[a]

Specific

    Modulus <0.5 times Ti6AI4V (H)

    Strength as high as possible (M)

    Endurance limit as high as possible (H)

    Corrosion/release rate as low as possible (H)

    Wear rate (against UHMWPE) lower than current rates (M)

    Color: yellow (L)

General

    Minimum cost per kilogram (L)

    No limit on source of supply (M)

    Simplicity in fabrication (M)

[a] Priorities: H, high; M, medium; L, low.

of what is wanted as an end product of the design process. The material's design team must now put its talents to work to understand these desires and to satisfy them. Some of these initial objectives may come from other sources: the engineering manager is always worried about the manufacturing costs of the designs that the group produces; the color was suggested by the sales manager since yellow is widely used in the company's packaging and has come to be identified with it.

The material's design team must go through two substeps to produce the refined set of goals, also shown in Table 15.1. The first is the initial creative act in the design cycle. The question is posed: "What should an improved material for a THR prosthesis look like?"

Creation of ideas is not an easy process for engineers. There is a tendency to "freeze," to be unable to produce ideas, or to have an initial thought and then to proceed to develop it. The general solution for the individual designer is to produce a situation that is both stimulatory and non-self-critical. (Because of the need for continuing review and creative stimulation, design is generally best played as a team sport. However, from here on, they will be referred to as a single individual for simplicity's sake. All of the comments here apply equally to design teams; however, the use of a team introduces additional interpersonal dynamics problems that are beyond the scope of this chapter.) In this case, the designer may decide, "I'm going to set the problem aside, go for a 2-kilometer run, and when I come in, write down the first 10 things that come into my head." Such a procedure, with variants, has been adopted by most creative persons and is sometimes referred to as "creative avoidance" of the problem: undertaking other activities to distract the conscious mind and then using the products of subconscious deliberation, without self-criticism or censoring.

The initial list is then reviewed for reasonableness and duplication and perhaps the process is repeated or extended, until there is a sense that all of the immediately possible options, in this case, design goals, have been acquired. Often the review of an initial list "triggers" new ideas not previously considered. The designer, in our example, has added two specific goals and no general goals to those that might be inferred from the general design objective and the other previously cited desires. Note that this is an abbreviated example; step 2 of an actual design cycle might produce dozens of specific and general goals.

The second substep is assigning a priority to each of the goals, to produce a set of refined goals. This is necessary since, in an actual design case, the number of goals very rapidly grows to the point where it is obvious, a priori, that all cannot be met. Thus, a ranking of importance is necessary. In this case, the designer employed a common practice and selected three priorities:

High (H): must be met for successful design

Medium (M): would like to meet during design cycle

Low (L): desirable to meet but may be sacrificed

Therefore, the material's modulus is identified as a much more important attribute than its color, although the desire to satisfy the sales manager is still considered as part of the later steps in the cycle. In a more subtle distinction, it is recognized that in the intended application, the endurance limit is a more important material attribute than the tensile strength, although both are important. Additionally, some goals may be restated for clarity.

Step 3: Set specifications   Setting specific and general goals and then refining the list produces considerable clarification of the problem in hand but does not provide the details necessary for later steps in the design cycle. To achieve this, it is necessary to translate the refined goals of step 2 into measurable quantities.

As an example, the specific goal "modulus less than half that of Ti6A14V" may be translated to a specification "modulus less than 50 GPa." The general goal "minimum cost" might be translated to "cost of less than $10 per kilogram."

In some cases, when the goals are specific, such as "The modulus must equal that of live cortical bone," there is also a need to apply a margin of error or variability to the specification. It is typical to select two types of margin: narrow for features critical to safety and efficacy and wider for those that are not.

Setting specifications produces the first significant constraint to the design process and thus the completion of step 3 is a good place for a formal review of the progress to date. This may be held with the "customers"; in this case, the device design team, the engineering manager, and the sales manager. In any case, the acts of reviewing and presenting the process and its results at this point are important to the material's designer and may produce new insights and revisions of previous ideas. Early feedback from a multidisciplinary team in reviewing the specifications can help avoid delays down the road. If specifications are set by the engineering team, but say without input from the sales team who may have on-the-ground feedback from the users, a device may be developed that does not meet the users' needs.

Step 4: Develop concepts   Development of design concepts is the heart of the design process and the point at which most fatal mistakes are made. It requires, again, a suspension of self-criticism and a source of external stimulation. For most people, design concepts evolve more readily in a group situation in which one person's ideas trigger another person's imagination. Nevertheless, the goal is the same as that in the first substep of step 2: developing as many essentially independent approaches to the problem at hand as is possible.

As an introduction to this step, the material's designer begins to gather supporting information on past and present materials used for THR prosthesis components as well as current progress in materials' design, and processing is started. Information acquired at this time serves the subconscious as a source of ideas. In addition, such information is needed for the next steps of the design process.

Table 15.2 presents a list of ideas that might arise from such a step 4 exercise. The initial list was developed in two creative sessions; the final list was developed some days later after review of the initial list.

In this hypothetical case, the "blue sky" idea sessions produced an initial list of 18 concepts (left-hand column), which could be grouped, with some ideas eliminated, into four concepts (right-hand column). Three focus on fabrication processes and might require full design cycles themselves, whereas the fourth, a new titanium-base alloy, is more restrictive and could be addressed by simple continuation of this cycle.

Step 5: Select approach   At this point, a very limited design development of as many final concepts as possible (all if time and resources allow) is performed to begin step 5. The goal is to provide just enough information to allow an estimate to be made of which one or two approaches seem best able to meet the ranked goals developed in step 2. It is also possible at this point to combine approaches that have aspects in common. This preliminary evaluation may result in the conclusion that a particular approach is unworkable or unable to meet a high priority (H) goal, and it may be abandoned. It is the general experience that one or at

Table 15.2 Hypothetical design concepts: new THR material

Initial list	Final list
Tusk	Modified natural material
Modified wood	Fiber-reinforced composite
Cloned tree with new properties	Powder composite
Petrified wood	Modified titanium alloy
Coral	
Metal impregnated coral	
Woven ceramic fiber/resin impregnated	
Carbon fiber/graphite	
Carbon/silicon carbide powder composite	
Carbon/polyethylene powder composite	
Hydroxyapatite/polyethylene powder composite	
Metal fiber–reinforced silicone nitride	
Alumina/polymer composite	
Woven sapphire fiber/metal impregnated	
Sapphire beads with spring connectors	
Whisker-reinforced polymer	
New titanium alloy	
Titanium/polymer power composite	

the most two approaches are seen to be clearly better than the rest. When this selection is made, the process moves on to step 6.

Step 6: Complete design   Completing the design of the approaches selected in step 5 is the final pure design step of the design cycle. Not much needs to be said in that it involves traditional engineering processes of analysis, calculation, and simulation and may even require some pilot experiments to verify design and manufacturing concepts. Parametric studies, in which the effects of varying controllable independent variables are tested, are of great value in later considerations.

When alternative approaches were selected (step 5), design completion usually results either in their being ranked in a pragmatic order of preference or in the elimination of one or more owing to inability to realize a complete design.

Step 7: Evaluate design   Design evaluation is a simple process of comparing the attributes of the final design to the specified values developed in step 3 and determining how well they are met. If no design conferences have been held since the one at the end of step 3, now is the ideal time to do so. Ideally, all high and most medium goals should be met, through satisfaction of the dependent specifications, for the design to be said to be acceptable and for it to advance to the next cycle of the overall design process.

If, in the opinion of the reviewers, the design is not acceptable, there are several options. They include reviewing the design concepts to see whether additional ones may be developed, reviewing the specifications to see whether they may be relaxed, and reviewing the goals to see whether they are all necessary and have appropriate priorities. If changes may be made at any of these three steps, then the cycle may be resumed to determine whether a satisfactory design results.

It is not obvious that such a design process will always yield a satisfactory result. Objectives may be unrealistic or even forbidden by basic physical principles or the goal may not be technologically achievable at the time. However, it is clear that in the majority of cases the process does produce satisfactory results with well-articulated foundations and justification. Thus, structured design is to be preferred to inspired guesses in designing biomaterials and medical devices, as in other areas of engineering.

PROBLEM 15.1

Generally speaking, what is the order of steps involved in the design of a material or device?

    A. Set goals

    B. Complete the design

    C. Select an approach

    D. Develop concepts

    E. Define objectives

    F. Test the design

    G. Set specifications

ANSWER:

The order is E, A, G, D, C, B, F. However, the design process is iterative in nature; therefore, it may require multiple cycles, not all of which necessarily involving all steps.

Regulatory requirements

Though the design cycle is described in detail above, what has not been considered is the quality system requirements mandated by the Federal Government of all manufacturers during the medical device design process. In 1997, the Quality System Regulation (QSR; 21 Code of Federal Regulations Part 820) replaced the 1978 Good Manufacturing Practices (GMP) for medical devices. This was to ensure that good quality assurance practices are used during the design process. One of the key elements of QSR is design controls, which make systematic assessment of the design an integral part of the development. This will help increase the likelihood that the design will be transferred to production as a device that is appropriate for its intended use.

Design controls can be applied to any design development process. A classic example is what is known as the "waterfall" model (Figure 15.2), whereby the design proceeds in logical sequences, similar to what has

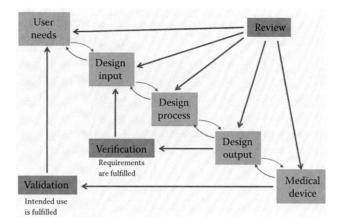

FIGURE 15.2 **(See color insert.)** The waterfall model for the design process.

been described above. This process involves the development of requirements and designing a material or device to meet those requirements. After the material or device has been assessed, it is then transferred to manufacturing. This process is iterative because there are feedback loops throughout the process, as well as evaluations by a review team to ensure that each step is performed sufficiently to avoid delays in the process and to limit the chance that a material or device may be developed without meeting its intended use.

Two of the key components of design controls are document control and change control. Document control relates to enumeration of design documents and tracking of their status and revision history. It also includes maintenance of a document index and history of document revisions. Change control involves documenting decisions for design change requests and identification of the possible design matter that the requester believes should be corrected. Any acceptances of changes should be documented, along with any assignment to members of the design team to further evaluate the change request and review the impact of the design change on the design inputs and intended uses.

Since the design cycle is an involved process, involving many design considerations and decisions, it is important to establish and maintain a *design history file*, which is a compilation of records that describe the design history of the finished product. This includes documentation that is necessary to demonstrate that the design was developed in accordance with the design plan and CFR 820 requirements. This tells the story of design development process from beginning to end, in a chronological order, providing a permanent record of the knowledge base. This is especially helpful when key employees leave or if the company reorganizes, and so on. All in all, the design history file contains the documentation necessary to assure that any changes to the device design or manufacturing process do not adversely affect the performance of the device, ultimately leading to an improvement in the device design and process.

Laboratory studies

Safety and efficacy
Once a material has been designed and sample quantities have been fabricated, a process to assure its safety and efficacy in its intended medical device application must be begun. The phrase "safety and efficacy" is an echo of the Medical Device Amendments of 1976 (PL 94-295, 21 USC 301), which amended the Food, Drug, and Cosmetic Act of 1923 to empower the US Food and Drug Administration (FDA) to regulate the production and sale of medical and surgical instruments and devices in the United States.

The meaning of "safety and efficacy" is not clear by statute, but may be understood in a commonsense fashion as follows:

A biomaterial is safe if it exposes a patient to no unreasonable or unexpected risk.

A biomaterial is effective if its use produces significant palliation or alleviation of the patient's condition it is used to treat or if it serves satisfactorily during the medical or surgical procedure in which it is used.

Although these points are obvious, they must be extended by the legal principle of the "reasonable man." That is, in addition to being safe and effective in its intended application, a biomaterial should also be safe and effective when used, not as intended, but in a manner that a mythical "reasonable man" might assume it would be used. Another way of thinking about safety and efficacy is whether the probable benefit to health from the use of the product outweighs the risk from its use.

Classes of devices

In an attempt to simplify regulation, the Amendments separate all medical and surgical devices (including implant materials by implication) into three categories or classes, reflecting both relative risk and intentions for regulation:

Class I, General Controls. Devices for which general controls, that is, other than special controls and premarket approval, are sufficient to assure safety and efficacy. These devices pose minimal potential harm to the user/patient.

Class II, General Controls with Special Controls. Devices for which general controls are insufficient to assure safety and efficacy but for which there is sufficient information for the establishment of a performance standard or special controls to provide such assurance. These special controls may include special labeling requirements, mandatory performance standards, or postmarket surveillance.

Class III, Premarket Approval. Devices for which insufficient information exists to assure that general controls and special controls would provide reasonable assurance of safety and efficacy and that are represented to be either life sustaining, life supporting, or implanted in the body in a manner that present a potential unreasonable risk of illness or injury. Clinical data are typically necessary for such devices.

All devices in commercial (interstate) trade before May 28, 1976, were exempted from the premarket approval provisions of these Amendments. However, as a guide for later regulation, in the late 1970s, the FDA, assisted by advisory panels of doctors and academic professionals, attempted to classify all so-called pre-enactment or pre-amendment devices. Not surprisingly, when final classifications for most orthopaedic devices were issued (Federal Register 52(172): 33686, Sept. 4, 1987), most implantable devices and materials were designated as class III. Although some devices may later be reclassified into class II, it is expected that any device containing a new material will most probably be viewed as a class III product. Thus, the balance of this discussion on the testing and introduction of new materials will consider that they are destined for a premarket approval process.

Equivalent materials

A section of the Amendments, 510(k), permits the FDA to authorize sale of "new" devices if they are essentially equivalent to ones that were in commercial trade before May 28, 1976. Although expert advice is used, this so-called 510(k) process is subjective and a bit paradoxical. Slight reflection would suggest that if a device (or material) is really superior to previous art, then it cannot be essentially equivalent to that same previous art. In practice, a certain amount of pragmatism is applied. Thus, an application seeking to use a new or modified stainless steel alloy in a device previously fabricated with cast stainless steel alloy A 286 might be expected to be successful, whereas one that proposes to alter corrosion behavior of an implant by use of a polyvinyl dip coating might be expected to fail. Nevertheless, the vast majority of 510(k) applications have been approved, suggesting that it is a viable route for modest changes in design, composition, or processing of materials. The FDA's guidance for when to submit a 510(k) is based on when the change or the sum of the incremental changes to a device could significantly affect the safety and effectiveness of the device. These changes can include changes to the labeling, performance specifications, and materials.

Selection of laboratory studies

By laboratory studies is meant the full spectrum of experiments that will be performed before trials in patients are begun. Simple engineering judgment dictates the selection of engineering studies needed to verify the results of the material's design cycle(s), to provide additional needed information for device designers and manufacturing engineers, and, finally, to verify the performance of materials in manufactured devices.

However, selection of appropriate biologic tests is a much more difficult and controversial process. There are no Federal regulations that dictate test selection, but there is an American Society for Testing and Materials (ASTM) consensus standard, F 748 (F 748-06 [2010]: Standard Practice for Selecting Generic Biological Test Methods for Materials and Devices. Volume 13.1, *Annual Book of Standards: Medical Devices.* American Society for Testing and Materials, Philadelphia). This guide considers implant applications in terms of general type of device, the principal tissue to be contacted, and, if implanted, the period of implantation. For chronically implanted devices intended to contact bone and tissue, but not blood, the following tests (listed in Table 15.3) are recommended. The overall philosophy of these recommendations is to establish a reasonable level of confidence concerning the biologic response to a material or device containing that material when it is introduced into clinical trials. A standard used throughout Europe is ISO 10993, which is for evaluating the biocompatibility of a medical device (ISO 10993: Biological evaluation of medical devices. International Organization for Standardization, Switzerland). This includes a series of 20 standards, covering aspects from identification and quantification of degradation products to a variety of biological tests. In 1995, the FDA issued its own version of ISO 10993-1 to provide guidance on biocompatibility testing and evaluations. Once the key categories of biological effects for the biomaterial have been identified, various sources of information can be used to confirm that each effect has been adequately addressed. For example, safety data from previous studies using the same material, data from raw material vendors, and data from prospective studies can all be used.

Table 15.3 Biologic tests suitable for biomaterials for chronic (>30 days) bone and soft tissue contact

Cytotoxicity (cell culture)
Short-term intramuscular implantation (animal)
Carcinogenicity (cell culture)
Long-term implantation (animal)
Systemic injection acute toxicity (animal)
Skin irritation or intracutaneous injection (animal)
Genotoxicity (cell culture)
Pyrogen test (animal)
Sensitization test (animal)
Immune response

Source: See F 748-06: Standard Practice for Selecting Generic Biological Test Methods for Materials and Devices. Volume 13.1, *Annual Book of Standards: Medical Devices.* American Society for Testing and Materials, Philadelphia.

Three typical biological tests are *in vitro*: cytotoxicity, genotoxicity, and carcinogenicity. Cytotoxicity is a well-established comparative test in which the ability (or lack of ability) of the material or extracts from it to impair multiplication or kill fibroblasts from standard cell lines is compared with positive and negative controls. A variety of techniques including agar diffusion and overlay and flask dilution are used. In addition to being used as an early screening test in development of new materials, cytotoxicity testing is routinely used in the medical device industry for quality control of polymeric materials' production. Both the genotoxicity and carcinogenicity tests are less well developed but tend to depend on observations of transformation of sensitive cells, such as Chinese hamster ovary cells or reversion of mutated bacteria, as in the Ames test. In general, a positive finding (response significantly above inert controls) in either test, if reproducible, is a reason for further investigation of the material in question, or at the least considering modifications in its composition or processing.

The next level of testing involves four relatively simple acute *in vivo* procedures: pyrogenicity, systemic acute toxicity, intracutaneous injection, and intramuscular implantation (less than 30 days). There are well-standardized methods for each of these procedures, and the results are comparative, with positive and negative controls.

The final level of testing requires chronic animal implantation. The "benchmark" for such studies is again an ASTM standard, F 981 (F 981-04 [2010]: Standard Practice for Assessment of Compatibility of Biomaterials for Surgical Implants with Respect to Effect of Materials on Muscle and Bone. Volume 13.1, *Annual Book of Standards: Medical Devices*. American Society for Testing and Materials, Philadelphia). This requires implantation in either rat or rabbit species and observation duration for 12, 26, and 52 weeks. Larger animals such as dogs, goats, or sheep may be used instead, as test hosts for bone implants. Negative controls (implant materials with a long history of experimental observation and clinical use) are used. This procedure calls for placing test specimens in either intramuscular or transcortical locations. Analyses include observations of the gross appearance of the tissue surrounding the implants and the corresponding histopathological examinations.

1. It is frequently assumed that the composition and processing of the biomaterial are well controlled by the time of chronic implantation studies and not to examine or characterize the actual test specimens, either preimplantation or postimplantation.

2. The test specimens used, although of standard, defined geometry, are relatively small and do not produce SA/BW (ratio of implant surface area to host body weight) exposures, even without adjustment for the test animals' higher metabolic rates, that patients would encounter with real implants.

3. The test locations are essentially passive ones and thus do not result in exposure of the test animals to wear debris, products of fretting, and so on.

4. Evaluation concentrates on examination of local host response and neglects study of systemic or remote site effects unless gross morbidity or mortality occurs.

5. It does not provide a comprehensive assessment of the systemic toxicity, immune response, carcinogenicity, teratogenicity, or mutagenicity of the material, which is covered by other standards.

6. This only applies to materials that are expected to reside in bone or soft tissue in excess of 30 days and will remain unabsorbed.

It is to be hoped that improved test procedures will come into use for evaluation of chronic (>30 days) biomaterials. There has been increased interest in recent years in the use of active prostheses, scaled for the test animal, to evaluate the performance of new materials, especially surface coatings adapted for fixation by tissue adhesion or ingrowth.

Tools for design: material testing

When seeking to introduce a new biomaterial, there are numerous standards that provide guidance to the design team to consider. The ASTM has published standards that cover various test methods including corrosion, wear, fatigue, degradation, aging, and strength. These methods utilize not only materials testing equipment but also microscopy and other chemical and physical characterization tools. Optical microscopy is one of the most readily available laboratory tools and is utilized for the close-up examination of an object surface. In particular, using light and a system of lenses, it allows the magnification of small features following testing of a particular material. One example would be the examination of witness marks on knee arthroplasty components whose non-articulating surfaces were contacting owing to impingement.

It may also be important to understand the chemical and physical properties of a material and how it may change in anticipated environments. Information that may be useful includes knowing the purity and constituents of a material, the impact of its temperature in a certain environment, its degradation state, and the condition of its surface.

Fourier transform infrared spectroscopy

Fourier transform infrared (FTIR) spectroscopy is a technique used to identify the constituents of a material through examination of how well the material absorbs and transmits infrared energy (wavelength longer than visible light) of differing wavelengths. After directing an input infrared spectrum onto a sample, the frequencies of the vibrations between the atomic bonds in the sample alter the spectrum output to a detector. On the basis of the resulting spectrum, FTIR can identify an unknown material, the amount of each constituent of a sample, or the quality of a substance. It has been described as exposing the unique "fingerprint" of a given sample. FTIR can be used to characterize the degradation of polymers caused by sterilization and aging (oxidation index) or to determine a material's potential to oxidize (hydroperoxide index). An indication of the degree of molecular cross-linking in a material, which is an important characteristic of wear performance, can also be assessed (trans-vinylene index).

Differential scanning calorimetry

Differential scanning calorimetry is a technique to measure how much heat flow is required to increase the temperature of a substance. This is particularly useful in measuring properties of phase transitions (transitions between solid, liquid, and gaseous states) or glass transitions (liquid–glass transition from a hard and relatively brittle state into a molten or rubber-like state) in a substance. This technique has wide applicability in determining the purity of manufactured substances, checking the composition of polymers, and analyzing curing processes for polymers and drug compounds. This can be useful in evaluating the effects of processing and manufacturing of the devices.

White light interferometry

White light interferometry can be used to measure the three-dimensional microstructure and topography of a specimen surface, otherwise known as the "roughness" of a surface. The method analyzes the interference pattern of a wave directed at a location of interest and a reference wave. Depending on the path traveled by each wave, they later combine and result in some degree of constructive or destructive interference, which is captured by a detector and processed to characterize the surface roughness. White light interferometry is often used to examine the surface roughness of components that articulate or rub against one another and can aid in determining wear mechanisms.

Gel permeation chromatography

Gel permeation chromatography (GPC) is a method for measuring the proportions of the constituents of a material, using the relative permeability of the constituents. The technique is carried out by pouring a solution of the sample (dissolved into a solvent) into a column with gel layers that are designed for a range of molecular weight. Depending on permeability, the gel will retain some constituents and will not retain others. Various detectors can then be used to analyze the separated sample. GPC can be used to determine a polymer's molecular weight distribution or to determine changes following degradation.

Tools for design: material modeling

Material modeling in the form of computer simulations can also be used to evaluate how a material will respond to certain loading conditions. Historically, computer simulation or finite element analysis (FEA) is used to solve complex structural problems in traditional fields such as civil and mechanical engineering. The foundation of the FEA approach is based on numerical modeling of physical systems using small interconnected building blocks (finite elements) that resemble the geometry of the structure. By breaking a single complex problem into numerous simple problems, the deformation, strain, and stress can be mapped throughout the entire structure (Figure 15.3). The utility of any FEA results depends on the validity of the model inputs. Key components of

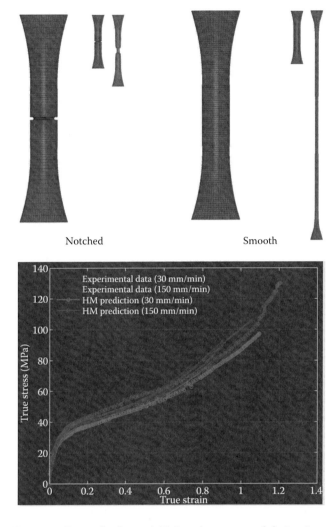

FIGURE 15.3   (See color insert.) Finite element models (top) to simulate tensile testing of smooth and notched rod biomaterial samples, with corresponding finite element results and physical experiments demonstrating good concordance.

an FE model include a clinically relevant representation of the geometry, material properties, applied loads, boundary conditions, and interface (contact) conditions. After validation of the FE model, virtual experiments can be performed to simulate conditions experienced by the biomaterial. Basic analyses can easily be extended in a parametric study to include considerations of expected variations in design, surgical, and patient factors. When developed and analyzed carefully, FE models can provide valuable insight into the clinical performance and potential failure modes of a biomaterial. In addition to analysis of the mechanical response, these models can be developed further to examine fluid and thermal responses.

FEA, when developed with scientific/technical rigor and used in an appropriate manner, can be a powerful tool. However, it is critical to recognize the limitations of FE models for biomedical applications. Biological structures such as bone, ligaments, tendons, and cartilage have highly complex mechanobiology. The biological interactions at the cellular and molecular levels are not typically incorporated into conventional bone-implant models. Bone density and architecture can vary dramatically between anatomic sites and also spatially within each site. For this reason, any FE model of human bone that does not incorporate the nonhomogeneity of bone properties (from QCT data, for example) is less able to capture the complex interactions between an implant and its supporting bony tissue. Models that include heterogeneous material properties also have limitations. These models tend to be representative of a single "patient" in terms of anatomy and bone quality. Therefore, analysts should be cautious of extrapolating the outcomes from a single model to the entire patient population. Although QCT data can be used to develop more "realistic" models, there are many models in the literature that do not link CT scan data to actual patient-specific models. In addition, there is often a lack of knowledge of the interface mechanical properties, which provide challenges in understanding how loads and stresses are transferred between the device and surrounding bone/tissue. Despite these limitations, careful FEA is a powerful tool for understanding the fundamental response of a biomaterial or implant design in a complex biomechanical environment.

Tools for design: 3D printing

Prototypes, individual functional models, are commonly used during the design process to allow the design team and the ultimate users to have a sample in their hands to try out. Construction of a prototype often leads to design simplification and thus can play a key role in design. One way to develop a prototype is through establishing a pilot manufacturing process. However, this can be expensive and slow, often due to the need to develop processes and tooling for fabrication. Alternatively, 3D printing provides an avenue to construct a relatively fast and inexpensive 3D prototype. As the name suggests, 3D printing is the process of making three-dimensional solid objects from a digital or computer-aided design (CAD) model of the device. The printer segments the CAD model into thin cross sections, which are deposited additively in successive layers of material to create a 3D composition of the object. A material printer is able to output layers of liquid, power, or sheet material. 3D printing has found utility at various points during the design process, from pre-production through full-scale production or post-production customization.

Three-dimensional printing is still in its relative infancy, having only been developed in the 1980s. As the technology is improved, the opportunities will continue to grow.

The technology is currently being explored as a possibility for tissue engineering applications, including in the construction of replacement organs and body parts. Living cells can be layered onto a gel medium and slowly built up to form 3D biological structures. There is also potential for the use of 3D printing to produce customized devices, such as "patient-specific" joint replacement components. However, this has yet to be explored on a commercial basis. Any such device would have to comply with standard regulatory requirements prior to implantation.

Clinical trials

Initial studies

The most exhaustive engineering and biologic tests of a new biomaterial can do no more than to remove the risk of gross adverse biologic response in clinical application. Qualification of a new material for routine clinical use in specific device types requires careful, controlled prospective clinical trials.

Ethical considerations prevent the isolated testing of new materials in patients as can be done in animals. Often, such clinical trials become an examination of the performance of a new material in a new or modified device for treatment of a particular clinical condition. As a result, "qualification" of implant biomaterials is not really possible: other applications may raise new questions and require additional preclinical and clinical testing. Appropriately, animal studies serve as surrogates in evaluations of new materials.

Therefore, initiation of clinical trials will require the production of some quantity of a device incorporating the new material. In the early stages of such evaluation, the devices may be made, one at a time, at the direct instruction of a physician with the intention that they be used on a specific patient. Such devices are said to be "custom devices" and are controlled by only two regulatory requirements:

1. They must be manufactured in a registered facility that meets the FDA's GMP regulations (21 USC 351, 352; 21 CFR Part 820).
2. Their use must be approved by the Institutional Review Board (IRB), which ordinarily controls experimental procedures on patients in the given institution.

These are relatively modest requirements that will permit the initial group of academic and clinical investigators to finalize aspects of design, fabrication, and clinical use of the material in question, with implantations in perhaps 5–15 patients, before embarking on a full-scale clinical trial.

Clinical protocol

Design of clinical protocols has become an art in itself and is the subject of many articles and books. Many institutions now employ specialists to aid in this, and similar services are available from a wide range of qualified consultants.

All trial protocols have in common the following features:

1. The patients to be treated display uniform and well-characterized clinical conditions.

2. Patients enter the study only after having its advantages and disadvantages explained and after giving informed consent to their participation. (For this reason, questions have been raised about the suitability and ethical justification of studies involving young children and the "old, old.")

3. Identities and medical histories of patients are kept confidential and protected from public view.

4. The procedures and types of treatment to be used are well defined and reasonably uniform.

5. There is a reasonable possibility of specific benefit to each patient involved.

The selection of the number of patients for a clinical trial is difficult and depends strongly on the condition to be treated. The present de facto minimum standard is as follows: at least 100 patients selected for a single condition and treated uniformly with a minimum follow-up of 2 years. This is a satisfactory minimum guideline for most new *device* designs, but is inappropriate as a general standard for three reasons:

1. Some conditions, such as fresh fractures or even nonunions, may be satisfactorily followed with shorter follow-ups.

2. On the other hand, observation of long-term effects of new materials may require 7–10 years, perhaps with some lower level of clinical surveillance, to provide reasonable assurance of clinical safety.

3. Although a minimum number of patients is required for overall statistical design, there is a hazard involved in spreading too few among too many investigators. To overcome "learning curve" problems, it is inadvisable for any investigator to perform less than 12–15 procedures. This "minimum" number of procedures will be dependent on a number of factors, such as the complexity of the procedure and the condition that is being treated.

Investigational device exemption

Before such trials are begun, with quantities of devices used in patients to a fixed protocol approved by IRBs in the participating institutions, additional review and approval by the FDA are required. This is achieved in the form of application for an Investigational Device Exemption (IDE) (Federal Register 45(13): 3732ff, 1980). This application states the full conditions of the design, conduct, and reporting of the proposed trial, as well as the supporting results of laboratory tests of safety and efficacy, and seeks exemption from the applicable sections of the Medical Device Amendments to permit the manufacture, sale, interstate shipment, and use of a specific number of the devices in question. (Information submitted to support claims of *safety* must be obtained in facilities operated in compliance with FDA Good Laboratory Practices regulations. See the Federal Register 43(247):59986, 1978.) In essence, it contains the information that will be required later for class III premarket approval, except for the specific results on safety and efficacy, which will be obtained from the proposed clinical trial.

If a good case can be made that the proposed trial will operate within the applicable standards and regulations and will expose the patient volunteers to no foreseeable exceptional risk, the IDE will be granted. The trial may then proceed under the surveillance of an independent quality control organization, which is charged with reporting both compliance to protocol and the results of the trial to its sponsors in a form satisfactory to the FDA. Changes in the protocol, including alterations of treatment indications, treatment procedures, and number of patients, may be necessary as the trial proceeds. Provisions in the IDE regulations permit such changes to be made, although frequently with some difficulty, by amendment of the original application.

Release for general use

After completion of the clinical trials, the entire body of information gathered must be submitted to the FDA for final approval (the so-called PMA or premarket approval) before the device containing the new material passes into general clinical use. The material will be reviewed by an advisory panel of academic and clinical experts in the field (in this case, orthopaedics). The advisory panel will recommend approval or disapproval, and the FDA will act on this recommendation.

Approval will generally be given if the findings suggest that the material in this application meets the conditions of safety and efficacy previously stated. However, there are a number of caveats to such approval:

1. The approval will only be given for the application that was the subject of the clinical trial. Other, expanded indications may be added at a later date through amendments to the original PMA or possibly through 510(k) applications, but may also require additional clinical trials. In particular, approval of a material in one device does not signify blanket approval for other device applications.

2. The indications and contraindications for use must be agreed to between the FDA and the manufacturer. In particular, they must appear in the packaging insert and in advertising material, and advertised claims must be restricted to agree with them.

3. Some form of long-term follow-up of the original study group may be required as well as surveillance of patients treated for some period after initial release (typically 2–4 years). Such a follow-up may produce additional information on clinical performance and may require changes in the previously agreed indications and contraindications for use.

4. Future questions may be raised that could result in re-evaluation of the premarket approval decision. Although the statutory basis for such re-review is unclear, it will readily come about in the face of reports of clinical problems related to device design or composition.

Standardization

Once a new biomaterial, or any other new material, for that matter, has entered into commercial use, it is desirable that its composition and properties become standardized. Such standardization does not infringe patented protection or proprietary rights but makes the material available as a part of the device designer's armamentarium. Furthermore, standardization of materials tends to produce a focus on a narrower range of materials rather than constant innovation for the sake of difference, yielding more rapid recognition of a particular material's strengths and weaknesses in various applications. A wide number of organizations are active in standardization of medical and surgical materials and devices, with the ASTM (Philadelphia) taking the lead role in standardization of evaluation methods for biomaterials in the United States and

Table 15.4 General timeline for new biomaterial introduction

Begin:	Concept
	Material design
End of Year 1:	Trial fabrication
	In vitro tests, engineering characterization
Year 2:	Acute *in vivo* tests
	Begin chronic in vivo tests
Year 3:	$\downarrow$
Year 4:	Begin device design
	Complete chronic in vivo tests
Year 5:	Complete device design
	Engineering tests of device
Year 6:	Initial patient trials ("custom device")
	Design protocol/apply for IDE
Year 7:	*Begin clinical trial*
Year 8:	
Year 9:	$\downarrow$
	Complete clinical trial (2-year follow-up)
Year 10:	Apply for premarket approval
	Release of biomaterial for first indications
Year 11:	Begin standardization, continue postintroduction surveillance (if required)

the International Standards Organization (ISO; Geneva, Switzerland) similarly in the European Community.

Schedule for introduction of a new material

The entire process of introducing a new biomaterial has been suggested to take as long as 8–11 years. The progression from concept to general clinical use is shown, for a typical situation, in Table 15.4.

Serendipity and friendly fortune may slightly shorten this progression. However, for chronic applications in which patients may be facing exposures exceeding 25 years, prudence suggests the need for care and thoroughness in developing and introducing new orthopaedic biomaterials.

Afterword

Adverse clinical experiences with some joint replacement components should serve to further temper enthusiasm for the rapid clinical introduction of novel materials or even of long used biomaterials in novel designs. Design and material properties are intimately related: new, improved materials permit new designs; new design approaches produce the need for new materials. The use of the careful stepwise process described in this chapter, combined with patience on the part of all stakeholders in that process, should permit the future evolution and clinical introduction of new devices fabricated from safe and effective biomaterials.

Annotated bibliography

1. Medical Device Amendments of 1976. Public Law 94-295, May 28, 1976.
   One of the last official acts of the Ford Presidency; the basic law regulating medical use of biomaterials in the United States.
2. ASTM F748–06 (2010): Standard Practice for Selecting Generic Biological Test Methods for Materials and Devices. Volume 13.1, *Annual Book of Standards: Medical Devices*. American Society for Testing and Materials, West Conshohocken, PA.
   A consensus guide for selection of appropriate biologic tests.
3. ASTM F981-04 (2010): Standard Practice for Assessment of Compatibility of Biomaterials for Surgical Implants with Respect to Effect of Materials on Muscle and Bone. Volume 13.1, *Annual Book of Standards: Medical Devices*. American Society for Testing and Materials, West Conshohocken, PA.
   Guide for experimental protocols for biological assays of tissue reaction to nonabsorbable biomaterials for surgical implants.
4. Blue Book Guidance G95-1, Use of International Standard ISO-10993, 'Biological Evaluation of Medical Devices Part 1: Evaluation and Testing,' FDA, May 1, 1995.
5. Design control guidance for medical device manufacturers. FDA, 1997. http://www.fda.gov/medicaldevices/deviceregulationandguidance/guidancedocuments/ucm070627.htm, U.S. Food and Drug Administration, Center for Devices and Radiological Health, Silver Spring, MD.

Guidance intended to assist manufacturers in understanding quality system requirements concerning design controls.

6. HENCH LL: Development of a new biomaterial–prosthetic device. In Ghista DN, Roaf R (eds): *Orthopaedic Mechanics: Procedures and Devices.* Academic Press, London, 1978.

    An article on the subject, with examples from the author's experience in developing and testing "bioactive" glass materials.

7. ISO 10993-1:2009—Biological Evaluation of Medical Devices—Part 1: Evaluation and Testing within a Risk Management Process, International Organization for Standardization, Geneva, Switzerland.

    The standard international guide for selection of host response studies before clinical testing, with distinctions made for period of exposure and tissues at implant site. Previous title is a useful guide to this sometimes opaque standard.

8. Medical Devices; Procedures for Investigational Device Exemptions. Fed Reg 45(13) (Part II):3732–3759, Jan. 18, 1980.

    Final proposal for Investigational Device Exemption (IDE) regulations, with useful discussion of objections to the original proposals of August 20, 1976. Explains how new biomaterials may move into clinical trials.

9. Orthopaedic Devices; General Provisions and Classifications of 77 Devices; Final Classification. Fed Reg 52(172) (part II):33686–33711, Sept. 4, 1987.

    Final classification of all but a very few diagnostic, prosthetic (implantable), and surgical (instruments) orthopaedic devices. No materials are classified as such; materials references are generic (e.g., 888.3310 Hip joint metal/polymer constrained cemented or uncemented prosthesis. Class III).

10. VON RECUM AF (ed): *Handbook of Biomaterials Evaluation.* MacMillian, New York, 1986.

    A collection of 50 chapters dealing with testing and evaluation of biomaterials. Sections 9 and 10 are especially useful in designing test protocols.

CHAPTER SIXTEEN

Materials retrieval
and analysis

With the exception of a very small number of studies, orthopaedic devices that "fail" in service are still not routinely or systematically collected and studied. Studies of those implants that are collected tend to concentrate on the physical findings obtained from the device itself, neglecting the patient and events of treatment. Clinical reviews and case reports of implant malfunction tend to focus on the patient, often to a near total exclusion of an engineering description of the device. Finally, both types of study concentrate on frank failures, with an absence of comparative data from successful or partially successful performance of similar or identical devices. Thus, much of what we think we know about orthopaedic device performance is drawn from a very small, non-random sample of the actual clinical experience. This is an error, in the same way that studies of criminology based solely on prison populations are.

This error is further increased by a failure to separate materials aspects from device aspects. In fact, with few exceptions, study of retrieved devices focuses on mechanical features of the devices and the local host response to these features. A more careful approach would yield useful information concerning biologic performance of biomaterials in clinical use.

An additional reason to become more thorough in studying devices in clinical experience is the increasing interest being shown by both lawyers and (in the United States) federal regulatory officials. The present system and practice of device removal make it difficult to account for particular devices, to establish that a particular device was removed from a patient, and to determine the device's condition at removal. The ability to deal with these questions is desirable and may in the future become mandatory.*

---

* Postmarket introduction surveillance orders by the FDA ("522" orders) frequently mandate such reporting in subsequently approved study plans.

The recommended analytic approach to the study of retrieved devices is that of the traditional medical case history study, marrying medical and engineering approaches. A careful accumulation of clinical findings, the development of a working hypothesis involving both modes and mechanisms, and the use of clinical and engineering test methods to substantiate preliminary impressions will result in a coherent view of device performance in cases with both satisfactory and unsatisfactory clinical outcomes. In addition, the use of an analytic (triage) system to establish the level of study of each device can provide results at a substantially lower cost than is possible through the use of a fixed recovery and analysis protocol. Finally, provisions should be made for permanent record preparation and controlled storage of retrieved devices.

Throughout this discussion, the parallel with examination of tissue removed from patients during surgery will be noted. This is deliberate; it is felt that the problems to be dealt with are essentially identical, although the device retrieval case is further complicated by the existence of patient's property and other rights associated with the manufactured and electively inserted implant. However, many of the same techniques are used and many of the same benefits result in each kind of study.

The increased enforcement of postmarket product surveillance has also been emphasized by regulatory agencies. The US Food and Drug Administration (FDA), for example, has developed initiatives for more active surveillance through data networks, such as the Sentinel System in 2008. In the orthopaedic world, implant registries have been in existence since the early 1970s, mainly pioneered by the Swedish joint arthroplasty registries. Efforts to develop a similar type of infrastructure in the United States began picking up steam in 2009. All these data systems or data networks provide additional resources to better understand the performance of materials in medical devices in the real world.

Significance of device retrieval and analysis studies

The development of orthopaedic implants has been more or less an empirical process. From the initial applications of ivory pegs, soft iron wire, and wood screws in fracture treatment to the use of modern high-strength alloy total joint replacements, devices have been built from concept to practice under the guidance of treating surgeons. Safety and performance have been measured against comparative and subjective criteria: Is the patient's condition improving? Is the patient satisfied with the results?

From modest beginnings, the use of orthopaedic implants has grown to enormous proportions. Between 5 and 10 million metallic, polymeric, or ceramic parts are implanted each year; perhaps as many as 100 million parts have been used and millions remain in patients permanently, either by design or by chance. The performance of a device in the field cannot be predicted with 100% certainty, since it is widely accepted that there are uncertainties in predicting the performance of present devices owing to the contributions from many factors. From that standpoint, some may view the medical device field as a vast experiment, involving millions of subjects and lasting far beyond the lifetimes of those who started it. But while it is also widely accepted that there are risks with any surgery and the use of any device, it is the implicit expectation of the medical professional, the patient, and the design team that the benefits of the device will outweigh its risks, even if such considerations are not explicit. In the normal course of such a widespread application of technology, we would expect a continual feedback from the user to the developer and the manufacturer that would lead to an evolutionary improvement and convergence of design and practice.

There has been some convergence, in the sense meant here, but in most device applications in orthopaedics, there appears to be an increasing divergence of design and materials with no real extension in the length of the design change cycle, which still seems to be less than 3–5 years, even for permanent implants such as total joint replacements. This is probably the case since the vast majority of evidence of device performance is neither obtained nor studied publically. This situation has arisen from two conditions.

First, devices only attract attention when they fail to fulfill their intended function. Such failure, of either the device or treatment plan, or both, is relatively rare, with clinical "success" rates generally exceeding 90% for periods of as much as 10 years. The most common, easily observable failure is the removal of a permanent device, such as a total hip replacement (THR). Even if defects in the device are suspected or recognized before or during revision, they are not generally studied in depth. Frankly broken or damaged devices often excite fears of legal action against surgeons, hospital, or manufacturers. Such devices may simply "disappear." Some devices are returned to the manufacturers for analysis. The knowledge gained from such study is often limited by a lack of access to clinical records and a resulting failure to understand the clinical aspects of the origin of the problem. Some devices are given to patients, either as a gift or on demand by the patient's lawyer. And many devices end up, unlabeled and unprotected, in a drawer in the surgical scrub area, or disposed of by the hospital.

Second, there is little or no effort made to study successful devices. Clinical studies that are performed focus on improvement in overall function and reduction in pain, along with temporal measures of retention of improvement. These studies are isolated; in fact, when a device gains a degree of clinical acceptance, it apparently rapidly ceases to be a suitable subject for study. Few clinical studies have included any strategies for examination of implant function and condition, other than by radiography, independent of the clinical condition of the patient. Furthermore, a device that is performing successfully provides no reason for it to be removed, providing no opportunity for investigation, except postmortem.

In some ways, the failure to study this other 90%–99% of devices is even more tragic. We know remarkably little about the normal host–implant interactions, either local or systemic, in patients. Autopsy samples are rarely available, with the declining rate of autopsy in the United States making such studies more difficult and rare. As indicated in earlier chapters, we have only very poor estimates of true *in vivo* corrosion and wear rates, even of long-used materials. With the exception of some isolated experiments with instrumented implants, we know almost nothing about the true stresses and strains in functioning devices or the effects of these conditions on growth, repair, and remodeling of surrounding tissues.

If we were able to study successful devices, functioning in patients, at routine removal and at patient death, in a systematic way, many of these unknowns could be resolved. The result would certainly be a better selection of materials and devices for specific patients as well as better prospective design of improved devices. In addition, there would be greater confidence in performance predictions of current and new designs.

Ultimately, the study of devices and their materials, regardless of whether they are successful or not, needs to consider all patient, surgical, and device/material factors. This approach considers the performance on a "whole case" basis. This means that the device, its history, the patient's history, the clinical and surgical details, and all engineering and clinical test data may contribute to the outcomes. It is the intent that the retrieval studies described here will provide a systematic approach to better understanding device performance.

Immediate aims of device retrieval and analysis studies

The systematic record developed by a uniform, mandatory (within an institution) device retrieval and analysis (DRA) program serves three more immediate aims:

1. Careful study of a device removed from a patient for cause may contribute directly to the patient's ongoing medical care. Some of the immediate outcomes may be helpful in choosing the material and design of a replacement device and resolving differential diagnoses on the basis of local inflammation or infection.

2. The completed record of the retrieval and examination of the device represent an "expert" study of the device aspects of the patient's treatment. Thus, they represent a unique resource available in the event of legal action associated with failure of the device to function or with medical treatment associated with its insertion or removal.

3. Device failures that are of a serious nature, are life threatening, or are associated with a mortality must be reported to the FDA through the Manufacturer and User Facility Device Experience (MAUDE) system.* A well-developed mandatory DRA system and record provide a mechanism for timely reporting while protecting the rights of all parties.

---

* The MAUDE database represents reports of adverse events involving medical devices. The data consist of voluntary reports since June 1993, user facility reports since 1991, distributor reports since 1993, and manufacturer reports since August 1996.

Institutional setting for DRA studies

DRA is an institutional responsibility that practicing physicians should insist on, as they insist on other forms of institutional support. Thus, this section is intended for the guidance of administrators in setting up DRA services and of physicians in measuring the performance of such services. It is not intended that individual physicians be encouraged to establish such studies in their own practices. In most cases, adequate resources are not available and liability might be incurred through poor conduct of studies.

Within a treating institution, the DRA service should be reasonably autonomous, with a structure and chain of responsibility parallel to that of the institutional clinical pathology service. Lack of resources may require one DRA service to serve several institutions or even to function on a regional basis. Such arrangements are possible but care must be taken to maintain appropriate professional oversight.

A professional with a PhD degree in bioengineering/biomedical engineering, materials science, or equivalent expertise with an engineering background and some experience in DRA should supervise the service and report to the institutional medical board. The service should be permanent, after an initial experimental period, and adequate funding must be provided. It should be physically housed within the institution and be given access to all normal institutional services (security, data processing, library, etc.) that other services enjoy. It renders clinical rather than research or administrative service and should be situated accordingly within the treating institution's management scheme.

A formal, continuing review board should be available to oversee the operation of the DRA service and ratify the decisions of the service chief, in much the same manner as a tissue committee. It should meet periodically, on a regular schedule, to maintain immediacy and retain disposition of cases. Major device-using services should be represented as well as external experts. Although it is strongly recommended that such DRA services encompass *all* removed devices in a given institution, the following comments focus specifically on orthopaedic devices.

Procedures for DRA studies

Beyond benefits to specific patients, the utility of DRA programs depends strongly on their ability to collect all but a narrowly excluded group of implants. The devices that should be recovered are as follows:

Metallic implants: all parts except for skin clips, isolated cancellous and cortical bone screws, and cerclage and suture wires.

Nonmetallic implants: all parts except for sutures, drains, packings, or other disposable items and fragments of bone cement smaller than 1 cm in the largest dimension.

However, any excluded device that shows frank damage by x-ray, computed tomography, magnetic resonance imaging, and so on, at surgery *and* in the treating surgeon's opinion has failed to fulfill its intended function should also be recovered and preserved. There may also be interest in collecting periprosthetic tissue if it exhibits a visibly different response, such as blackened or darkened tissue or fluid accumulation. Another reason for examining periprosthetic tissue would be if the device involves the frank wearing away of its material. In this case, the tissue could contain wear particles that can provide histological examination of the inflammatory response. Finally, in some cases, there may be a need to recover contemporaneous patient-derived fluids (blood, serum, urine, etc.) in a controlled manner for later study.

Such a collection program requires either the full-time services of a clinical technician or the identification of a member of the regular operating room staff who will receive special training and for whom this will become a first priority. Experience has shown that failure to provide such a person results in loss of devices to a greater or lesser degree and in degradation of the quality of the clinical information acquired.

Under the direction of the DRA service chief, the designated individual is responsible for the following initial steps:

1. Prospective identification of scheduled surgical procedures involving or possibly involving nonexcluded device removal.
2. Attendance during removal to receive, identify, and package the device parts as well as to take intraoperative photographs when necessary to document the case.
3. Follow-up on analyses ordered at surgery on tissue and fluid specimens.

The device parts are carefully washed, with care not to remove adherent corrosion evidence, and packaged in containers suitable to protect them and to permit gas sterilization. Alcohol and dilute hydrogen peroxide solutions may be useful; however, their use should be controlled by prospective protocol. All devices should be regarded as contaminated and, immediately after primary examination, ethylene oxide sterilized for worker protection. Tissue specimens or device components with adherent tissue, such as ingrowth fixation surfaces on joint replacements, should be packaged in chemical fixatives to preserve the tissue from degradation and to maintain the cellular structure. Formaldehyde (or formalin) is a commonly used and generally suitable fixative.

Initial evaluation

As soon as possible after device retrieval, the DRA service chief should perform an initial review. This includes examination of the device and other materials recovered at surgery, review of the patient's medical history, and study of the results of intraoperative clinical studies. The goal of this initial review is to assign the case to one of three removal classes:

Class I: Devices removed for probable cause or displaying probable evidence of frank failure.

Class II: Devices removed for probable cause but without evidence of frank failure.

Class III: Devices removed for other than probable cause (routine removal, secondary procedures, autopsy, etc.).

Figure 16.1 shows two examples of class I devices. From Figure 16.1a, an early radiograph (left side, 18 months postoperation) shows an essentially normal femoral component with a neck–stem angle measured to be 128°. A later view (right side, 36 months postoperation) obtained immediately before removal shows a reduced neck–shaft angle of 119° and an apparent crack on the medial side of the stem (arrow). Such a radiographic history is useful in later study and analysis. From Figure 16.1b, a radiograph taken at 2 years (left side) shows probable narrowing of the femoral neck after hip resurfacing arthroplasty. At 3 years and 4 months

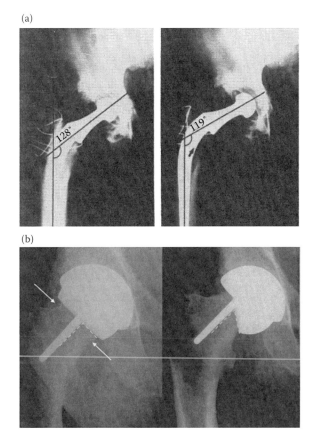

(a)

(b)

FIGURE 16.1 (a) Class failure, detected *in vivo*. Left: 18 months postoperation. Right: 36 months postoperation (immediately before removal). (b) Left: narrowing of the femoral neck at 2 years postoperation. The angle between the peg and head is 90°. Right: collapse of the femoral head at 3 years and 4 months postoperation with a relative tilt of the head with respect to the peg to approximately 55°.

follow-up, there is tilting of the femoral head about the short stem, providing appearance of a collapsed head (dashed lines).

Postretrieval testing

On the basis of this initial classification or triage scheme, a series of diagnostic tests will be ordered. Other tests may be desired for the purposes of research or special studies; however, those described here fall within the scope of normal diagnosis and should be chargeable to the base costs of patient treatment. It is recommended that a single charge be used that averages the costs of all studies (of removal class I, II, and III devices) and that it be adjusted periodically on the basis of experience. This strategy will tend to limit testing to essential studies only.

Table 16.1 outlines the possible procedures, on a case-by-case basis, associated with DRA studies under this triage scheme. The normal expectation is that 1%–2% of orthopaedic devices will fall in class I, less than 10% in class II, and the balance in class III. The final deposition should be made by the review board, on the recommendation of the service chief.

DRA disposition

After the results of all tests are available, the DRA service chief should prepare a note describing the examination and his conclusions. This note

Table 16.1 Conduct of DRA studies

Steps	Class I	Class II	Class III
Retrieve			
Package			
Identify			
Sterilize			
Classify			
Evaluate			
Photographs	X	X	X
Culture reports	X	X	
Histology	X	X	
Metallography	X		
Dimensional analysis	X		
Mechanical analysis	X		
Chemical analysis	X		
Special tests	X	X	
Mechanical testing (device portions)	X		
Hardness	X		
Specific histology stains	X		
Metal analysis (AAS) (fluids, tissues)	X		
Case disposition	X	X	X
Prepare report	X	X	X
Store device	X	X	X

The "Removal class" header spans the Class I, Class II, and Class III columns.

should specifically address the initial removal classification, changing it if necessary and, if the device is found to be a removal class I device, making recommendations for change, in both this specific case and in future use of the device. This note, with the supporting materials, should be presented to the DRA review board. After discussion, when affirmed by this board, the note should then be placed in the patient's medical record and be communicated, without patient identification, to all interested parties. A permanent record should also be preserved that links the note with all observations and test results, either by inclusion or by reference, and the location of the device, including its final disposition. This, as well as the device, should be maintained by the DRA service in a secure manner.

In addition, the results of study of removal class I cases should probably be presented to the institution's periodic morbidity and mortality conference. Periodic summaries of all retrieval studies, with patient identification protected, should be made to treating physicians within the institution. In exceptional cases, reports may be made to appropriate manufacturers and to the FDA, depending on institutional policy.

Questions and answers concerning DRAs

Numerous special points have been raised concerning the design and execution of DRA studies. They are presented here with appropriate responses. (These questions and responses have been of particular value in instructing lay persons concerning DRA.)

1. What is an implant?

    Answer: An implant is any manufactured material or part of a device that (1) must penetrate the epithelium or mucosa during installation and (2) remains, by design, in the body of the patient after completion of the initial surgical procedure.

2. Why should implants be retrieved and studied?

    Answer: The study of retrieved devices is necessary and vital since even the most extended clinical testing program will involve a small number of patients compared with those who will eventually receive the device. If the results of the use of devices in patients can be studied continuously on a statistical basis, then the body of information about each particular device will continue to grow. In addition, examination of a retrieved device yields information about a particular patient's condition and thus contributes to diagnosis and treatment of the patient's problems in the same way as any other laboratory test.

3. Why should a standard procedure (protocol) be used for retrieval and study of implants?

    Answer: Such a protocol provides a framework in which the following benefits may be realized:

    i. The user (patient) will be assured as to the cause for device removal and that necessary corrective measures, if possible, are being taken.

    ii. The surgeon or doctor involved will be assured that causes of removal are being investigated in a systematic way that will tend to contain any possible liability within the bounds of actual medical malpractice and reduce the risk of transmittal of liability of others to him.

    iii. The treating institution will be assured that the best possible care is being provided, that patients' rights are being preserved, and that liability is being contained.

    iv. The manufacturers will be assured that maximal effort is being made to determine whether either singular or generic failures, referable to engineering factors, have occurred in a manner that will permit rapid corrective action to be taken if it is indicated.

    v. Both academic investigators and regulatory agencies will be assured that collection of clinical data, in a uniform and controlled manner, is being facilitated so that identification of failure modes and mechanisms will be possible.

4. What are the necessary elements of a DRA program?

Answer: The American Society for Testing and Materials (ASTM) has been examining this issue through their F 4 Committee and have identified the following general requirements for DRA programs:

    i. A general definition of implant failure (when programs are restricted to study of "failures")

    ii. A classification system of clinical and engineering failure indications specialized for the medical discipline involved

    iii. A standard protocol for recovery of implants at surgery with associated tissue and fluid specimens

    iv. Identification of recommended clinical (intraoperative and other) tests results to be obtained

    v. A standard form (or computerized format) for reporting patient history, observations at surgery, and immediate associated test results, to be designated as the retrieval form

    vi. Standard protocols for the study of retrieved devices and tissues referenced to suitable standard (ASTM or other) procedures and recommended practices

    vii. Division of the investigation into three stages from essential minimum analysis for routine examination (Stage I) to nondestructive but more detailed studies (Stage II) to destructive and material-specific evaluations (Stage III)

    viii. A scheme for analysis of data

    ix. A classification system for assignment of failure mode and mechanism

A standard practice for retrieval of medical devices has been developed (F 561-05: Standard Practice for Retrieval and Analysis of Medical Devices, and Associated Tissues and Fluids; American Society for Testing and Materials, Philadelphia). The recommendations made elsewhere in this chapter are in general agreement with this practice.

5. Who is responsible for initiating the retrieval and analysis of a particular implant?

Answer: A workshop was held at the National Bureau of Standards in March 1976, in conjunction with a symposium on the retrieval and analysis of orthopaedic implants. The members of the workshop, drawn from industry, government, and the sponsoring organizations (including the National Bureau of Standards, the Orthopaedic Research Society, the ASTM, the American Academy of Orthopaedic Surgeons [AAOS], the American College of Surgeons [ACOS], and the FDA) recommended to both the AAOS and ACOS that this responsibility be recognized to be that of the senior treating physician.

6. What implants should be retrieved?

Answer: In general, all implants should be retrieved (as previously described), with exceptions being made only for small, isolated, noncritical devices such as skin clips, cerclage wire, and so on. However, any excluded device that shows evidence of frank failure, either preoperatively or intraoperatively, or, in the surgeon's opinion, has failed to fulfill its intended function, should also be retrieved.

7. Who owns retrieved implants?

Answer: The weight of expert and legal opinion is that the implant belongs to the patient despite any role of third-party payers or insurers. The practical requirements for accountability and the impact that analysis of implants may have on diagnosis and treatment suggests that the hospital should routinely retain custody of the implants for a period exceeding the statute of limitations in its jurisdiction after retrieval. Release before this time, either to the patients or their agents or for the purpose of research and teaching, should be only at the specific written direction of the patient.

8. Who should pay for DRA studies?

Answer: Study of retrieved implants is part of the process of diagnosis and treatment in the same way that radiography and laboratory studies are. Thus, the responsibility for payment for retrieval and initial studies should reside with the patients and such third-party insurers that they may retain. Initial studies are defined as those indicated by and contributing to the treatment of the patient's condition and specifically excluding tests desirable for research and teaching purposes. On the other hand, researchers may decide to fund such studies, with patient permission, to

Table 16.2 Materials-associated findings in THR arthroplasty

Finding	Mechanism	Potential implication
Radiographic		
PMMA fragments (early)	Operative debris	Third-body accelerated wear
	Single-cycle fracture	
PMMA fragments (late)	Fatigue	Third-body accelerated wear
		Cup loosening
PMMA mantle fracture (late)	Fatigue	Stem subsidence
Broken cerclage wire	Fatigue	(Early) trochanteric loosening, nonunion
		Wire migration
Stem deformation	Plastic yielding	Change in bony support?
		Inadequate stem size?
		Impending failure?
		Stem positioning?
		Manufacturing defect?
		Chronic overload
		Change in bony support?
		Stem/cup positioning?
Stem or cup fracture	Fatigue	
Local lytic lesion[a]	Immune response?	Metal sensitivity?
		Excess wear debris?
		Progressive failure?
Progressive dissecting lesion[a]	Osteoclasis	Excessive wear debris?
		Metal sensitivity?
		Neoplasm?

Loose metallic debris	Wear	Third-body accelerated wear
		Fretting (loose THR)
		Fretting (modularity e.g., between head and stem taper)
	Fatigue ± corrosion	Inadequate processing of porous coating?
Clinical		
Intraoperative hypotension	Central control	Methyl methacrylate monomer sensitivity?
		Fat embolism?
Hip pain[a]	Immune response?	Metal sensitivity?
		Implant positioning?
Ectopic calcification	Wear debris nucleation?	Excessive wear
Dermatitis/eczema/bronchospasm	Delayed hypersensitivity	Metal sensitivity?
Histologic		
Fibrous capsule	Local host response	Normal
Hystiocytosis with multinuclear cells	Chronic inflammation	Manufacturing issues?
		Wrong material?
		Excess wear debris
Lymphocytic infiltration with plasma cells (aseptic lymphocytic vasculitis-associated lesions; ALVAL)	Delayed hypersensitivity	Metal sensitivity?
Fibrosarcoma/rhabdomyosarcoma/osteosarcoma	Neoplastic transformation	Chemical neoplasia?

[a] In absence of infection.

advance science and research related to medical device design, surgical optimization, and patient selection.

9. What is the relationship between DRA and implant registries?

Answer: The modern development of implant registries and their growing utility depend on a continuing flow of reliable statistical data concerning implant performance in the clinical setting. An important part of any DRA effort should be the provision for creation of a minimum data set and its routine anonymized transfer to a suitable implant registry. Thus, removal of an implant, either for cause or if intended to remain in place chronically, should produce a public data "event," in much the same way that human births and deaths universally do.

Recognizing biomaterials-related problems

In the context of this book, the important purpose of DRA studies is to recognize biomaterials-related problems in device performance. This is a large field of inquiry and cannot be easily summarized here. However, the specific case of THR arthroplasty may be used as an example of the relationship between clinical findings and possible biomaterials-related problems.

Failure of THR arthroplasty has been discussed frequently in the orthopaedic and bioengineering literature. Both frank failure and less than satisfactory ("fair" and "poor") outcomes have a variety of patient-, procedure-, and device-related origins. The purpose of this section is to try to separate those that may have a primary materials-related origin and to discuss their detection.

Table 16.2 summarizes the indications, mechanisms, and possible implications of adverse materials-associated findings in THR arthroplasty.

Additional considerations for DRA studies

This brief chapter can do no more than scratch the surface of an important and rapidly evolving aspect of clinical practice. The following sections of this chapter deal with additional considerations that should be addressed in any institution during the establishment and conduct of DRA studies.

Biohazard management

Since DRA studies of implantable devices will involve devices that are removed from the patient, protocols need to be in place to provide precautions for handling explanted components until they have completed a detoxification protocol. For example, a potential protocol could involve ultrasonic cleaning in soap and deionized water, rinsing, and sterilizing using a 10% Clorox solution. All participants in the DRA study should also be trained in biohazard safety. Such treatment is primarily for protection of hospital staff involved in patient care and should be followed with more rigorous procedures, as previously noted, before others, such as lay persons, lawyers, students, and so on, may come in contact with retrieved devices

Patient protection and informed consent

The study of the devices and the corresponding clinical information, beyond the immediate needs of diagnosis and treatment, will require informed consent from the patients. It should be routine practice to ask patients on admission to donate their devices and tissue for research and educational uses outside the DRA program. For implantable devices, since the devices are normally retrieved during the course of revision surgery, the collection process will pose no additional risks than those associated with the revision surgery itself. As part of the informed consent process, the patient should be asked to agree to share anonymized clinical data, records, and radiographs with researchers. In accordance with patient protection policies, based on law,* patient identifiers are safeguarded by all research investigators and not made publicly available. The retrieval facilities should also have controlled access.

Tools for characterizing retrieved implants and tissue

Nondestructive documentation and retrieval evaluations

An initial triage step is recommended to determine what level of nondestructive and destructive evaluations, if any, is performed. However, prior to any destructive testing, every implant will be photodocumented for its macroscopic appearance, using digital photography and optical microscopy. Additional imaging tools such as micro-computed tomography or scanning electron microscopy (SEM) can also be used to visualize the presence of different damage modes such as burnishing, abrasion, pitting, surface deformation, delamination, scratching, embedded debris, and cracks.

Destructive testing

After nondestructive testing has been completed, various forms of destructive tests can be performed, depending on the type of materials comprising the explant. These tests may include protocols for detailed failure, microstructural and chemical analyses, and the determination of physical and mechanical properties.

For metallic devices, the specimens can be etched to allow microscopic examination of inclusion content, grain size, grain boundary constituents, microporosity, and corrosion. Fractographic analysis from SEM imaging can be used to identify the presence of fatigue striations, evidence of ductile overload, and defects associated with crack initiation. If the device has a metallic coating, any missing sections of coating should be examined microscopically. Coating thickness and void content may be also determined. Energy dispersive x-ray is also a useful tool for

---

* Health Insurance Portability and Accountability Act of 1996; U.S. Department of Health and Human Services Privacy Rule; 45 Code of Federal Regulations (CFR) Part 160 and Part 164, Subparts A and E.

evaluating the chemical composition or changes to the elemental distribution on coating surfaces.

Destructive testing of polymeric devices involves microscopy and chemical analyses. Microscopic examination may be used to find evidence of surface damage or degradation. Inclusions or porosity and changes in density or crystallinity can be assessed using thin sections of approximately 5 to 10 microns and optical microscopy using reflected and transmitted, polarized and nonpolarized light. There is a wide variety of methods for the material characterization of polymers. Options for molecular weight of the specimen include gel permeation chromatography, osmometry, light scattering, viscometry, and melt index. Density can be determined from displacement or gradient methods, while thermal properties are also commonly characterized using differential scanning calorimetry for glass transition and melt temperatures. The presence of oxidation or degradation, as well as the chemical composition, can be analyzed using infrared analysis, Fourier transform infrared spectroscopy, nuclear magnetic resonance spectroscopy, and electronic spin resonance.

For retrieved tissues, there may be an interest in understanding if there are elemental particles contained in the tissue. This can be investigated with the use of chemical analysis tools such as inductively coupled plasma mass spectrometry (ICP-MS), which helps identify essential metals, metalloids, or non-metals in the tissue.

In all situations, care must be taken to ensure that any analysis must be done so as to not destroy any features that may become the subject of litigation. The choice of tests may be dependent on the reason for removal of the device, rather than selecting to perform all tests as this can be an expensive and time-consuming process.

Device evaluations using registries

In addition to establishing a DRA program on an institutional basis, efforts to collect implants on a regional or national basis require significant coordination and planning. Because the cost, complications, and outcomes of revision surgery are generally worse than in the initial primary surgery, there is motivation to try to improve the longevity of implants and to reduce the incidence of complications and the need for implant removal. As a result, starting in the 1970s, orthopaedic registries were developed in Scandinavia to track revisions on a national basis as a function of surgeon, patient, and implant characteristics. Over the past decade, orthopaedic registries have expanded across Europe, Canada, Australia, and New Zealand. Efforts to create a national orthopaedic registry are still in the early stages in the United States through the American Joint Replacement Registry. These registries provide additional resources to better understand the performance of medical devices in the real world.

A registry is not merely a data repository containing basic clinical, patient, and implant data regarding the implantation and revision of total joint replacements. In countries in which an implant registry has been established, the data are used as a tool to drive health care improvement by continuous feedback to the clinical community about procedure outcomes. The ability to identify factors that are important in achieving successful outcomes may improve standards and cost savings to the health care system.

Device monitoring by the FDA

Historically, the FDA has relied on spontaneous reporting systems to monitor the safety of medical products after they have been released in the marketplace. Hospitals, health care professionals, and patients can voluntarily report adverse events directly to the FDA through the MAUDE database, which was mentioned earlier in this chapter. Medical device manufacturers are also legally required to report to the FDA certain adverse events that they receive.

In 2008, the FDA launched the Sentinel System to leverage existing health care information to conduct active product surveillance to augment the existing spontaneous reporting systems. The data sources can include administrative and claims databases, electronic health care records, and existing registries to monitor outcomes in near real-time. At this time, the initial efforts have been implemented through the Mini-Sentinel pilot project to assist the FDA on scientific and technical issues related to the development of the Sentinel System.

The FDA has also proposed that all medical devices distributed in the United States carry a unique device identifier (UDI). The intention is to have a unique code that includes a device identifier, which is specific to a device model, as well as a production identifier with lot or batch information and expiration information. The purpose of the UDI is to help improve the quality of information for a medical device adverse event report, in terms of helping the FDA identify products more accurately and quickly. The ultimate goal is to improve patient safety by making postmarket surveillance more robust. The FDA is also creating a database with pertinent safety information that can be accessed by the public. Adoption and integration of the UDI system by manufacturers, hospitals, and health care professionals will be essential for the system to work effectively.

Conclusions concerning DRA

By and large, modern biomaterials as used in modern clinical implants are satisfactory and produce material and host responses superior to those experienced in the early days of implant surgery. Vigilance and attention to detail will permit these materials to continue to serve the patient well in established applications while increasing knowledge is gained about their few shortcomings. Despite the tradition for innovation in orthopaedics, care must be taken not to hazard these achievements in the search for new solutions to clinical problems. Well-designed, competently performed DRA studies complementing more traditional clinical studies will permit solid progress to continue to be made.

Annotated bibliography

1. ASTM F561-05: Standard Practice for Retrieval and Analysis of Medical Devices, and Associated Tissues and Fluids, American Society for Testing and Materials, West Conshohocken, PA.
   A consensus implant retrieval and analysis protocol.
2. COLANGELO VJ, HEISER FA: *Analysis of Metallurgical Failures*. John Wiley & Sons, New York, 1974.
   A discussion of study methods and observations of metallurgical failure. Of particular interest are Chapters 10–13, which discuss the contribution of manufacturing problems to failure.
3. DUMBLETON JH, MILLER EH: Failures of metallic orthopaedic implants. In *Metals Handbook*. 8th ed. American Society for Metals, Metals Park, OH, 1975.
   Overall review, with examples, emphasizing analytical techniques.
4. FDA Manufacturer and User Facility Device Experience (MAUDE) system. http://www.accessdata.fda.gov/scripts/cdrh/cfdocs/cfmaude/search. cfm.
   Database with reports of adverse events involving medical devices.
5. LANGTON DJ, JAMESON SS, JOYCE TJ, GANDHI JN, SIDAGINAMALE R, MEREDDY P, LORD J, NARGOL AVF: Accelerating failure rate of the ASR total hip replacement. *J Bone Joint Surg* (Br) 93B:1011–1016, 2011.
   Retrieval analysis of revised metal-on-metal hip replacements.
6. PIEHLER HR: Clinical environmental and the law: Product liability. In Caceres CA, Yolken HT, Jones RJ, Piehler HR (eds): *Medical Devices: Measurements, Quality Assurance, and Standards*. STP 800. American Society for Testing and Materials, Philadelphia, 1983.
   Device failure often leads, unfortunately, to litigation. Piehier discusses principles of tort liability, with special reference to the process of assigning liability to the various parties. Two appendices outline standards of reporting and of evaluation of professional opinions concerning devices.
7. ROBB MA, RACOOSIN JA, SHERMAN RE, GROSS TP, BALL R, REICHMAN ME, MIDTHUN K, WOODCOCK J: The US Food and Drug Administration's Sentinel Initiative: Expanding the horizons of medical product safety. *Pharmacoepidemiol Drug Saf* 21(S1):9–11, 2012.
   Background on the FDA Sentinel System to leverage existing healthcare information to conduct active product surveillance to augment the existing spontaneous reporting systems.
8. ROSTOCKER W, DVORAK JR: *Interpretation of Metallographic Structures*. 2nd ed. Academic Press, New York, 1977.
   Combined metallographic and scanning electron microscopic approach to the study of defective structure in metals. Many of the clear photographs can be compared with those obtained during the study of retrieved implants. Chapter 6 on quantitation of structure has broad applications.
9. U.S. General Accountability Office: Medical devices—FDA should enhance its oversight of recalls, 2011. http://www.gao.gov/assets/320/319569.html.
   Historical review of recalls in the United States.

10. WEINSTEIN A, GIBBONS D, BROWN S, RUFF W (eds): *Implant Retrieval: Material and Biological Analysis.* NBS Special Publication 601. US Printing Office, Washington DC, 1981.

An un-refereed conference proceedings volume for device retrieval and analysis methodology. Includes the results of a workshop on implant retrieval programs with sample retrieval protocols.

CHAPTER SEVENTEEN

Self-test

Instructions

This self-evaluation exercise is intended to be done in about 1.5 hours without reference material. No complex calculations are required. Individual point values for each question are given at the bottom right. Maximum score = 200.

Questions 1 and 2 refer to Figure 17.1

1. The forces exerted on the bar produce which type of stresses at point *A*? (select the best answer[s])

Tensile	_____
Torsional	_____
Compressive	_____
Shear	_____
Bending	_____
	(5)

2. If pin P is removed, the bar will (select the best answer)

A. Remain stationary	_____
B. Translate to right	_____
C. Translate to right and rotate clockwise	_____
D. Translate to left	_____
E. Translate to left and rotate clockwise	_____
	(5)

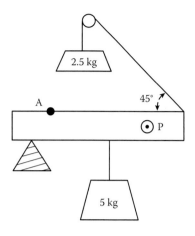

FIGURE 17.1

Questions 3 and 4 refer to Figure 17.2

3. From Figure 17.2, select the letter or combination of letters that are best identified with the following terms (write "X" if none apply):

Ductility	_____
Elastic strain energy	_____
Hysteresis	_____
Modulus	_____
Strength	_____
Toughness	_____
0.2% offset stress	_____
Ultimate stress	_____
Work of fracture	_____
Work hardening	_____
	(20)

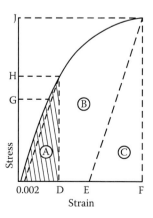

FIGURE 17.2

4. If the material represented by the stress–strain curve in Figure 17.2 is loaded to produce a stress between *H* and *J* and then completely unloaded, which of the following statements are *true*?

The material becomes more ductile.	___
The residual (unrecovered) strain is greater than 0.002.	___
The material becomes less tough.	___
	(3)

5. A viscoelastic material (*true* or *false*)

Can be represented by a Hooke body	___
Appears stiffer as strain rate increases	___
Contains mostly metallic bonds	___
Demonstrates hysteresis	___
Has a well-defined yield stress	___
	(5)

6. Stress relaxation (check the phrase that best completes the sentence)

A. Is the same as "cold flow"	___
B. Increases with increasing temperature	___
C. Is the same as creep	___
D. Occurs in tissues	___
E. May cause breaks in cerclage wires	___
	(5)

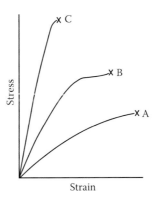

FIGURE 17.3

Question 7 refers to Figure 17.3

7. From Figure 17.3, select the letter or letters that best answer the queries:

Strongest material is?	_____
Stiffest material is?	_____
Most ductile material is?	_____
Material most likely to be a ceramic?	_____
Material most likely to be a polymer?	_____
	(10)

8. A 2.1-mm-diameter Steinmann pin, when compared with a 1.4-mm-diameter pin, both made of the same material, is (select the best answer[s])

A. 50% stiffer in bending	_____
B. 50% stronger in tension	_____
C. 125% stronger in tension	_____
D. 250% stiffer in bending	_____
E. 400% stiffer in bending	_____
	(15)

9. Rank the following materials from 1 (lowest) to 5 (highest) for indicated properties:

	Elastic modulus	Ductility	Strength
UHMWPE	_____	_____	_____
Cortical bone	_____	_____	_____
Cancellous bone	_____	_____	_____
Co-base alloy	_____	_____	_____
Ti-base alloy	_____	_____	_____
			(15)

10. The following are known to affect the efficacy of electric stimulation of bone fracture repair (*true* or *false*):

Electrode positioning	____
Current density	____
Fracture gap size	____
Electric field	____
Implant porosity	____
	(5)

11. Cortical bone (*true* or *false*)

Is stiffer if more highly mineralized	____
Is weaker if more highly mineralized	____
Is weaker in older individuals	____
Is elastic–plastic	____
Contains no important stress risers	____
	(5)

12. Articular cartilage (select the best answer[s])

A. Is viscoelastic	____
B. Has almost identical relaxed and unrelaxed moduli	____
C. Is a uniform material	____
D. May be represented by a standard linear model (for small deformations)	____
E. Displays creep for times less than t_{min}	____
	(5)

Questions 13–16 refer to the following paragraph

A 19-year-old male pedestrian was struck by a car, sustaining a tibial fracture at the junction of the mid and distal third. The fibula was intact; the tibia had an incomplete "butterfly" on the medial aspect (as seen in an anteroposterior [AP] view). The fracture was fixed with a stainless-steel eight-hole compression plate, placed laterally. The patient was discharged fully weight bearing.

The following clinical observations were made:

1 month postoperation (PO): Patient complains of pain over distal aspect of plate.

2 months PO: Continued complaint of pain, localized erythema.

6 months PO: Fracture nonunited in AP radiograph.

9 months PO: Patient presents with acute onset of pain "in leg"; AP radiograph reveals broken plate, nonunited fracture.

13. On surgical exploration, which is (are) the most likely finding(s)?

A. Plate broken between two screw holes	____
B. Plate broken at level of screw hole	____
C. Soft tissue discoloration over most distal screwhead	____
D. Soft tissue discoloration over most screwheads	____
E. None of the above	____
	(5)

14. The physical process most likely producing the early localized pain is: (select best answer[s])

A. Fretting	___
B. Failure of boundary lubrication	___
C. General corrosion	___
D. Galvanic corrosion	___
E. Crevice corrosion	___
	(5)

15. The plate fracture is due to (select the best answer[s])

A. Stress relaxation	___
B. Creep	___
C. Corrosion	___
D. Fatigue	___
E. Hysteresis	___
	(5)

16. The plate fragments can be almost perfectly fitted together. Mark the following statements *true* or *false*:

The plate broke because stainless steel is too weak to be used in internal fixation hardware.	___
The plate failure was a brittle fracture.	___
The plate failure was a high-stress, low-cycle failure.	___
The plate was probably damaged during insertion.	___
"Contouring" the plate might have contributed to its failure.	___
	(10)

17. Corrosion products from implants (*true* or *false*)

Produce elevated metal concentrations in plasma and urine	___
Are trapped in the implant site	___
May produce remote site immune responses	___
May be the result of manufacturing errors	___
Are bacteriostatic	___
	(5)

18. Dynamic coefficients of friction (select the phrase that best completes the sentence)

A. Are predictive of wear rates	___
B. Are larger than static coefficients	___
C. Are larger for prosthetic joints than for natural ones	___
	(3)

19. Wear debris (select the phrase that best completes the sentence)

A. Are unimportant *in vivo*	___
B. May contribute to device "loosening"	___
C. May produce "third-body" wear	___
D. Are trapped in situ	___
E. None of the above	___
	(5)

20. Consider the following wear–debris–response relations (*true* or *false*):

A. In a metal-on-polymer articulation, the polymer component will more likely wear.	___
B. In a ceramic on metal articulation, the ceramic component will more likely wear.	___
C. Metallic wear particles are generally smaller than polyethylene wear particles.	___
D. A particle size greater than 100 µm is required to induce osteolysis.	___
E. Like pairs of materials tend to show higher wear rates than unlike pairs.	___
	(5)

21. Poly(methylmethacrylate) bone cement (PMMA) (*true or false*)

Has a higher tensile modulus than cortical bone	___
When newly mixed, sticks to old PMMA in situ, *in vivo*	___
Is notch sensitive	___
Can be used to bear load in bone defects	___
Is naturally radiopaque	___
	(5)

22. Composite materials (select the phrase that best completes the sentence)

A. Combine the properties of their phases	___
B. Have the wear properties of their major phase	___
C. Have isotropic mechanical properties	___
D. Can mimic mechanical properties of hard and soft tissues	___
E. None of the above	___
	(5)

23. The goal(s) of fixation of joint replacement components are (*true* or *false*)

A. To eliminate or minimize relative motion between the implant and the bone during loading	____
B. To reduce resultant stress in the surrounding bone to levels below implantation of the device	____
C. To provide an interface between the implant and bone that is much stiffer than the surrounding bone in order to absorb forces generated during postoperative loading	____
D. To produce stresses on bone within a normal, acceptable range	____
	(4)

24. Fixation by biologic ingrowth (*true* or *false*)

Is generally caused by bone growing into under 10 μm pores	____
Occurs in patients in femoral but not tibial components of TKRs	____
May produce local "stress shielding"	____
Occurs more rapidly for polymeric than for metallic components	____
Is an FDA-approved design feature of some THRs	____
	(5)

25. "Micromotion" is the same as (select the term that best completes the sentence)

A. Creep	____
B. Stress relaxation	____
C. Hysteresis	____
D. Fretting	____
E. None of the above	____
	(5)

26. Immune responses to metals (select the phrase that best completes the sentence)

A. Are more common in men than in women	____
B. Are caused by organometallic complexes	____
C. May occur at sites remote from metal implants	____
D. Are due to the amount of metal present rather than its elemental composition	____
E. May play a role in TJR "loosening"	____
	(5)

27. The Device Amendments of 1976 empowers the FDA to (select the phrase that best completes the sentence)

A. Design implants	___
B. Prevent interstate shipment of devices	___
C. Regulate the treatment of individual patients	___
D. Adopt performance standards for devices	___
E. Examine all retrieved implants	___
F. Review results of clinical tests of devices	___
G. Prescribe the conduct of tests of device safety	___
H. Limit the clinical testing of devices	___
I. Classify devices on a generic basis	___
J. Require recertification of physicians	___
	(10)

28. Tissue engineering (*true* or *false*)

A. Is used to repair tissue	___
B. Uses stem cells to produce tissue	___
C. Alters genetic makeup of the organism	___
D. Restores living tissue	___
E. Regenerates living tissue	___
	(5)

29. The classes (Class I, II, and III) of medical devices are intended to (*true* or *false*)

A. Reflect the relative risk of the device	___
B. Indicate what type of controls are required	___
C. Assure safety and effectiveness of the device	___
D. Reflect the level of complexity of the device	___
E. Reflect whether it is implantable or not	___
	(5)

30. What evidence/clinical experience is generally required before a new material is introduced into clinical practice (*true* or *false*)?

A. Cost	___
B. Biocompatibility data	___
C. Background of design team members	___
D. Alternative materials that were considered	___
E. *In vitro* testing	___
F. Development timeline/schedule	___
G. Engineering test data	___
H. Sterilization information	___
I. Manufacturing method	___
J. Prototypes considered	___
	(10)

Answers

1. Compressive
2. E
3. F, A, X, H/(D-0.002), J, A+B+C, H, J, A+B+C, X
4. False, True, True
5. False, True, False, True, False
6. B, D
7. C, C, A, C, A
8. C, E
9. Elastic modulus: 2, 3, 1, 5, 4
   Ductility: 5, 1, 4, 3, 2
   Strength: 2, 3, 1, 5, 4
10. True, True, True, True, True
11. True, False, True, False, False
12. A, D
13. B, C
14. D, or E, or both
15. D
16. False, True, False, False, True
17. True, False, True, False, False
18. C
19. B, C
20. True, False, True, False, True
21. False, False, True, False, False
22. A, D
23. True, False, False, True
24. False, False, False, False, True
25. E
26. B, C, E
27. B, D, F, G, H, I
28. True, False, False, True, True
29. True, True, False, False, False
30. False, True, False, False, True, False, True, True, True, False

Index

Page numbers followed by f and t indicate figures and tables, respectively.

Printed and bound by CPI Group (UK) Ltd, Croydon, CR0 4YY

18/10/2024

01776271-0014